Handbook of cosmeceutical excipients and their safeties

Related titles

Therapeutic risk management of medicines
(ISBN 978-1-907568-48-0)

An introduction to pharmaceutical sciences: Production, chemistry, techniques and technology
(ISBN 978-1-907568-52-7)

Formulation tools for pharmaceutical development
(ISBN 978-1-907568-99-2)

Woodhead Publishing Series in Biomedicine: Number 65

Handbook of cosmeceutical excipients and their safeties

Yu Heng Kwan, Yee Kei Tung,
Jaspreet Singh Kochhar,
Hairui Li, Ai-Ling Poh
and Lifeng Kang

ELSEVIER

AMSTERDAM • BOSTON • CAMBRIDGE • HEIDELBERG • LONDON
NEW YORK • OXFORD • PARIS • SAN DIEGO
SAN FRANCISCO • SINGAPORE • SYDNEY • TOKYO
Woodhead Publishing is an imprint of Elsevier

WP WOODHEAD PUBLISHING

Woodhead Publishing is an imprint of Elsevier
80 High Street, Sawston, Cambridge, CB22 3HJ, UK
225 Wyman Street, Waltham, MA 02451, USA
Langford Lane, Kidlington, OX5 1GB, UK

British Library Cataloguing-in-Publication Data
A catalogue record for this book is available from the British Library

Library of Congress Control Number: 2014938531

ISBN 978-1-907568-53-4 (print)
ISBN 978-1-908818-71-3 (online)

For information on all Woodhead Publishing publications visit our website at http://store.elsevier.com/

Typeset by RefineCatch Limited, Bungay, Suffolk

Printed and bound in the United Kingdom

Contents

List of figures and tables

Figures

Tables

List of abbreviations

ACD – allergic contact dermatitis
CAGR – compounded annual growth rate
CFR – Code of Federal Regulations
DNA – deoxyribonucleic acid
EC3 – effective concentration 3
ECETOC – European Centre for Ecotoxicology and Toxicology of Chemicals
EECDRG – European Environmental and Contact Dermatitis Research Group
eLog P – experimental Log P
F – fraction of absorption
FDA – Food and Drug Administration
FD&C Act – Food, Drug and Cosmetic Act
HD – hypothetical dosage for humans that causes cancer
HRIPT – human repeat insult patch test
ICDRG – International Contact Dermatitis Research Group
J_{ss} – steady state flux
LLNA – local lymph node assay
LOEL – lowest observed effect level
M16SS – Minitab 16 Statistical Software
MCF-7 – Michigan Cancer Foundation-7
MI/MCI – Methylisothiazolinone and Methylchloroisothiazolinone
QSAR – quantitative structure–activity relationship
RNA – ribonucleic acid
ROAT – repeated open application test
ROS – radical oxygen species
SA – body surface area
US – United States

Preface

The terms cosmetics and cosmeceutics are becoming more prevalent with the increased market penetration of the products, in part influenced by the growing demand among consumers to enhance their aesthetic appeal. Cosmeceutics consist of a subset of cosmetics, intended for their skincare actions, without exerting any significant systemic or pharmacological action. Although quality research is being pursued with regards to the cosmetic ingredients, regulations on these products are not as stringent as drug products. Hence, many spurious or substandard products do exist on the market which may lead to dermatological problems.

Recently, we surveyed 257 skincare products from a local hospital pharmacy in Singapore. The labels were archived and their ingredients were entered into a database, which formed the basis of this book. The book intends to create awareness amongst cosmetic manufacturers and end users alike, highlighting important aspects such as the history of cosmetics, the regulation of cosmetics in various countries, permeation of cosmetics through the skin and potential local and systemic effects of cosmetic ingredients with an upper limit of usage for more than 502 of their ingredients. We provide monographs of these compounds with the emphasis of their physicochemical properties, rank of popularity, intended cosmetic function, and their carcinogenic and allergenic potential.

Since consumers are becoming increasingly aware about their needs and the products that they purchase, it is important that the manufacturers heed consideration to the science behind the products. While a lot of products show promising results when being used at the required dose, excessive use may result in adverse effects. As such, cosmetic testing becomes pertinent and critical to ensure product safety. We highlight this by providing recommendations for permeation testing of cosmetics to ensure cosmetic ingredients are used in limited amounts not eliciting any adverse effects. We believe this will pave the way for development of cosmeceuticals in times to come.

Y. H. Kwan, Y. K. Tung, J. S. Kochhar, H. Li, A-L. Poh and L. Kang
Singapore, August 2013

About the authors

Kwan Yu Heng graduated with a Bachelor of Science (Pharmacy) with first class honours from the National University of Singapore and is currently a Doctor of Medicine-Doctor of Philosophy candidate and an affiliate of the Centre of Quantitative Medicine at the Duke-NUS Graduate Medical School, Singapore. He is actively involved in clinical research at various restructured hospitals in Singapore including Khoo Teck Puat Hospital, KK Women's and Children's Hospital, Changi General Hospital, Alexandra Hospital and Tan Tock Seng Hospital. His research interest lies in community studies and one featured study was the first Asian-based community rehabilitation for patients with cardiovascular disease that was featured in the mainstream Mandarin newspaper *Lianhe ZaoBao* in Singapore. He has published many papers and has presented at international and local conferences and was awarded the Undergraderate Outstanding Researcher Prize in 2013 by the National University of Singapore.

Lifeng Kang is a lecturer at the Department of Pharmacy, National University of Singapore. His laboratory is focused on micro- and nano-scale technologies for tissue engineering and drug delivery. In drug discovery and delivery, miniaturized platforms are used to precisely control the fluid flow, enable high-throughput screening, and minimize sample or reagent volumes. In tissue engineering, micro-scale technologies are used to fabricate scaffolds with increased complexity and vascularization. Furthermore, these technologies are also used to control the cellular microenvironment, i.e., cell–cell, cell–matrix and cell–soluble factor interactions. Dr. Kang has published 33 peer-reviewed papers and book chapters, 40 abstracts and filed five patent applications. His work has been published in journals such as *Journal of Controlled Release*, *Pharmaceutical Research*, *Molecular Pharmaceutics*, *Journal of Pharmaceutical Sciences*, *Journal of Biomedical Materials Research* and highlighted in *Drug Delivery and Translational Research*.

Tung Yee Kei is currently in her final year of undergraduate studies at the National University of Singapore, majoring in Pharmacy. Not only was she an awardee in the Ministry of Health Scholarship Singapore for undergraduates (2010–2014), but she was granted an employment status in the midst of her studies at one of the largest psychiatric hospitals in Singapore, the Institute of Mental Health. She is actively involved in research which focuses on formulation of skin care products and medications.

Jaspreet Singh Kochhar graduated with a PhD from the National University of Singapore (NUS) and is currently working with a healthcare company in Singapore. He has a Bachelor of Pharmacy from University of Delhi and is a registered pharmacist with Delhi Pharmacy Council, India. During his PhD, under the supervision of Dr. Lifeng Kang and Associate Professor Sui Yung Chan, Jaspreet developed and patented innovative methods to fabricate microneedles and *in vitro* skin permeation testing apparatus. He has been actively involved in microneedle-based delivery of drugs and cosmetics through the skin. He has authored nine articles and a book chapter during his PhD and was awarded the Best Graduate Researcher in Pharmacy for 2013 by the Faculty of Science, NUS.

Hairui Li is currently a PhD student at the National University of Singapore. Her research focuses on microneedle-assisted drug delivery and cosmetic delivery. She obtained both her Bachelor and Master degrees from the China Pharmaceutical University and then she worked in the pharmaceutical industry as a research scientist for three years. Before she studied as a Ph.D student, she also worked as a research assistant on a polymeric drug delivery system development and topical gel development in Dr Lifeng Kang's laboratory. She has authored 5 articles and filed 5 patent disclosures.

Ai-Ling Poh received a BSc (Pharm) Hons degree in 2005 and a PharmD in 2012 from the National University of Singapore (NUS). Her research then focused on transdermal drug delivery technology. After graduation, she resumed the role of adjunct lecturer for Pharmacy Science at the Ngee Ann Polytechnic (Singapore). Currently, she is working as a senior clinical pharmacist in the Pharmacy Dept, Parkway Hospital (S) Pte Ltd. Her research interests include drug delivery and clinical pharmacy.

1

History of cosmeceutics

DOI: 10.1533/9781908818713.1

Abstract: The rapid increase in usage and varieties of cosmeceutics has brought about a wide impact and change in the life of consumers. Cosmeceutics, being in between the spectrum of an active pharmaceutical product and cosmetics, are very complex and need to have new regulations and guidelines to ensure safe usage of these products. Ways of testing of these products also need to be redefined so that consumers can be better informed to make decisions on usage of cosmeceutics. This chapter will give a brief introduction of the history of cosmeceutics and the impact they have on the economy, regulation and testing methods.

Key words: carcinogens, cosmetics, impact, history, regulation, testing, economy.

1.1 Introduction

Cosmeceutics is one of the fastest growing fields in cosmetics with about US$ 124 billion market size (Kumar, 2005). Cosmeceutics is a subset of cosmetics, but while cosmetics are intended for pure aesthetic purposes, cosmeceutics usually exert a minimal amount of systemic effect if not applied excessively on the skin. In this sense, cosmeceutics can also be synonymously defined as skincare products. Preparations such as hand lotion and sunscreens are considered cosmeceutics as they do not contain active pharmaceutical drug compounds that we will be prescribed with if we are ill. On the other hand, some products that contain pharmacologically active ingredients, such as antifungi and hydrocortisone preparation are not considered cosmeceutics because they may be harmful if applied excessively as they contain active pharmaceutical drug compounds. Cosmeceutics is a very new field and definitions may change accordingly due to different regulation context.

1.2 The rise of cosmeceutics

In 1962, Mr Raymond E. Reed (President of the Society of Cosmetic Chemists) coined the term 'cosmeceutics'. A cosmeceutic is further defined as: a product that produces a useful and desired effect; gives desirable aesthetic properties; meets fixed chemical, physical and medical standards; and is a scientifically designed product to apply to the human body externally.

The definitions give rise to a product which is of higher quality than cosmetics, but lower in standards than pharmaceuticals. Cosmeceutics is in fact a marriage between cosmetics and pharmaceutics, bringing therapeutic effect to mankind.

In 1993, Professor A. M. Kligman further augmented the idea of cosmeceutics being a hybrid of cosmetics and pharmaceuticals. This brought about discussions among physicians, scientists, experts and organizations to further explore this concept and its impact on the industries, regulations and mankind (Saint-Leger, 2012).

1.3 Impact of cosmeceutics

Being the fastest growing type of products in the cosmetics field, the impact of cosmeceutics on mankind will be greater than ever (Kaushik et al., 2005). The compounded annual growth rate (CAGR) of the cosmetics industry had been at 4.88% from 1997 to 2001 with the growth shifting from Western to Eastern countries. In 2002, the global cosmetics and toiletries were worth US$ 175 billion. The top three markets are haircare, skincare and colour cosmetics. The colour cosmetics segment accounted for 14% of the market and was the fastest growing segment with a growth rate of 12.9%. L'Oreal, being the top ranked company worldwide, had a strong output in terms of research and development with laboratories creating more than 3000 formulae a year (Kumar, 2005).

The latest report by GCI® mentioned that the markets in the US, UK, France, Germany, Italy, Japan and Spain were estimated to be worth about US$ 31 billion in 2011 and are projected to be around US$ 42 billion in 2018 with a CAGR of 4.6%. Mainly a few large companies (such as L'Oreal, Procter & Gamble, Unilever and Beisersdorf who own brands such as Olay, L'Oreal, Garnier and Nivea) control the market. It was expected that growing affluent countries such as India and China would attract an even wider audience due to a larger demand for such products (GCI, 2013).

1.3.1 Types of cosmeceutics

Cosmeceutic companies have designed many novel and practical products over the years and made them available in local pharmacies and cosmetics shops. These products are skin whitening or de-pigmenting agents, moisturizing agents, antiwrinkle agents, sunscreens, antiphotoageing agents, etc. They serve both therapeutic and aesthetic purposes for mankind (Gao et al., 2008).

1.3.2 Concept of excipient safety

Cosmetics were not under regulation in the US until there were cases of blindness in 1930. Currently, more is known regarding the structure and function of the skin. Cosmetics are generally perceived as safe, however, there are more substances coming to the market that could affect the skin structurally and functionally.

The US Food and Drug Administration (FDA) requires a safety warning to be labelled on the product as long as the final product or its ingredients are untested. However, one should know that the rigour, adequacy and types of tests are at the discretion of the manufacturers. The FDA is also authorized to regulate cosmetics advertising and prevent adulteration of products. It has issued Good Manufacturing Practice guidelines to ensure products are made under appropriate conditions (Kaushik et al., 2005).

In the past, cosmetics were thought to be just for aesthetic purposes. Currently, society holds the view that cosmeceutics have therapeutic value, although they contain no recognized drugs. The simple example, Vaseline®, made from petroleum, is actually used to protect the skin against chemical and physical traumas. It is also a very good moisturizer. An experiment in Professor Kligman's laboratory realized that Vaseline® can assist in suppressing UV-induced rays. For compounds with antiseptics or even added sunscreen agents, the matrix used to formulate the compound will determine the success or failure of that particular product. The ingredients of the matrices may unknowingly cause allergy, inflammation and maybe cancer (Kligman, 1993).

Because of the impact of the excipients on the overall product outcome, more attention has to be put into testing and regulating these products.

1.3.3 Regulation

The similarity of cosmeceutics to drugs requires a change in the regulation framework. Cosmeceutics should not just fall under the regulation framework of cosmetics. This is due to the fact that more potent compounds are added and there is a claimed effect by manufacturers (Saint-Leger, 2012). This will be addressed in greater detail in Chapter 2.

1.3.4 Testing

Cosmeceutics testing is non-compulsory and is at the manufacturers' discretion. When there is a conflict of interest, tests for adverse effects, such as genotoxic tests, may not be done. However, we should also note that the proving of claims might be done so as to gain a marketing advantage, but these are very expensive and may not make economical sense for cosmeceutics companies to carry out. For example, Johnson & Johnson was one of the few companies that had published a paper (in March 2010) regarding their new formulation of infant cleansers (Dizon et al., 2010).

T. Joseph Lin, an author for the *Journal of Experimental and Clinical Medicine*, has mentioned that testing is a matter of ethics (Lin, 2010). An evidence-based approach can allow the public to discern the pros and cons of their cosmetics. As more consumers become educated, better marketing of cosmeceutics requires giving consumers product knowledge that is accurate and easy to understand (Lin, 2010).

1.4 Conclusion

In summary, cosmetics and cosmeceutics have come a long way and have evolved into many new and innovative products. As the impact of cosmeceutics changes, we need to adapt our regulatory and testing frameworks. This is to allow consumers to better understand what they are buying and to assess the long-term effects of the products they use. A cosmeceutic with once unknown ingredients needs to be further explored using a scientific approach.

Regulation of cosmetics

DOI: 10.1533/9781908818713.7

Abstract: Cosmetic providers, be it a manufacturer or a distributor, have legal responsibility to ensure the safety and quality of the merchandise. Compliance to the regulation is highly recommended because it ensures product safety and minimizes unintended adverse effects, benefitting both the manufacturers and the consumers. In this chapter, the cosmetic legislation and regulation in major markets will be reviewed to facilitate a greater understanding of the different requirements in the respective markets and the subsequent adoption of the recommendations provided by the respective legislatures.

Key words: legislation, comparison, compliance, restriction, requirements.

2.1 History

The first cosmetic legislation – known as the United States Federal Food, Drug, and Cosmetic Act (FD&C Act) – was implemented in 1938 in order to extend control of cosmetics, provide a safety limit for inevitable poisonous substances and authorize factory inspection in the cosmetic industry. In 1960, the Color Additive Amendment was effected which required manufacturers to establish the safety of colour additives in foods, drugs as well as cosmetics. This was followed by the enacting of the Fair Packaging and Labeling Act (FP&L Act) in 1966 with the obligation for honest and informative labelling on all products within the interstate commerce while enforcing provisions on foods, drugs, cosmetics, and medical devices by the FDA (USFDA, 2012b).

In Europe, the first cosmetic legislation was enacted much later than in the US. This was the European Council Directive 76/768/EEC, comprising the main regulatory framework to ensure the safety of cosmetic products and free circulation of the products in the domestic market. Later, this regulatory framework was simplified for the interest of economic activities in the European Union (EU). The simplification was in the form of a recast to 'codify legislative text and its amendments and introduce substantive improvements'. Adaptations to the new legislative act and its amendment were carried out regularly until the replacement of the Cosmetic Directive with EU Regulation 1223/2009 – an internationally recognized robust regime to reinforce product safety with the consideration of modern technological developments (EC, 2013)

Significant alterations of the cosmetic regulation and legislation in the US and Europe are summarized in Figure 2.1. With the implementation of cosmetic regulations by these two major markets (US and Europe), emerging markets such as China began to adopt similar protocols to their respective cosmetic industries.

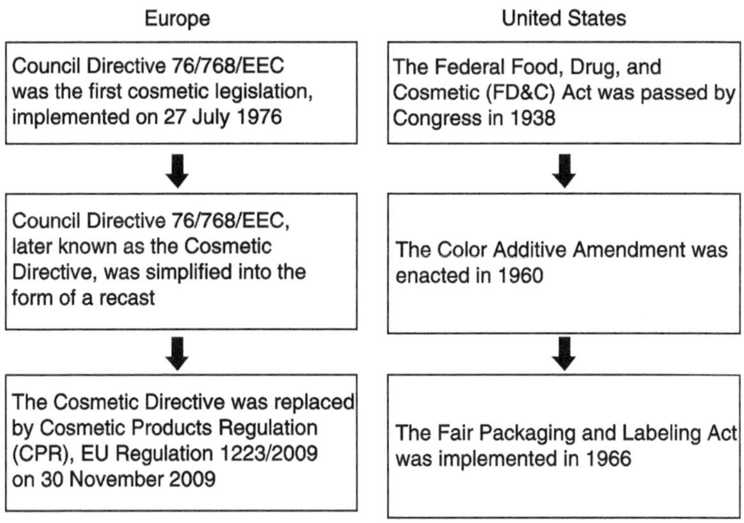

Figure 2.1 History of cosmetic legislation in Europe and the US

2.2 Comparative study of cosmetic legislation and regulation

Despite having different origins, the legislations in the two major cosmetic markets share certain similarities, which will be elucidated in this section. The comparative study will also include the cosmetic regulation in Singapore to provide information on the local situation for those interested. A comparative study of cosmetic legislation and regulation was conducted across Europe, the US and Singapore and is shown in Tables 2.1 to 2.5.

2.3 Similarities in cosmetic regulation or legislation among the developed countries

In general, these are some of the similarities of the cosmetic regulation among the three countries:

- no premarket approval by the authority is required;
- in-market surveillance is conducted by the authority;
- cosmetic providers have full responsibility in ensuring product safety and quality;
- compliance to the restriction and prohibition of substances is mandatory;
- compliance to the requirements on product claims is necessary;
- violation of the law will be subject to penalty.

Much similarity can be seen between the European CPR and ASEAN Cosmetic Directive as Singapore has adopted the cosmetic regulation from Europe. These are:

- the definition of cosmetic;
- the classification of cosmetic according to the product formulation and function;
- a distinct classification of restricted and prohibited substances such as colourants, preservatives and UV filters;
- product notification is mandatory;

Table 2.1 **General differences in cosmetic regulation in Europe, the United States and Singapore**

	Europe	United States of America	Singapore	Reference
Authority	European Commission (EC)	Food and Drug Administration (FDA)	Health Science Authority (HSA) Cosmetic Control Unit (CCU)	
Legislation	(a) European Union (EU) Cosmetic Directive (76/768/EEC) (b) EU Regulation (1223/2009) (latest, adopted on 30 Nov 2009)	(a) Federal Food, Drug, and Cosmetic Act (FD&C Act) (b) Fair Packaging and Labeling Act (FP&L Act) (c) Title 21, Code of Federal Regulations (21 CFR)	(a) Health Products Act (Amendment of First Schedule) (No.2) Order 2007 (b) Health Products Regulations (Cosmetic Products – ASEAN Cosmetic Directive) (2007 and 2010)	
Definition of cosmetics	*Any substance or mixture intended to be placed in contact with the external parts of the human body (epidermis, hair system, nails, lips and external genital organs) or with the teeth and the mucous membranes of the oral cavity with a view exclusively or mainly to cleaning them, perfuming them, changing their appearance, protecting them, keeping them in good condition or correcting body odours*	*Articles (other than soaps consisting of an alkali salt of a fatty acid and making no claims other than cleansing) intended to be rubbed, poured, sprinkled, or sprayed on, introduced into, or otherwise applied to the human body or any part thereof for cleansing, beautifying, promoting attractiveness, or altering the appearance*	*Any substance or preparation that is intended to be placed in contact with the various external parts of the human body (epidermis, hair system, nails, lips, eyes and external genital organs) or with the teeth and the mucous membranes of the oral cavity with a view exclusively or mainly to cleaning them, perfuming them, changing their appearance, correcting body odours, protecting them or keeping them in good condition*	Nwaogu and Vernon, 2004; HSA, 2011

	A substance or mixture intended to be ingested, inhaled, injected or implanted into the human body shall not be considered to be a cosmetic product			
Classification of cosmetics	Based on the formulation and function of the cosmetic products	Based on the function of the cosmetic products only	Based on the formulation and function of the cosmetic products (adopted from the EU)	Nwaogu and Vernon, 2004; HSA, 2011
Premarket approval	Not required as 'free movement' is being practiced, but notification to the Commission is required prior to placing the product on the market	Not required except for: (a) colourants (b) products that are violated	Not required, but notification using the online and acknowledgement of the notification from HSA must be received before the product can be marketed	USFDA, 2005; EC, 2009; HSA, 2011
Responsibility of ensuring product safety	A 'responsible person' which includes: (a) manufacturer established within the Community (b) a person within the Community who is designated by the manufacturer within the Community (c) a person within the Community who is designated by the manufacturer which is not within the Community	Responsibility of product safety assurance lies on: (a) manufacturer (b) packager (c) distributor	The company or person who is placing a cosmetic product in the market: (a) manufacturer (b) assembler (c) importer (d) distributor	EC, 2009; HSA, 2011; USFDA, 2012a

(*continued*)

Table 2.1 General differences in cosmetic regulation in Europe, the United States and Singapore (*continued*)

	Europe	United States of America	Singapore	Reference
	(d) an importer who is responsible for imported cosmetics (e) a person within the Community who is designated by the importer (f) a distributor with the marketed cosmetic product under his name or tradename or with products which have been modified and comply with the applicable requirements of the regulation			

Table 2.2 Differences in the restriction or prohibition of ingredients in Europe, the United States and Singapore

	Europe	United States	Singapore	Reference
Prohibited substances	Yes	Yes	Yes	CFR, 2004b; CFR, ASEANCD
Restricted substances	Yes	Yes	Yes	CFR, 2004b; CFR, ASEANCD
Colourants	Yes	Yes	Yes	CFR, 2004b; CFR, Act, 1993
Preservatives	Yes	Not applicable	Yes	ASEANCD
UV filters	Yes	Not applicable	Yes	
Provisionally allowed substances	Not applicable	Not applicable	Yes	ASEANCD
Carcinogenic, mutagenic and toxic to reproduction (CMR)	Yes	Not applicable	Not applicable	
Nanomaterials	Yes	Not applicable	Not applicable	
Traces of prohibited substances	Yes	Not applicable	Not applicable	

Table 2.3 Differences in the prohibition of cosmetic products in Europe, the United States and Singapore

	Europe	United States	Singapore	Reference
Adulterated product	Not applicable	Yes	Yes	2008, USC, 1993
Misbranded product	Not applicable	Yes	Not applicable	USC, 1992
Counterfeited product	Not applicable	Not applicable	Yes	USC, 1993
Tampered product	Not applicable	Yes, under adulterated product	Yes	USC, 1993
Unwholesome product	Not applicable	Not applicable	Yes	USC, 1993

Table 2.4 **Differences in the requirement for compliance to product safety in Europe, the United States and Singapore**

	Europe	United States	Singapore	Reference
Good manufacturing practice (GMP)	Mandatory	Voluntary	Mandatory	USFDA, 2008; ASEANCD
Safety assessment	Mandatory	Voluntary. Inspection of cosmetic firms without prior notice and cosmetic review by the Cosmetics Ingredients Review (CIR)	Voluntary	ASEANCD
Compliance to the requirements in labelling and packaging	Mandatory	Mandatory, on ingredients and warning statements for domestic and imported products	Mandatory	CFR, 1983; CFR, 1996; CFR, 2004a; ASEANCD, 2007a
Product notification	Mandatory	Voluntary	Mandatory, with notification fees which differ among different cosmetic products; product re-notification is required for subsequent year	
Product information file	Mandatory, to be kept for 10 years after the date on which the last batch of product is marketed	Not required	Mandatory, to be kept at least three years after the product is last placed on the market	

Sampling and analysis of cosmetic products and ingredients	Mandatory	Mandatory, for domestic and imported products whereby a violation of the FD&C Act may exist	Mandatory	
Compliance to the restriction or prohibition for substances	Mandatory	Mandatory, including colourants for domestic and imported products	Mandatory	CFR, CFR, Act, 1993
Compliance to the requirements in product claims	Mandatory	Mandatory as of product labelling, focuses on drug claims for domestic and imported products	Mandatory	ASEANCD, 2007b
Reporting of adverse event	Mandatory	Voluntary, follow up of consumer and trade complaints for domestic products	Mandatory	
Record keeping	Not required	Not required	Mandatory, to be kept for two years after the date of supply. Name and notification number of the product, name and address of supplier, and the batch number, date and quantity of product supplied are to be recorded	
Compliance to microbiological limit	Mandatory	Mandatory, for domestic and imported products	Mandatory	

(*continued*)

Table 2.4 **Differences in the requirement for compliance to product safety in Europe, the United States and Singapore (*continued*)**

	Europe	United States	Singapore	Reference
Compliance to requirements for information on substance	Mandatory	Voluntary, on product safety usage for domestic and imported products	Not required	
Information transparency to the public	Mandatory	Not required	Not required	
Compliance to the requirements for imported or exported goods	Voluntary	Mandatory, for imported products only	Not required HSA regulatory guideline is not applicable for: (a) imported products solely for re-export (b) manufactured in Singapore solely for export	
Penalty implementation	Mandatory	Mandatory	Mandatory	

Table 2.5 Differences in the labelling requirements in Europe, the United States and Singapore

	Europe	United States	Singapore	Reference
General requirement for labelling	Indelible, easily legible and visible lettering	Prominent and conspicuous	Prominent and conspicuous on the product at the point of sale	USFDA, 1991
Language	To be determined by the law of the Member States in which the product is made available to the end user	(a) English language statements: all label or labelling statements required by law or regulation must be in the English language unless the predominant language is one other than English (b) Foreign language statements: if the label contains any foreign language representation, all statements required by regulation must also appear on the label in the foreign language. If labelling bears foreign language representations, the required statements must appear on the label or other labelling as required in English	(a) English and/or (b) national language and/or (c) a language understood by the consumer where the product is marketed	
Contact details	Name or registered name and the address of the 'responsible person'	Name and place of business of manufacturer, packer, or distributor	Name and address in Singapore of company responsible for placing the product on the market	

(continued)

Table 2.5 **Differences in the labelling requirements in Europe, the United States and Singapore (*continued*)**

	Europe	United States	Singapore	Reference
Identity statement	Function of the cosmetic product unless it is clear from its presentation	Nature and function of the product	Name and function of cosmetic product unless clear from product presentation	
Content quantity	Nominal content at the time of packaging in terms of weight or volume	Net quantity of contents, in terms of weight, measure, numerical count or a combination of numerical count and weight or measure	Contents (weight or volume in either metric or both metric and imperial system)	
Expiry date	The date until which the cosmetic product stored under appropriate conditions will continue to fulfil its initial function and in conformity with Article 3	Not required	As required (including the manufacturing date)	
Warning and precautionary information	As required	As required	As required	
Product batch number	Batch number of manufacture or the reference for product identification	Not required	Batch number given by the manufacturer to the batch of cosmetic products	

List of ingredients	Except impurities in the raw materials used, subsidiary technical materials used in the preparation but not present in the final product, perfume and aromatic compositions unless mentioned as required under the column 'Others' in Annex III	Except flavour, fragrance and trade secret ingredients	Except impurities in the raw material used, subsidiary technical materials used in the preparation but not present in the final product and materials used as solvents or carriers for perfumes and aromatic compositions
Instructions for use	As required, including instruction for disposal	As required	As required unless clear from product presentation

- a Product Information File (PIF) is required for the product upon marketing;
- language used for labelling is to be understood by the end user;
- expiry date and product batch number are required on labelling.

2.4 Differences in cosmetic regulation or legislation among the developed countries

2.4.1 General differences

The definition of cosmetic in the US focuses on the intended usage of the product. On the other hand, Europe and Singapore are more specific in the definition as they include the site of application of the product. In the US and Singapore, the responsibility of product safety assurance lies with the person who is conventionally named – manufacturer, importer, etc; hence, the duty of this 'responsible' person is defined by any ordinary dictionary. European CPR, on the other hand, devises its own definition of the 'responsible' person.

Product notification is not made compulsory in the US, unlike Europe and Singapore. Europe is the only one among the three markets that has banned animal testing on cosmetic products.

2.4.2 Restriction and prohibition of ingredients and products

In the US, there are three broad categories for restricted and prohibited substances while Europe has a more sophisticated classification which includes Carcinogenic, Mutagenic, Toxic to Reproduction (CMR), nano-materials and traces of prohibited substances.

Unlike the legislation in the US and Singapore, there is no specification in the European CPR with regards to the product prohibition. The US FD&C Act prohibits the marketing of adulterated or misbranded cosmetics in interstate commerce while Singapore's Health Products Act prohibits the marketing of adulterated, counterfeited, tampered and unwholesome cosmetic products.

Overall, Europe emphasizes on the inclusion of substances in the product within its safety limits whereas the US and Singapore focus on the exclusion of substances as well as products in the market.

2.4.3 Compliance to product safety

Good manufacturing practice (GMP), safety assessment of the cosmetic products, product notification before marketing and reporting of adverse effects are voluntary actions, according to the FDA. Moreover, sample analysis is conducted only when the product is suspected of law violation. However, the FDA continues to stress the importance of complying with these guidelines to attain product safety assurance. In general, compliance to product safety is achieved if the cosmetic is not found to be adulterated or misbranded.

In the US, guidelines or legislation pertaining to the compliance to product safety is less unambiguous compared to that in Europe or Singapore. The origin of the product, domestic or imported, has been taken into consideration by the FD&C Act.

2.4.4 Requirements for labelling

The FDA is more stringent in their language used in labelling compared to the HSA and the European Commission. Conversely, expiry date and batch number are required in the labelling as stated in the Fair Packaging and Labeling Act (FP&L Act), unlike Singapore or Europe. The FP&L Act particularly sets requirements for various labels on the product such as the principal display panel and the information panel. In addition, listing of ingredients, similar to Europe and Singapore, is needed in the US but with the exemption of flavour, fragrance and trade name of ingredients.

A major difference that distinguishes US cosmetic legislation from the other two countries is that the former has an additional specification on the labelling for cosmetics if a drug or 'active ingredient' is present in the product. Listing of the drug name is prior to that of other cosmetic ingredients.

2.5 Conclusion

The implementation and enforcement of cosmetic legislation is essential in ensuring consumer safety. The imperatives of each emerging cosmetic market (and hence its cosmetic legislation) might vary slightly or significantly, as apparent from the above discussion. The differences among the myriad of legislations might not always be obvious to the cosmetic dealer. To reduce confusion and ease the operation of cosmetic dealers, an international cosmetic legislation may be consolidated, perhaps with reference from existing legislations by the FDA and EC.

3

Skin permeation of cosmetics

DOI: 10.1533/9781908818713.23

Abstract: In this chapter we provide a brief overview of skin's anatomy and various mechanisms that have been postulated for percutaneous absorption. The concept of flux, a parameter used to quantify absorption, will be described in detail with mathematical formulae to calculate flux and determine the permeability of a particular compound. We will also discuss *in vitro* permeation experiments using diffusion cells and their relevance in pre-formulation studies, using excised animal and human skin. An overview of the correlation between animal and human skin's permeability will be provided to enable the formulator to predict human absorption. Finally, we will discuss briefly the calculation of limits of cosmeceutical excipients, to prevent adverse effects and to lead the readers into the next two chapters which specifically deal with systemic and topical adverse effects of cosmetic ingredients.

Key words: formulation, permeation, absorption, flux.

3.1 Introduction

Advancement in physiological understanding about skin, hair and nails over the past few decades has influenced the design of cosmetic formulations. Until the 1960s, it was believed cosmetic ingredients did not permeate the skin. However, with the development of newer formulations containing a diversity of ingredients and intended actions, experts now believe that permeation of these chemical compounds cannot be ruled out. As such, it is imperative for the formulator to have a basic understanding of permeation profiles of cosmetic ingredients to ensure the safety of the final product. Since cosmetic products do not require regulatory approval, it is also important to have a system in place for necessitating sufficient pre-formulation studies to generate safety data for cosmetic products. With this view in mind, we aim to introduce the cosmetic formulators with the basic principles in transdermal absorption.

3.2 Human skin, barrier properties and challenges to absorption

The skin, also known as integument, is a complex multi-layered organ that comprises approximately 7% of total body weight (Marieb and Hoehn, 2007) and is made up of five different cell types, with other cells of the immune and nervous systems residing in the skin transiently (Menon, 2002; Proksch et al., 2008). It varies in thickness in different parts of the body, ranging from being thinnest at the eyelids to being thickest at the sole of the feet (Lee and Hwang, 2002). The primary function of the skin is to provide a rigid structural barrier for protecting the underlying tissues rather than being an amenable passage for chemicals to permeate. In addition, skin is a major contributor in thermoregulation and maintenance of body temperature. It also performs some endocrine functions such as synthesis of vitamin D and conversion of prohormones (Menon, 2002).

The skin has three basic layers: epidermis, dermis and hypodermis (Marieb and Hoehn, 2007). The epidermis, which is the outermost layer, is comprised of the following five layers which from top to bottom are as follows: *stratum corneum*, *stratum lucidum*, *stratum granulosum*, *stratum spinosum* and *stratum basale* (Marieb and Hoehn, 2007). The outermost layer of the epidermis is the *stratum corneum*, so called because the horny layer presents a strong permeation barrier. The barrier properties of *stratum corneum* were proved as early as in 1924 by Rein and supported by several subsequent studies (Blank, 1964; Scheuplein, 1965). This compacted mass of dead corenocytes interspersed with a lipid-rich matrix resembles 'brick and mortar' architecture and is primarily essential to prevent the transepidermal water loss, the egress of other endogenous substances and ingress of foreign particles (chemicals and drugs) (Bouwstra and Honeywell-Nguyen, 2002; Brown, 2003), maintaining the internal homeostasis of the body.

Apart from being a structural barrier, skin also acts as a chemical barrier due to its highly organized multi-layer overlapping cells which are sealed by tightly packed intercellular lipid multi-lamellae (Cevc, 1997), as well as a biological barrier due to the presence of dendritic cells and macrophages (Marieb and Hoehn, 2007). This complex organization of cells and lipids offers resistance to most cosmetic and pharmacological agents, making it a hurdle for topically administered products to exert their effect. This has limited the number of cosmetic and drug candidates that can be delivered transdermally and the commercial transdermal products that are available for human use are only limited to a certain category of molecules.

Considerable research on skin barrier properties and ways to overcome them has been carried out in the past 50 years, evaluating parameters that govern the permeation of a molecule. A detailed description of various factors affecting transcutaneous absorption was provided as early as 1974 by Brisson (Briston, 1974). As a general rule, molecules smaller than 500 Da are able to passively diffuse through the skin (Bos and Meinardi, 2000). A thorough study on various topically used compounds revealed that beyond 500 Da there is a rapid decline in passive permeability due to molecular size, and active permeation techniques such as use of chemical enhancers (Kang et al., 2007), microneedles (Kochhar et al., 2012, 2013), iontophoresis (Dubey and Kalia, 2011), electroporation (Zhao et al., 2006), etc., may be needed to enhance drug diffusion. Parameters including the formulation vehicle, Log P and the skin's hydration also play a critical role in determining the permeation of a compound (Hadgraft and Lane, 2005). Occlusion helps to hydrate the keratinocytes and increases the water content in the intercellular lipid domains, helping to increase the partition coefficient of hydrophilic drugs. Enzymes present in the viable epidermis may catalyse some oxidation, reduction or hydrolytic reactions, rendering the compound inactive even before absorption. Certain drugs such as nicotine, β-blockers and steroids have been reported to be retained in the skin, possibly due to interaction with *stratum corneum* lipids. The skin's age, density of appendages and region of the body are other biological factors influencing permeation of a compound.

For cutaneous absorption, four different mechanisms have been postulated (Prausnitz et al., 2004). Compounds which are lipophilic in nature can either pass transcellularly (through the keratinocytes and lipid-rich matrix) or intercellularly (through the lipid-rich matrix interspersed between the keratinocytes). In both cases, the compound has to be sufficiently lipid soluble as well as small in size. This path becomes more relevant in the presence of chemical enhancers that solubilize and extract the intercellular lipids (Kang et al., 2007; Mah et al., 2013). On the other hand, other small molecular weight compounds can pass through the appendages (such as hair follicles or sweat ducts) all by themselves or on application of little voltage, as in iontophoresis (Illel, 1997) (see Figure 3.1). However, since appendages are not very ubiquitous and only form up to 0.1% of skin surface area, this route of absorption is not widely studied (Moser et al., 2001). Highly water soluble ionic compounds need to be repelled from the skin by application of higher voltage and ultrasound to disrupt the lipid bilayer structure. Macromolecular compounds such as proteins and peptides cannot diffuse through the intact skin and hence creation of micron-scale channels using thermal poration or microneedles is used to deliver these compounds (Kochhar et al., 2012, 2013).

Most of the currently available cosmetic compounds, active ingredients and excipients are small molecular weight entities and hence diffusion through the layers of skin is the predominant pathway for absorption although some biotechnological products are currently being developed

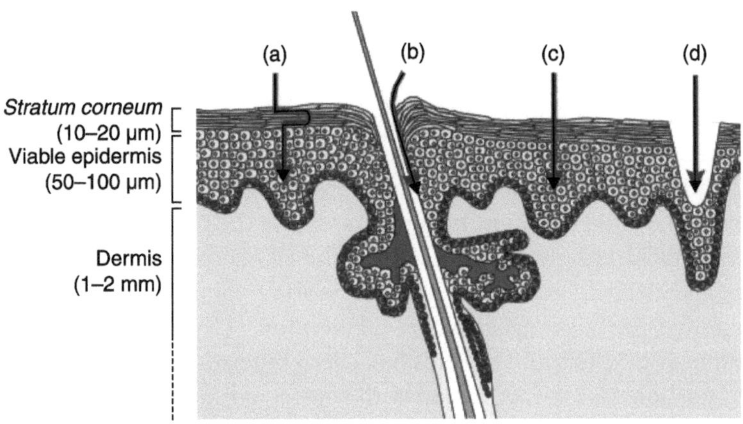

Figure 3.1 **Schematic representation of a cross-section through human skin**

Note: (a) Transdermal diffusion, possibly in the presence of a chemical enhancer, takes place by a tortuous route across the *stratum corneum,* winding around cells and occurring along the interfaces of extracellular lipid bilayers. (b) Low-voltage electrical enhancement by iontophoresis can make transport pathways through hair follicles and sweat ducts more accessible. (c) High-voltage enhancement by electroporation has been shown to occur via transcellular pathways made accessible by disrupting lipid bilayers. The application of ultrasound seems to make pathways (a) and (c) more permeable by disorganizing lipid bilayer structure. (d) Microneedles and thermal poration create micron-scale holes in skin to provide pathways for drug transport. Adapted from Prausnitz et al., 2004.

for cosmetic applications that would require active disruption of skin for efficient transdermal delivery. For this chapter, we will focus on the small molecular weight entities as they comprise over 99% of the compounds in the database of cosmeceutical excipients described at the end of this book.

This makes determination of absorption of cosmetics particularly relevant from two standpoints: efficacy and safety. A particular cosmetic compound may not be efficacious if the required amount of it is not absorbed and does not enter its site of action in the skin, leading to suboptimal performance of the product. On the other hand, significantly high amounts of absorption may lead to excessive build-up of chemicals in the skin and beyond, which may have systemic side effects, jeopardizing the health of consumers and leading to product failure due to health risks. Since pharmacological and toxicological assessment of a skincare product depends on its percutaneous absorption, it becomes important to evaluate the relative amounts of permeation for cosmetic compounds. An important parameter, widely used in the pharmaceutical industry during the pre-formulation characterization of transdermal products, called 'flux', helps to evaluate the relative absorption of a compound through skin, both in *in vitro* and *in vivo* models.

3.3 The concept of flux

Flux (J) is defined as the amount or number of molecules (m) moving across a defined cross-sectional area (A) in a given period of time (t). It is usually expressed in the units of $\mu g\ cm^{-2}\ hr^{-1}$.

$$J = \frac{m}{At} \qquad [3.1]$$

Since diffusion is the major mechanism of transport across a membrane for transdermal absorption, Fick's first law can be used to describe diffusional flux by using the following equation:

$$J(x,t) = -D\frac{\partial C(x,t)}{\partial(x)} \qquad [3.2]$$

Given by German physiologist, Adolf Fick, the equation describes a differential concentration gradient over a path length in a given period of time. D represents the diffusion coefficient in cm^2/s and can be defined by the Stokes-Einstein equation:

$$D = \frac{RT}{6\pi\eta Nr} \qquad [3.3]$$

where *R* is gas constant, *T* is absolute temperature in Kelvin, η is the viscosity of the solution, *N* is Avogadro's number and *r* is the radius of the solute.

In vitro diffusion experiments across biological membranes are usually carried out in a typical apparatus consisting of a donor compartment (which holds the formulation) and a receptor compartment (which holds or has a continually flowing buffer solution mimicking body fluids). In an *in vivo* setting for transdermal diffusion, the permeated drug is rapidly cleared by the highly vascularized dermis, practically maintaining sink conditions, with receiver concentration negligible with respect to the donor. In such a case, flux becomes a function of the concentration gradient and Fick's law can be simplified to:

$$J = -D\frac{KC}{h} \qquad [3.4]$$

where C is the concentration in the donor vehicle or formulation, *h* is the diffusion path length and *K* is the diffusion coefficient of the compound between the formulation and skin.

Since an exact estimation of *D* and *h* is not possible due to the tortuous path taken by the drug in a heterogeneous membrane like skin (Friend, 1992), a term known as the permeability coefficient can be introduced in Eq. 3.4:

$$P = D\frac{K}{h} \qquad [3.5]$$

$$J = PC \qquad [3.6]$$

where *P* is the permeability coefficient given in cm/s. Equation 3.6 is a simplified time independent version of Fick's law that can enable calculation of the permeability of a molecule across a membrane, at a particular concentration gradient. Such experiments are critical in designing effective and safe cosmetic formulations, by providing the formulator with enough information about the dose that is both functionally active and safe to administer. The data thus derived may also allow the formulator to choose between similar compounds. However, caution must be observed in comparing permeability data, especially when it is acquired from different sets of tissues, as inter-sample variability may lead to markedly different results.

3.4 Mathematical modelling of flux

Although experimental permeation studies have been used widely to compute flux, they do not provide much information about the molecular factors that govern permeation of drug compounds (Karadzovska et al., 2013b). Moreover, with growing ethical and animal welfare concerns, mathematical modelling provides a viable alternative, provided that models are robust and inclusive of all parameters that govern permeation. In the 1970s and 1980s, research was focused on studying the effect of individual parameters such as molecular weight, partition coefficient, molecular size, solubility, etc. on permeation. Seminal work in this area was done by Scheuplein and Blank in 1971 to find a linear correlation between the hydrophobicity and permeability for a series of alcohols and alkane vapors. Since then, significant interest has been generated, particularly after the development of multifactorial quantitative models, by Flynn (1990) and Potts and Guy (1992) in the early 1990s. These *in silico* methodologies, collectively called quantitative structure permeability relationships (QSPeRs) (Kupczewska-Dobecka et al., 2010) are gaining prevalence with the increasing number of products being available for topical use. These methodologies not only aid in determining drug permeation properties, but also provide critical information for discovery of new chemicals whose properties can be customized and modified to enhance their transdermal absorption (Moss et al., 2012).

Although desirable, it is difficult and sometimes impractical to assess the permeation properties of each compound experimentally. Hence, researchers have developed some comprehensive mathematical models to predict permeability of drug compounds based on their structure and other physico-chemical properties including lipophilicity, molecular weight and melting point, among others. Flynn prepared a dataset of 94 compounds and demonstrated that the permeability was a function of octanol water partition coefficient and molecular size (Flynn, 1990). In this work, Flynn reported hydrophobicity could be used to predict the permeation of small and large molecular weight compounds. However, the model lacked statistical model fitting (Moss et al., 2002). Potts and Guy (1992) elaborated this knowledge further, by using 93 compounds in the Flynn dataset, and derived a simple equation to correlate permeability P, with molecular weight (MW) and octanol–water partition coefficient $K_{o/w}$

$$\mathrm{Log}P = -6.3 + 0.71 \log K_{o/w} - 0.0061\,MW \qquad [3.7]$$

Later, Cleek and Bunge (Cleek and Bunge, 1993; Bunge and Cleek, 1995; Bunge et al., 1995) further improved this model by incorporating the variables for hydrophilic resistance of viable epidermis to lipophilic compounds as well as exposure time of the compound on skin. Other researchers have incorporated parameters such as melting point (Barratt, 1995), hydrogen bonding (Abraham et al., 1995, 1997), linearity of a molecule (Patel and Cronin, 2001) and L-α-dimyristoyl phosphtidyl choline (DMPC)–water partition coefficient (a compound having similarity to lipids in biological membranes) (Patel et al., 2002a) so as to have better predictive models. Patel et al. (2002b) incorporated some of the above mentioned parameters and predicted the permeability of 158 chemicals, proposing the following equation to have a better fit than the Potts and Guy model:

$$\mathrm{Log}P = 0.781 \log \mathrm{K}_{o/w} - 0.01115M - 2.19 \qquad [3.8]$$

A shortcoming from these models is that all models assume infinite doses being applied using water as a vehicle. A recent report by Karadzovska and colleagues included the effect of vehicle, compound and its dose (both finite and infinite) in modelling of permeation of compounds across pig skin. Another factor, termed as mixture factor (MF) accounting for the properties of compound/vehicle mixture, was also incorporated. This factor, which is the inverse of melting point, significantly contributed to flux and absorption, as did the vehicle and its saturation level (Karadzovska et al., 2013b). They also reviewed and compared various other studies, highlighting the increased body of knowledge in prediction of skin permeability from a mixture of vehicles (Karadzovska et al., 2013a). Another recent study also found positive correlation between transepidermal water loss, skin integrity and percutaneous absorption (Hui et al., 2012).

A collective model based on several different approaches has been formulated as an online permeability calculator for the use of formulators. The calculator makes use of molecular weight, log $\mathrm{K}_{o/w}$, concentration (mg/ml) to calculate flux and permeability. This online calculator can be accessed as the skin permeator calculator at the Centers for Disease Control and Prevention website: *http://www.cdc.gov/niosh/topics/skin/skinpermcalc.html.*

Another term known as '*skin notation*' has been applied to estimate the dermal permeation of occupationally absorbed compounds, where fluxes are correlated to occupational exposure limits (OELs) and evaluated for potential toxicity. The readers are recommended to read an important review on this topic by Kupczewska-Dobecka and colleagues (2010) for further details.

3.5 *In vitro* skin permeation testing

Experimental evaluation of transdermal diffusion is mostly carried out using diffusion cells that have been fabricated in a variety of designs, but have a certain commonality in their elements, including donor and receptor chambers, having a piece of excised skin or equivalent membrane sandwiched between two. Such studies are important in highlighting the behaviour of a dosage form *in vitro* or *ex vivo* and its likely performance *in vivo*. These permeation set-ups make the drug development process shorter and more economical (Godin and Touitou, 2007). In the next section, various skin models are described that will enable the formulators to choose the skin system that fits their needs best.

3.6 Skin models for permeation testing

During the development of a new dosage/cosmetic form, however desirable it may seem, testing directly on human subjects is unethical due to the unknown absorption and toxicity profile of the formulation components. Ideally, skin from human cadavers or donors from cosmetic surgery could be used to closely mimic the natural conditions. However, access to human skin tissues is not readily available to all researchers and skin from various anatomical sites and diseased state cadavers may lead to large variations in the results. Animal skin models, ranging from mouse, rat, rabbit, guinea pig and snake to membranes of poly (dimethylsiloxane) and, more recently developed, cultured human skin substitutes have been used to obviate the issues surrounding the use of human skin. These skin models vary differently in their physical and biological properties as well as permeation characteristics as compared to human skin, and the researchers have looked at extrapolating results from these substitutes to predict the permeation across human skin. The difference between animal and human skin primarily lies in the intercellular lipid composition of the *stratum corneum* (Netzlaff et al., 2006). Although other parameters such as the type of diffusion cell, temperature of skin, applied dose and diffusion area may affect the results, these diffusion cell models are nonetheless critical in the estimation of absorption of a compound as well as excipient characterization in transdermal dosage forms and cosmetics.

Pig skin has been shown to most closely resemble human skin properties (Simon and Maibach, 2000), particularly with respect to permeation, skin thickness and lipid composition, and is available in abundance, usually from abattoirs. Specific research on pig skin lipid properties has revealed that *stratum corneum* in particular breeds, especially Hampshire and Yorkshire pigs aged 1–14 weeks, resembles that of man (Simon and Maibach, 2000). In a study comparing the permeation of hydrophilic and lipophilic compounds across various animal models, pig ear skin showed the closest correlation to human abdominal skin, especially for lipophilic compounds (Dick and Scott, 1992). Another study demonstrated the comparable flux achieved across newborn pig skin and human epidermis for a particular class of drugs (Cilurzo et al., 2007). These results have been supported by several others as well (Gore et al., 1998; Singh et al., 2002; Jacobi et al., 2007).

Rat skin, on the other hand, shows significantly higher permeability than human skin owing to difference in lipid compositions, water uptake and variation in skin thickness (Morimoto et al., 1992). However, they are used predominantly in permeation studies because of economy, ease of handling and housing as well as maintenance of hairless genetic variants of these rodents (El-Kattan et al., 2000). The same is true for hairless mouse skin, although it has been reported to be 30–40 times more permeable than human skin (El-Kattan et al., 2000). One of the studies reported hairless skin to be more permeable than hairy skin for all polar compounds (Lauer et al., 1997), possibly due to the presence of cysts and enlarged sebaceous glands, which take the place of mature hair follicles, providing polar pathways. Van Ravenzwaay and Leibold (2004) compared the permeation through rat skin and human skin *in vitro* and *in vivo*. Permeation through rat skin was found to be higher in both *in vitro* and *in vivo*, and it was suggested that extrapolation to percentage absorption in humans could be calculated using the following equation:

$$\%\ \text{Human absorption} = \frac{\%\ \text{Absorption in rat}\ (\textit{in vivo}) \times \%\ \text{Absorption in human}\ (\textit{in vitro})}{\%\ \text{Absorption in rat}\ (\textit{in vitro})} \quad [3.9]$$

This approach of using data from three sources has been officially adopted as a ‘triple pack’ by the Organisation for Economic Co-operation and Development (OECD), in their guidelines on dermal absorption (OECD, 2010). It has also been reported that inter-individual variation is less in Sprague Dawley rat skin as compared to human skin samples and frozen samples had similar permeation properties as fresh samples, indicating the possibility of harvesting and storage of skin samples when readily available (Takeuchi et al., 2011).

With advancement in tissue engineering technologies, human skin equivalents have been developed by co-culturing cells with matrix proteins and skin lipids. These models are available as epidermal skin substitutes consisting of a layer of differentiated keratinocytes or full-thickness skin substitutes in which keratinocytes are grown at the air–liquid interface over a layer of collagen matrix containing dermal cells, thus providing keratinocytes an environment to differentiate (Mak et al., 1991). While the epidermal constructs are chiefly used in burn patients to replace the superficially injured tissue (Riva et al., 2007), full-thickness skin equivalents can be used for severe burn injuries as well as a substitute for transdermal absorption studies (Huang et al., 2009; Egles et al., 2010). These skin equivalents provide an alternative to animal testing, and as they are constituted chiefly of human cells, they are expected to behave in a similar manner to human skin, with similar barrier properties. However, due to a lack of similar amounts of fats and lipids as well as sweat glands, hair follicles and improper or partial differentiation of keratinocytes, these systems are usually more permeable than human skin. Many of these, such as Graftskin® and Skinethic®, are commercially available but have been shown to be 800–900 times more permeable than split-thickness human skin, particularly for hydrophobic compounds. But a similar permeation profile was found for less hydrophobic compounds (Schmook et al., 2001). Thus, these skin equivalents may not be suitable for testing of all compounds. Excellent reviews on various commercially available human skin substitutes and their applications are provided by Groeber et al. (2011) and Zhang and Michniak-Kohn (2012). These models are still not widely used, owing to their cost, relative difficulty in fabrication and handling and lack of reproducibility (Godin and Touitou, 2007). They are however used in skin irritation testing (Ahn et al., 2010) and have been endorsed by COLIPA, the European agency for cosmetics and toiletries.

Apart from these animal and cultured skin equivalents, use of synthetic membranes has also been envisaged as an economical alternative. Though these artificial membranes are devoid of the complicated histology of native human skin, and hence they may not provide the perturbation effect due to skin lipids, they may be helpful in providing critical information in drug–skin partitioning as well as diffusion behaviour of compounds. Wang and colleagues used three artificial membranes, including low density polyethylene (LDPE), low fouling composite (LFC) and mixed cellulose esters (MCE) to evaluate the permeation of *N*, *N*-diethyl-*m*-toluamide (DEET) and oxybenzone from commercial insect repellent and sunscreen preparations. It was found that permeation was significantly higher than that achieved with piglet skin. Variations amongst test membranes with respect to rate and extent of absorption were attributed to the physico-chemical properties of the membranes, test compounds and their formulations (Wang et al., 2006). Loftsson and colleagues developed a membrane similar to the lipid bilayer membrane structure of the biological membranes, where the hydrophilic membrane was composed of a hydrated semi-permeable cellophane membrane and the lipophilic membrane was made up of n-octanol in a nitrocellulose matrix. The membrane was shown to have similar permeation properties to hairless mouse skin and eye cornea for cyclodextrin-containing formulations (Loftsson et al., 2006). Polydimethyl siloxane (PDMS) and its derivatives have also been used widely in percutaneous absorption studies (Gu et al., 2004; Frum et al., 2007; Gu and Chen, 2009; Rao and Zhang, 2012), although the permeability through PDMS has been found to be significantly higher than human epidermis. Cellulose nitrate impregnated with lauryl alcohol has also been used as a lipophilic membrane (Mura et al., 2007). Merck Millipore launched a synthetic multilayered polyethersulfone membrane (Strat-M™), with permeation properties similar to human skin. The samples do not require any special storage or preparation prior to use (Merck Millipore, 2012).

With a wide range of membrane models available, it is the prerogative of the cosmetic formulator to choose the one which closely represents human skin for that particular formulation. Ideally, among animal models pig ear skin bears resemblance to human models and wherever possible should be the membrane of choice. Human skin substitutes are currently being researched and developed at a fast pace, and are expected to provide reliable alternatives in the near future.

3.7 Conclusion

With an ever-increasing demand for cosmetic products and heightened desire amongst humans to look aesthetically elegant, manufacture of products with ensured safety and efficacy is called for. Regulatory guidelines pertaining to cosmetics need to be evaluated periodically by the relevant bodies and implementation of testing of products through *in vitro* and *in vivo* methods be made a norm. Permeation testing provides a platform which can be tapped upon to reveal basic properties such as extent of absorption and retention in the skin, which could be used for further toxicology studies. This would provide a higher degree of consumer safety, by ensuring excipients are used in the right amounts, thereby avoiding potential undesirable side effects.

4

Systemic effect of cosmeceutics – cancer

DOI: 10.1533/9781908818713.35

Abstract: Currently, no database is available to monitor the number of skin products in a pharmacy or functions of the ingredients used and there is no central platform whereby information on the safety and carcinogenicity of the ingredients is available. There is no guide on the ability of the compounds to permeate the skin and there are no guidelines issued on the recommended limits that should be used on probable carcinogens in the cosmeceutics. This chapter will summarize the procedures done to establish the limits to be proposed.

Key words: database, guidelines, carcinogens, compounds, categories.

4.1 Introduction

Excipient safety is a concern in general for oral and transdermal drugs. This is also true for cosmeceuticals, whereby excipients may diffuse through the skin and cause various harmful effects to the body (Pifferi and Restani, 2003). However, most consumers have limited knowledge of the ingredients inside the cosmeceuticals. A study from Gokdemir and co-workers showed that 42.5% of the participants in their study did not consult anyone when purchasing a skin product. Nine out of ten subjects did not receive professional consultation and purchased the skin product according to their own knowledge (Gokdemir et al., 2008). Hence there is an urgent need for public health workers to conduct research on the adverse effects of cosmeceutics and to educate the public to protect the health of consumers.

Besides the lack of knowledge in consumers, the regulations and controls are limited in the cosmetic industry. The United States Food and Drug Administration (USFDA) is less stringent when it comes to regulating skin products (Karstadt, 2010). The Personal Care Products Council, a national trade association representing the global cosmetic and personal care products industry, set up the Cosmetic Ingredient Review (CIR) for reviewing ingredients in the market (Ross, 2006). However, cosmetic companies make up the council, which may create a conflict of interest.

Harvey and Darbre called for further research to determine the link between cosmetics and cancer as there was evidence showing increased breast cancer. Environmental factors such as cosmetics may play a big role in these cases (Esteve, 1996; Harvey and Darbre, 2004). Furthermore, there is currently no evidence on long-term, low-dose carcinogens and its implications on cancer when used in cosmeceutics. Also, cancer is one of the top killers in the world (WHO, 2008). Therefore, among all the adverse effects of cosmeceuticals, the ability to cause cancer calls for greater attention. There are databases created by voluntary groups such as the Environmental Working Group from the US (Group, 2013). However, its database only provides general information on carcinogenicity but does not further elaborate on the significance of these cosmeceuticals on humans. Currently, no database is available to monitor the number of skin products in a pharmacy or functions of the ingredients used and there is no central platform whereby information on the safety and carcinogenicity of the ingredients is available. Lastly, there is no guide on the ability of the compounds to permeate the skin and there are no guidelines issued on the recommended limits that should be used on probable carcinogens in the cosmeceutics.

This chapter will summarize the procedures done to establish the limits to be proposed. Skincare products were collected from a hospital pharmacy to form a database that encompasses the number of ingredients, the ingredients' functions, permeability data, carcinogenicity and concentration limits. The skin permeation rate of a compound determines the total amount of it that can enter humans after a certain period of time. Potentially, carcinogenic compounds can only induce cancer when they permeate in sufficient amounts through the skin. By calculating their skin permeation rates and comparing this with their carcinogenic doses, we can determine the percentages that can be used in a certain skincare product. With this database, consumers and healthcare professionals can be made aware of the potential danger of cosmeceutical products on the market.

4.2 Methodology

4.2.1 Collection of products

Labels of 257 skin products were collected in the first half of 2010 from a local hospital pharmacy in Singapore. Tabulation showed that these products were imported from 13 countries, mainly from the US, France and Australia at 36.6%, 19.8% and 15.6% respectively. Products were manufactured by 39 companies across the globe with L'Oreal®, Pierre Fabre® and Dermo-Cosmetique® as the top manufacturers producing 18.7%, 9.3% and 7.4% of the skin products collected. The labels were archived and their ingredients were entered into a database.

Natural products were subsequently removed from the database as there was limited documentation of their effects and exact composition in current literature. Natural product was defined as a compound or mixture of compounds extracted from plant, animal or (rarely) mineral substances (ACS, 1974). The remaining ingredients were then ranked according to their prevalence and subjected to further analysis.

4.2.2 Carcinogenicity of ingredients

The carcinogenicity of the ingredients was determined using PubMed® and Web of Science® databases. The keywords used were 'compound name AND cancer' or 'compound name AND mutation'. Compounds that showed evidence of carcinogenicity were recorded. Carcinogenic compounds were defined conservatively whereby if evidence of conflicting conclusions were presented, the compound involved would be regarded as carcinogenic as long there is evidence proving its potential carcinogenicity. Studies that mentioned carcinogenicity include clinical, animal and cell line studies. Types of cancer assessed were not restricted to skin cancer but were considered for any form of cancer that can be produced by the carcinogens when they enter the body. The number of carcinogenic compounds and the number of products containing these carcinogenic ingredients were tabulated using Predictive Analytics SoftWare Statistics 18. In-depth analysis of the mechanism of increasing risk of each carcinogenic compound was carried out.

4.2.3 Human transdermal per day doses derived from animal studies

Based on animal studies which reported per day oral doses, a hypothetical oral dosage for humans that causes cancer (HD) was calculated by using a dose translation formula by Reagan-Shaw et al. (2008). Further, to convert the human per day oral dose into transdermal dose, bioavailability of 57% was used for calculations (Andrews et al., 2000). For example, in the case of triethanolamine's human transdermal dose calculations, *F* refers to bioavailability:

$$\text{Animal oral dose}\left(\frac{\text{mg}}{\text{kg}}\right) \times \text{Conversion factor} \times \text{Human weight (kg)} \times F$$
$$= 100 \times 3/37 \times 60 \times 0.57$$
$$= 277\,\text{mg} \qquad [4.1]$$

4.2.4 Flux of carcinogenic ingredients through skin

After the transdermal per day dose is known, the flux of the compound needs to be calculated to find out if the hypothetical transdermal dose can actually permeate through a certain skin surface area. The flux of carcinogen through skin was calculated by using the skin permeation calculator provided by the National Institute for Occupational Safety and Health in the US (Frasch, 2010). To calculate the flux, data on solubility, Log P and molecular weight were gathered from SciFinder® Web's database. For compounds with no Log P value reported, its component (such as its weak acid or base's data) was used instead. For example, in the case of triethanolamine, its MW is 149.2 and Log P is –1.0, thus its flux is 8.44×10^{-3} mg/h/cm^2.

Once the fluxes are obtained, it is possible to calculate the amount of compounds that can permeate through a certain area of skin in 24 hours. The result is then compared with the transdermal per day dose to decide if a compound can permeate through skin enough to induce a cancerous response. For example, in the case of triethanolamine, its human transdermal per day dose is 277 mg while its permeation in 24 hours is 3240 mg. Permeation of triethanolamine in 24 hours is calculated by:

$$J\ (\text{mg/h/cm}^2) \times t\ (\text{h}) \times A\ (\text{cm}^2)$$

$$= 8.44 \times 10^{-3} \times 24 \times 13440$$

$$= 3240\,\text{mg} \qquad [4.2]$$

Where J refers to flux, t refers to time and A refers to area applied.

4.2.5 Maximum percentage in a product

To find out the maximum percentages of those compounds in a formulation such as gel or creams, the general application amount needs to be known, which was reported to be 2 mg/cm^2 (Hayden CGJ, 1997). Therefore, for a certain body surface area, the total amount of product can be obtained. Body surface area (SA) of the different body parts was proposed by Livingston and Lee (2000). The SA used to calculate the amount of flux that permeated the skin was 13440 cm^2, 216 cm^2 and 640 cm^2 on body (excluding the hair, buttocks, perineum and feet), face and hands respectively.

4.3 Results

In total, 257 skincare products were collected. There were a total of 63 body products, 9 hand products, 58 sun care products and 127 facial products. The summary of the results of this study is shown in Figure 4.1. There were 520 ingredients, excluding natural compositions used in these cosmeceuticals. The top 100 compounds are listed in Table 4.1. There were 87 potential carcinogens (16.7%) out of 520 ingredients. The 87 compounds were categorized into seven groups based on their mechanisms, which were compounds causing cancer via generation of active species (22 compounds), altering the cell genetics (22 compounds), estrogenic effect (13 compounds), altering the cell environment (10 compounds), altering cellular mechanisms (8 compounds), other mechanisms to cause cancer (7 compounds) and no mechanism proposed (5 compounds). The majority (56.8%) of the carcinogenic compounds can permeate the skin well.

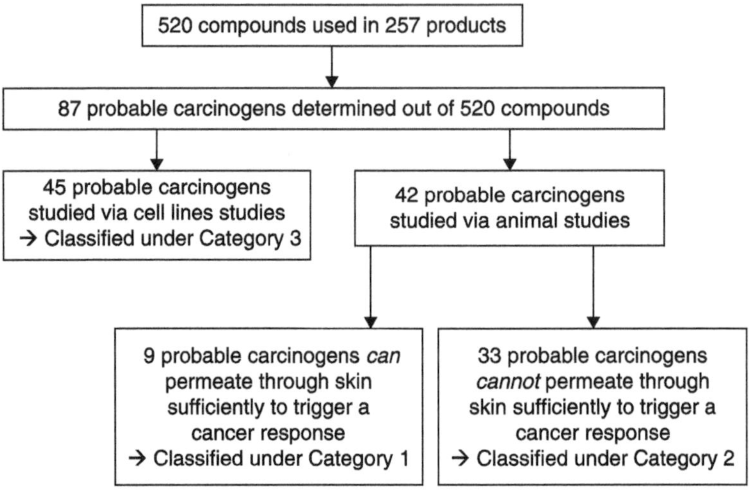

Figure 4.1 Summary of the skincare products and their ingredients

Based on the calculations of flux and dosage used for carcinogenic experiments in animals, the potentially carcinogenic compounds were grouped into three categories as shown in Table 4.2. Out of 87 potential carcinogens, 42 had animal studies carried out on them while 45 had cell line studies done. Nine of 42 potential carcinogens were found to be able to reach HD by permeating through the skin, thus they are classified in Category 1. The other 33 potential carcinogens were classified in Category 2 because they were determined to be safe to use on the skin as they were not able to reach HD. The last 45 potential carcinogens were categorized into Category 3 and were given recommendations to exercise caution when using them.

Concentration limits of the nine potential carcinogens are shown in Table 4.3. For example, triethanolamine was recommended to be formulated at less than 0.86 %w/w in body products and the calculations were: Human transdermal per day dose (277 mg) / Body area to be applied (13 440 cm^2) / (2 mg/cm^2) × 100%.

Table 4.1 The top 100 compounds in the database and their prevalence (520 compounds in total)

Compound	%	Compound	%	Compound	%	Compound	%
Water	87	Cyclomethicone	14	C13-14 isoparaffin	7	Arginine	4
Methylparaben	54	Ethanol	14	Hydroxyethyl cellulose	6	Isopropyl myristate	4
Glycerine	54	Diazolidinyl urea	14	Zinc oxide	6	Gluconolactone	4
Vitamin E	44	Cetearyl alcohol	13	Sorbitol	6	Lactic acid	4
Propylparaben	43	C12-15 alkyl benzoate	12	Lecithin	6	Cyclohexasiloxane	4
Fragrance	37	Butylene glycol	11	Chlorphenesin	6	Isononyl isononanoate	4
Phenoxy-ethanol	33	Acrylates/ C10-30 alkyl acrylate crosspolymer	10	Trisodium EDTA	5	Sodium carbomer	4
Dimethicone	33	Oxybenzone	10	Imidurea	5	Sodium chloride	4
Propylene glycol	32	Cyclopentasiloxane	10	Laureth-7	5	Aluminium starch octenylsuccinate	4
Glyceryl stearate	30	Butylated hydroxytoluene	10	Sorbitan stearate	5	Bisabolol	4
Triethanolamine	28	Tetrasodium EDTA	9	Potassium cetyl phosphate	5	Polymethyl methacrylate	4
Disodium EDTA	26	Isobutylparaben	9	Drometriazole trisiloxane	5	Palmitic acid	4
Stearic acid	25	Avobenzone	9	Ecamsule	5	Benzyl alcohol	4
Cetyl alcohol	23	Octocrylene	9	Salicylic acid	5	Sodium lactate	4
Liquid paraffin	21	Soft white paraffin	9	Iodopropynyl butylcarbamate	5	FD & C blue N1	4
Carbomer	20	Sodium hyaluronate	8	PVP /Eicosene copolymer	5	Cetyl palmitate	4

(continued)

Table 4.1 The top 100 compounds in the database and their prevalence (520 compounds in total) (*continued*)

Compound	%	Compound	%	Compound	%	Compound	%
Octinoxate	19	Sodium citrate	8	Aluminium hydroxide	5	Potassium sorbate	4
Butylparaben	18	Squalane	8	Glycolic acid	5	Myristic acid	4
Titanium dioxide	18	Isopropyl palmitate	8	FD & C yellow N5	5	Ammonium hydroxide	3
Vitamin B5	18	Polyacrylamide	8	Dimethiconol	5	Sodium benzoate	3
PEG-100 stearate	17	Magnesium aluminum silicate	8	Sodium PCA	5	Emulsifying wax	3
Citric acid	16	Sodium hydroxide	7	Ceteareth-20	5	PEG-40 stearate	3
Stearyl alcohol	16	Vitamin A	7	Silica	5	Zinc gluconate	3
Xanthan gum	16	Allantoin	7	Isohexadecane	5	Magnesium sulphate	3
Ethylparaben	15	Polysorbate 20	7	Sodium lauryl sulphate	4	Vitamin B3	3

Table 4.2 Compounds that fall into the three different categories

Categories	Carcinogenic compounds
1. Compounds which can permeate sufficiently to trigger a cancer response (9 compounds)	Triethanolamine, retinyl palmitate, glycolic acid, myristic acid, isopropylparaben, chlorhexidine digluconate, T-butyl alcohol, alpha hydroxyl acid, butylated hydroxyanisole.
2. Compounds which cannot permeate sufficiently to trigger a cancer response (33 compounds)	Glycerine, glyceryl stearate, butylparaben, titanium dioxide, ethanol, diazolidinyl urea, octocrylene, sodium citrate, zinc oxide, silica, sodium chloride, polysorbate 80, benzoyl peroxide, guar gum, paraffin, coal tar, iron oxides, cholesterol, FD & C green No. 3, octyl dimethyl para-aminobenzoic acid, barium sulphate, talc, copper gluconate, bentonite, elastin, beta carotene, silicon dioxide, glyceryl distearate, nitriloacetic acid, potassium phosphate, amaranth, lemonene (biphenyl), serine.
3. Compounds which only had data available from cell lines studies but not animal studies (45 compounds)	Methylparaben, propylparaben, ethylparaben, oxybenzone, sodium hyaluronate, sodium hydroxide, arginine, gluconolactone, lactic acid, benzyl alcohol, potassium sorbate, vitamin C, homosalate, sodium bisulfite, sorbic acid, 4-methylbenzylidene camphor, sodium sulfite, phenylbenzimidazole sulfonic acid, kojic acid, sodium metasulfite, copper sulphate, biotin, resorcinol, benzaldehyde, ammonium chloride, sodium methylparaben, sodium dehydroacetate, sodium ascorbate, zinc sulphate, phenol, benzyl salicylate, glucose, urea, benzoic acid, chloroxylenol, arbutin, eugenol, butylphenyl methylpropional, menthyl anthranilate, triglycerides, calcium panthothenate, caramel, methylene blue, triclosan, sorbitan oleate.

Table 4.3 Percentage limits of Category 1 compounds in application to the body, face and hands

Compound	Flux (mg/h/ cm^2)	Transdermal per day dose (mg)	Max percentage (% w/w)		
			Body	Face	Hands
Triethanolamine	0.008	4.86×10^{2}	1.0	64.2	21.6
Retinyl palmitate	0.626	1.66×10^{-1}	6.2×10^{-4}	3.8×10^{-2}	1.2×10^{-2}
Glycolic acid	0.024	–	10.0*	–	–
Myristic acid	0.135	7.00×10^{3}	26.0	>100	>100
Isopropylparaben	0.902	5.84×10^{3}	21.8	>100	>100
Chlorhexidine digluconate	0.097	1.33×10^{1}	5.0×10^{-2}	3.0	1.0
T-butyl alcohol	0.212	3.24×10^{2}	3.4	>100	72.2
Alpha hydroxy acid	–	–	10.0*	–	–
Butylated hydroxyanisole	0.007	1.38×10^{3}	5.2	>100	>100

Notes
Max percentage: Dividing the transdermal per day dose by the total amount of skin product that can be applied on certain body surfaces (body, face and hands). Limits above 100% indicate that it is safe for the product to consist wholly of that compound.
* Values were obtained directly from skin application studies with the stated concentration

4.4 Discussion

4.4.1 Large number of products, less stringent regulations

The great number of skin products on the market with cancer as a potential side effect calls for greater concern. The regulation on skin products has been relatively less stringent as compared with oral drugs which needed a whole myriad of tests before market launch (Karstadt, 2010). Therefore, more resources should be allocated towards understanding the side effects of skin products.

Out of the four types of skin products (body, facial, hand and sun care), facial and sun care products, representing 72% of all skin products, deserve more attention and regulation. Facial products are designed for the face as the face has more sebaceous glands (Martini, 2006), which increases the permeability of lipophilic components. Sun care products contain active ingredients which are potentially more reactive, likely resulting in more damage to skin integrity (Serpone et al., 2007). Hence, these products may pose a greater risk to consumers so more attention should be paid to them.

4.4.2 Prevalence of carcinogenic compounds in skincare products

Out of 257 products, 239 (93%) contained at least one or more of the 87 potential carcinogenic compounds reported. This information may be contrary to consumers' assumption that most cosmeceuticals are safe (Sautebin, 2008). Nearly two-thirds of the ingredients did not have published data on carcinogenicity. Should they be found carcinogenic, the risk to consumers may increase even more. Many of the compounds stated in the label were mixtures, such as fragrance, C12-14 alkyl benzoate and C12-15 alkyl octanoate. These mixtures should be further defined so that their safety profile can be better understood. Hence, it is important that more studies be done for such compounds to prevent consumers from being harmed unknowingly.

4.4.3 Mechanism of potential carcinogenic compounds

The 87 potential carcinogens are categorized into the following seven mechanisms based on postulations made by other authors as shown in Figure 4.2.

4.4.4 Compounds that generate active species

There were 22 compounds that had been found to be able to generate active species that can cause cancer. Sixteen of these compounds involved generation of radical oxygen species (ROS). They were titanium dioxide (Msiska et al., 2010), vitamin A (Gulkac et al., 2004), silica (Msiska et al., 2010), arginine (Shephard et al., 1987), vitamin C (Philips et al., 2007), benzoyl peroxide (Sharma and Sultana, 2004), alpha hydroxyl acid (Kornhauser et al., 2009), menthyl antranilate (Beeby and Jones,

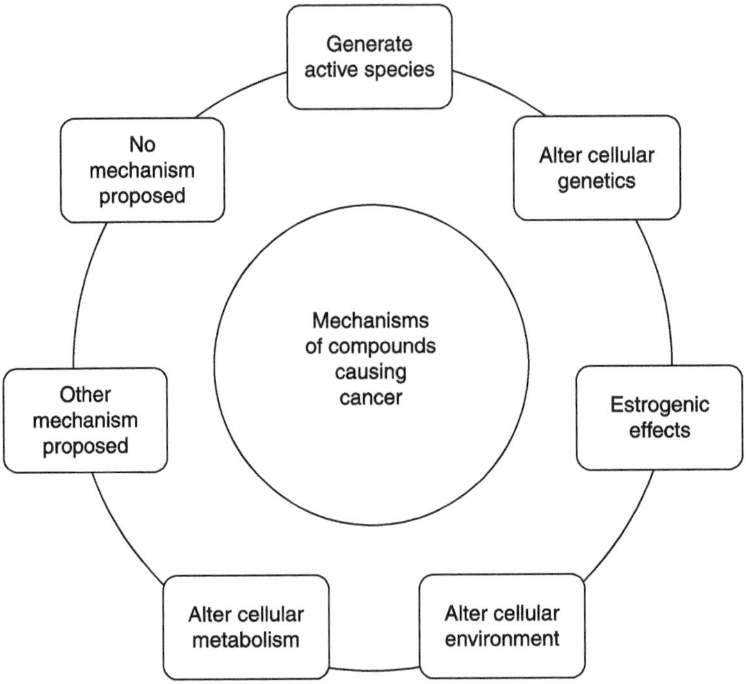

Figure 4.2 **Summary of mechanism of potential carcinogenic compounds**

2000), chloroxylenol (Malaveille et al., 1994), 4-phenylbenzimidazole-5-sulfonic acid (Inbaraj et al., 2002), copper sulphate (Villela et al., 2006), talc (Baan, 2007), resorcinol (Walles, 1992), phenol (Someya et al., 2008) and beta carotene (Gulkac et al., 2004). It had been found that ROS can increase oxidative stress to cells, hence increasing cancer formation (Scibior-Bentkowska and Czeczot, 2009).

Gluconolactone produces gluconate radical and this may result in proliferation of aberrant cells (Merch Index, 2001). It was also found to modify proteins and ribonucleic acid (RNA) by inhibiting the incorporation of uracil into RNA and threonine into protein. This resulted in a massive reproduction of cells, and hence increased the risk of cancer (Villa et al., 1976).

Five compounds produced mutagenic metabolites. They were ethanol, diazolidinyl urea, benzaldehyde, arbutin and eugenol. They produced different compounds in the form of acetylaldehyde (Jelski and Szmitkowski, 2008), formaldehyde (Pfuhler and Wolf, 2002), N-nitroso-N-methylbenzylamine (Demir et al., 2008), hydroquinone (Blaut et al.,

2006) and eugenol-2,3-oxide (Someya et al., 2008), respectively. These compounds may result in aneuploidogenic, mutagenic, clastogenic and genotoxic effects on the DNA and cells, and hence increase the risk of cancer.

4.4.5 Compounds that alter cellular genetics

There were 22 compounds that alter the genetics of cells. They were divided into a further nine categories of base substitution, frameshift mutation, alkylation of DNA bases, direct binding of compound onto DNA, altering gene cycle, hyperplasia, chromatic aberrations, DNA damage and altering gene expression. All these factors had been proven to increase the risk of cancer directly (Whitcomb and Greer, 2009). The compounds that fell under this category were kojic acid (Cheng et al., 2006), biotin (Scheerger and Zempleni, 2003), elastin (Pocza et al., 2008), silicon dioxide (Gao et al., 2009), benzoic acid (Demir et al., 2008), sodium sulfite (Jagiello et al., 1975), chlorhexidine digluconate (Ribeiro et al., 2004), FD & C green No. 3 (Giri and Mukherjee, 1990), octyl dimethyl para-aminobenzoic acid (Gulston and Knowland, 1999), butylated hydroxyanisole (Sasaki et al., 2002), caramel (Stich et al., 1981), amaranth (Sasaki et al., 2002), biphenyl (Sasaki et al., 2002), glycerine (Witschi et al., 1989), sodium metabisulfite (Rencüzogullari et al., 2001), glyceryl distearate (CIR, 2007), zinc sulphate (Takano et al., 1993), methylene blue (Webb and Hass, 1984), potassium sorbate (Mamur et al., 2010), sorbic acid (Mamur et al., 2010), sodium bisulfate (Popescu and DiPaolo, 1988) and coal tar (Culp et al., 2000).

4.4.6 Compounds with estrogenic effects

There were 13 compounds that had been found to increase estrogenic effects on Michigan Cancer Foundation-7 (MCF-7) human breast cancer cell lines. They were parabens (Byford et al., 2002), oxybenzone (Coronado et al., 2008), octocrylene (Matsumoto et al., 2005), benzyl salicylate (Charles and Darbre, 2009), butylphenyl methylpropional (Charles and Darbre, 2009), triclosan (Gee et al., 2008), homosalate (Schlumpf et al., 2001) and 4-methylbenzylidene camphor (Mueller et al., 2003). These compounds act on target cells by binding to estrogen receptors, ERα and/or ERβ. They function as ligand-activated transcription factors, regulating gene expression at specific response elements in the deoxyribonucleic acid (DNA). They fit into the ligand binding pocket of the ligand binding domain, increasing the proliferation of MCF-7 cells, hence increasing the formation of tumors (Byford et al., 2002). This is especially so for breast cancer patients where applying large amounts of these compounds results in a great increase in systemic concentration, thus proliferating the cancerous cells further. These patients should be advised to avoid these compounds. Should there be a need, they should avoid large quantities and direct application of the product to the breast (Harvey and Darbre, 2004).

4.4.7 Compounds that alter cellular environment

There were ten compounds under this category. Sodium citrate (Fukushima et al., 1986), sodium hydroxide (Kurien and Scofield, 2007), lactic acid (Morita et al., 1990), urea (Wangenheim and Bolcsfoldi, 1988), guar gum (Harris and Ferguson, 1999), glucose (Wangenheim and Bolcsfoldi, 1988), ammonium chloride (Ishidate Jr et al., 1984), sorbitan oleate (Setala, 1956) and sodium dehydroacetate (Ishidate Jr et al., 1984) were found to increase the risk of cancer via altered environment. They either involved changing pH or osmotic pressure, thus predisposing the cell to DNA changes. Hence, the risk of cancer is increased.

Sodium hyaluronate was found to be able to alter the cellular matrix. This increased the motility of tumour cells mediated CD44 receptor. Tumour cells can also break down hyaluronic acid to oligosaccharides to stimulate angiogenesis. Hence, this increased cell proliferation and metastases (Tan et al., 2001).

4.4.8 Compounds that alter cellular metabolism

There were eight compounds altering cellular metabolism. They were divided into three groups – chelation, choline deficiency and changed metabolism. Nitrilotriacetic acid was found to chelate divalent cations, thus resulting in *in vivo* DNA damage (Nesslany et al., 2008).

Bentonite (Stott et al., 2004) and triethanolamine (Stott et al., 2004) were found to cause choline deficiency. This resulted in decreased choline, phosphotidylcholine and betaine levels, thus causing a deficient amount of S-adenosylmethionine, which is critical for DNA maintenance. This increased the chances of DNA damage and thus increased the risk of cancer (Stott et al., 2004).

Cholesterol (Larking, 1999), T-butyl alcohol (Bunge and Cleek, 1995), triglycerides (Ulmer et al., 2009), calcium pantothenate (Sivak and Tu, 1980) and potassium phosphate (Shibata et al., 1992) altered cellular metabolism directly in different ways. Their individual mechanisms were described in published journals.

4.4.9 Other compounds that cause cancer

There were seven compounds sorted under this category. Copper gluconate caused cancer by increasing oxidative stress, resulting in cell and tissue damage (Abe et al., 2008). Myristic acid and sodium chloride are precursors to forming mutagens such as ruminant fats (Mannisto et al., 2003) and 2-chloro-4-methylthiobutanoic acid (Chen et al., 1996). Paraffin may result in an increased number of mitoses and tumours. Benzyl alcohol suppressed natural killer cell activity to eliminate cancer cells (Chapman et al., 1973). Glycolic acid altered the skin sensitivity to UV light, thus increasing DNA damage (Ali and Konishi, 1998). Glyceryl stearate inhibited growth of *Bacillus Calmette-Guerin* which was needed to perform cytotoxic functions in the treatment of bladder tumour (Bohle et al., 1996). Hence, patients with bladder tumours are advised to avoid this compound so as to avoid a drop in therapeutic efficacy.

4.4.10 Compounds that had no mechanism proposed

Zinc oxide (Someya et al., 2008), polysorbate 80 (Program, 1992), serine (Hiasa et al., 1984), iron oxides (Goldberg et al., 2001) and barium sulphate (Wagner et al., 1973) were found to be carcinogenic with cell and animal studies but no mechanism was proposed for their carcinogenicity.

4.4.11 Potentially carcinogenic compounds

The percentages of excipients inside a product were mostly unknown. Therefore, to minimize the risk of potential carcinogenicity of cosmeceuticals, a tabulation of the limits of carcinogens that are being used was developed to assist formulators in reducing the risk of cancer to consumers. The animal studies published in the literature were done via continuous exposure to the probable carcinogens over long durations as stated in the studies. The types of animals used involved mice and rats whose skins are considered similar to human skin (Godin and Touitou, 2007). These limits were then calculated from doses that gave a statistical significance in animal and correlation studies. As these carcinogens may cause an increase in risk even at low doses, these compounds were recommended to be avoided as far as possible in formulation. However, if there is a genuine need in using these carcinogens, formulators should use them within the limits recommended.

As shown in Table 4.2, the potentially carcinogenic compounds were grouped into three categories. Category 1 comprised nine compounds that had flux that allowed HD to be attained and had animal studies carried out to allow the determination of HD. Currently, there is no guide for formulators to follow regarding the possible limit to prevent an adverse effect from happening. This guide, as shown in Table 4.3, allows formulators to choose a compound of interest and decide on its limit for a particular skin product. Body and sun care products typically have lower limits as they are spread to a much larger surface area compared to the face and hands. Percentage weight-in-weight over 100% indicates that it is safe for the product to consist wholly of that compound only. It must be noted, however, that consumers may apply skin products that contain a particular compound to other parts of the body other than the face and hands. This means that the compounds in the product may permeate through a larger area than assumed.

Category 2 comprised 33 compounds and their skin permeation cannot attain HD. However, one should take note that many formulations contain penetration enhancers. These penetration enhancers can bring about increased permeation which may otherwise trigger a cancer response.

Category 3 comprised 45 compounds. The carcinogenicity studies of these compounds were done on cell lines, thus the limits cannot be calculated as the dose translation formula does not apply. Also, volume of distribution cannot be accurately determined to safely calculate the dosage needed in milligrams to trigger a carcinogenic response. Hence, with these constraints in mind, a warning to minimize use of compounds in this category is advised.

Some limitations such as the keywords used to search for carcinogenic evidence may not be all-encompassing and may exclude unpublished work. The flux was assumed to be the same regardless of the presence of sebaceous glands. The area of application of sunscreen and body products was assumed to be 13 440 cm^2, which may vary with different consumer habits. Assumption was made that consumers only apply skin products once daily at 2 $mg{\cdot}cm^{-2}$. Some carcinogens were mentioned to have more than one cancer-causing mechanism, but this project classified them into clear categories based on the main mechanism found in the literature. The evidence obtained in this study were mainly limited to animal and cell-lines studies.

Going forward, the results of this research should inspire more researchers to conduct animal studies on compounds that currently have only cell-line studies. More research can also be done on the majority of the compounds that have no publications on their carcinogenicity.

Lastly, research on animal studies can be controlled by using the same species of animal for the permeation study. This can allow formulators to understand their materials better and to design products that are safer for consumers.

4.5 Conclusion

In conclusion, this chapter has shown evidence that potential carcinogens are present in cosmeceuticals and has given recommendations on reducing cancer risk from cosmeceuticals. Its implications can be found in areas such as product formulations and consumers' selection of skin products. The chapter has quantified the limits of carcinogenic compounds that can be used in skin products, bringing the message to consumers' attention that some skin products may cause adverse effects in the long run. Regulators can do more in ensuring the safety of future market cosmeceuticals.

Local effect of cosmeceutics – allergic contact dermatitis

DOI: 10.1533/9781908818713.53

Abstract: Cosmeceutical firms are accountable for ensuring the safety of their products. However, the safety of products and ingredients are often overestimated. Ingredients that can cause allergic contact dermatitis are found in a wide range of products. To address this issue, scientists and dermatologists have initiated various approaches to identify allergens in the cosmeceutics.

Key words: cosmecuetics, allergic contact dematitis, allergens, allergenic potency, flux.

5.1 Introduction

Unlike drugs, biologics and medical devices, cosmeceutics are not required to seek premarket approval from the Food and Drug Administration (FDA). According to the code of Federal Regulations (CFR) title 21, it is the prerogative of cosmeceutical firms to be accountable for ensuring their product safety. However, without the necessity to report the safety profile before marketing, the safety of products and ingredients are often overestimated and overlooked by manufacturers. An example is the cosmetic ingredient, Methylisothiazolinone and Methylchloroisothiazolinone (MI/MCI). Regardless of the warning issued by the European Environmental and Contact Dermatitis Research Group (EECDRG) on ingredients causing allergic contact dermatitis (ACD) as described in Figure 5.1, allergens or sensitizers such as MI/MCI can be readily found in 55 000 tons of

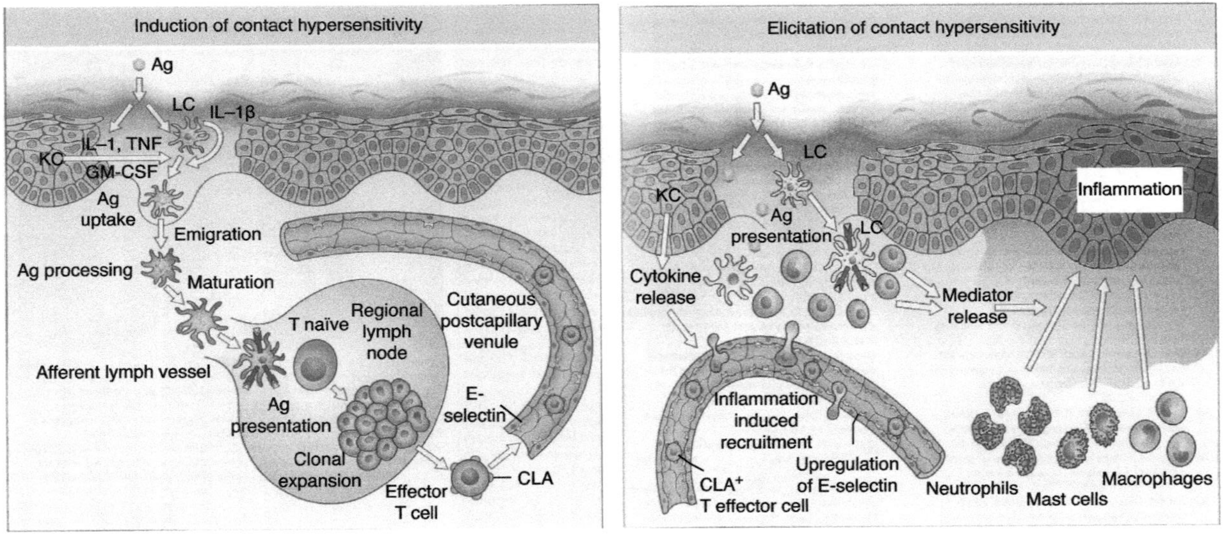

Figure 5.1 **Hypothesized diagram of sensitization and elicitation phase of ACD (Bolognia et al., 2003)**

Note: ACD or cosmetic dermatitis (CD) is a delayed-type IV hypersensitivity reaction on the skin upon direct contact with allergens. In the sensitization phase, the allergens undergo haptenization with the endogenous proteins to form hapten-protein complexes (HPC). Recognized as antigens, the complexes induce the release of cytokines mainly by keratinocytes and Langerhan cells (LC) within the epidermal layer of skin, which thereby activates LC in the uptake of the complexes. While LC are migrating to the proximal peripheral draining lymph nodes, the antigens are being processed, transforming LC into antigen-presenting cells (APC). Within the lymph nodes, APC will activate the specific T naïve cells which proliferate clonally and mature into effector T cells. The mature T cells bear surface markers such as the cutaneous lymphocyte antigen (CLA) that interact with E-selectin located at the inner walls of the cutaneous capillaries, guiding the cells back to the periphery. Upon subsequent epi-cutaneous application of allergens, APC will be detected by the peripheral effector T cells and cytokine release is initiated. As a result, leukocyte migration is promoted, causing cutaneous inflammation during the elicitation phase of ACD.

products on the European market (Toxicology, 1992). With the rapid rise in cosmeceutic consumption (Weber and Villebonne, 2002) and the emergence of a greater variety of products on the market (currently a database of 5500 skincare products from the Mayo Clinic) (Preventice, 2012), these exacerbating factors have also contributed to the increasing prevalence of ACD (Mehta and Reddy, 2003) from 7.2% in 1995 to 12.9% in 2010 in Denmark (Broeckx et al., 1987; Kohl et al., 2002; Mortz et al., 2012).

To address this issue of ACD, scientists and dermatologists have been actively initiating various approaches (Christfnsen and Wall, 1987) to identify allergens in the cosmeceutics. Confirmatory tests have been intensively conducted for the reported allergen via animal (Robinson et al., 1990, Marzulli and Maibach, 1975), *in vitro* and clinical tests (Beck and Wilkinson, 2008) for reproducible results. Subsequently, classification of the allergens is done so as to place greater emphasis on certain ingredients causing ACD. Known to be a dose-dependent reaction on the skin (Andersen et al., 2001), potency is one of the approaches to classify the allergens. Qualitative risk assays such as visual examination on the severity of the clinical symptoms of ACD in Figure 5.2 is one of the methods to determine allergenic potency (Griem et al., 2003). Although being recognized as an appropriate assessment (Marks Jr et al., 1998; Kimber et al., 2003), it has unfortunately contributed to the

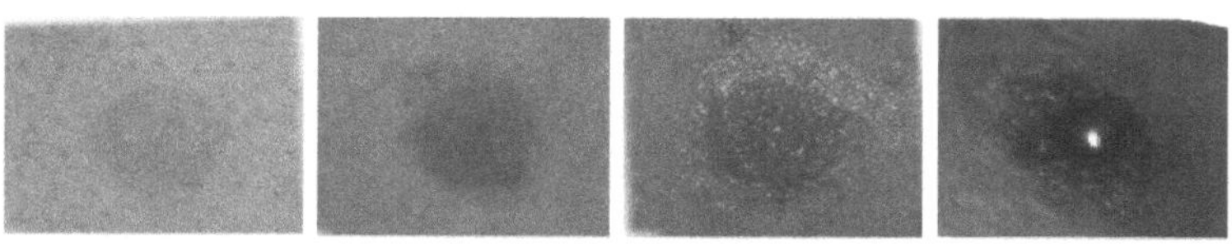

Figure 5.2 **Severity of the symptoms of ACD (Bolognia et al., 2003) and standard recording of patch test reactions recommended by the International Contact Dermatitis Research Group (ICDRG) (Marks Jr et al., 1998)**

Note: Quantification of visual examination on clinical symptoms of irritant reaction (IR) is as follows: no erythema (negative result or – sign); faint erythema (doubtful result or +/– sign); palpable erythema, infiltration (weak positive result or + sign); erythema, infiltration, papules vesicles (strong positive result or ++ sign); intense erythema and infiltration and coalescing vesicles (extreme positive result or +++ sign).

increasing prevalence of ACD due to pre-exposure to the allergen during the diagnostic tests (Anonymous, 2005).

Concurrently, quantitative risk assays such as the murine local lymph node assay (LLNA) and quantitative structure–activity relationships (QSAR) have been established. The former risk assay, LLNA, is an *in vivo* test (Basketter et al., 2000) which analyses the proliferation activity of the excised murine lymph node upon topical exposure to various concentrations of the test substance. The proliferation activity is then quantified and a certain threshold known as the effective concentration 3 (EC3) is obtained to identify any dermal sensitizers. Allergenic potency of the test substances is subsequently determined by their respective EC3 as well. With increasing concern of ethical issues on laboratory animal experiments (Clarkeburn, 2002), predictive tests emerge henceforth to implement the three Rs (i.e., Refinement, Reduction, and Replacement of animal tests). One such test is the QSAR; a computational modelling to predict the dermal allergenic potential of the test substances based on its specific physical–chemical properties (Moss et al., 2002) (hydrogen bonding, molecular weight, Log P, etc.) and molecular structure. Although QSAR is a potential predictive tool, there is still a lack of database on the dermal sensitizers as this assay is inclined towards the prediction of systemic toxicity (Harder et al., 2003) and skin irritation potential of topically applied substances (OECD).

The initial part will be focusing on the analysis of the prevalence of allergens within the cosmeceutics to show the significance of ACD. This is to stress the importance of the need for more stringent cosmeceutic evaluation and regulation. Next, we also aim to develop a potential quantitative risk assessment to overcome some controversial issues regarding conventional assays such as LLNA and QSAR. Based on the positive correlation of murine LLNA and human clinical data (Griem et al., 2003) as well as the mechanism of ACD, flux (defined as the rate of substance that permeates through a unit of skin across the *stratum corneum*) is proposed as a predictive parameter to quantify dermal absorption of allergens and classify their allergenic potency. This promising approach serves as a platform to promote more percutaneous studies, not only on drugs but also on cosmeceutics as well. Lastly, a formulation guideline is proposed for the cosmeceuticals to limit the amount of allergenic ingredients in the products. This will be a novel strategy to substantiate the safety of cosmeceutics and serve as a preventive measure of any possible ACD.

5.2 Methodology

5.2.1 Classification of the products and ingredients

According to the guideline from the European Cosmetic, Toiletry and Perfumery Association (COLIPA) and the US Food, Drugs and Cosmetics Act (FD&C Act) (Nwaogu and Vernon, 2004), 257 internationally available cosmetic products bought from a local pharmacy were classified into their intended usage, such as moisturizer or sunscreen. The functions of 502 cosmetic ingredients from these products were retrieved from the International Cosmetic Ingredient Dictionary and Handbook (Tara and John, 2012).

5.2.2 Identification of allergens

Before the allergens were identified from 514 ingredients, a thorough search on the different types of clinical assays employed for ACD was done. Keywords of 'assays' and 'allergic contact dermatitis' or phrases such as 'methods to test for allergic contact dermatitis' were keyed into the search engine of Google Scholar®, PubMed®, and Scopus®. Six clinical tests were then identified: patch test (Wetter et al., 2005), photo-patch test (European Multicentre Photopatch Test Study, 2012), open test (Christfnsen and Wall, 1987), repeated open application test (ROAT) (Hannuksela and Salo, 1986), human repeat insult patch test (HRIPT) (McNamee et al., 2008) and intradermal test (Herbst et al., 1993). Next, a systematic search on allergenic profiles of these 514 cosmetic ingredients was carried out by the same search engines with the use of keywords 'name of the cosmetic ingredient' and 'name of the clinical assay', e.g. for 'oxybenzone' and 'human patch test'. Published data from the *International Journal of Toxicology* on the safety assessment of these cosmetic ingredients was used for examination of similar profiles, when available. The allergenic profile of each ingredient had to be validated by all six clinical tests as variations in results for individual tests were observed. A general scheme in Table 5.1 was employed to classify the ingredients as 'known allergens', 'possible allergens' and 'unknowns'.

Table 5.1 General scheme to determine allergens

Compound	Patch test	Photo-patch test	Open test	ROAT	HRIPT	Intradermal test	Results
A	+	–	–	NIL	–	–	Known
B	–	–/+	–	–	–	NIL	Possible allergen
C	NIL	NIL	NIL	NIL	NIL	NIL	Unknown

Note: The cosmetic ingredient was considered as a known allergen as long as there was one positive result (+) in any of the clinical assays. On the other hand, those without any positive results, which included negative results (–), no search result (NIL) or unconfirmed results (–/+) would be classified as possible allergens. This was because results from other tests such as animal and *in vitro* assays were not taken into consideration and the tests might not be conducted at a concentration at which positive results would be observed. Lastly, cosmetic ingredients were classified as unknowns if the search engine on all six assays failed to provide any results.

5.2.3 Properties of the allergens

The next approach is to find out the chemical and physical properties of the cosmetic ingredients which could be allergenic in nature. Experimental Log P (ęLog P) and molecular weight (MW) of respective allergens were obtained from the database of Scifinder®. EC3 of the allergens was also acquired from published data (Kimber et al., 2001; Gerberick et al., 2004, 2005) so as to examine the correlation of this pharmacological property with flux.

5.2.4 Steady-state permeation rate of the allergens

The volume of allergen, area of skin in contact with the allergen and the duration of contact were some of the parameters required to calculate the steady-state permeation rate of the flux. These parameters, derived from the clinical assays, have standard requirements which are summarized in Table 5.2.

Flux is defined as the rate at which a certain dose of substance permeates through a unit area of skin. In order to derive flux mathematically, the minimum concentration of the cosmetic ingredients to acquire an allergenic profile and the parameters volume, area and time were used.

Table 5.2 **Standard requirements on the volume of allergen, area of skin in contact and time of contact in the six clinical assays (Christfnsen and Wall, 1987; Beck and Wilkinson, 2008; McNamee et al., 2008)**

Test	Volume of the test material (ml)	Area of the skin contact (cm^2)	Duration per application (hr)
Patch test	0.015–0.02[b]	0.5	24–48[c]
Photo-patch test	0.015–0.02	0.5	24–48
ROAT	0.1	5×5	12
Open test	0.085	1.75	48
HRIPT	0.015–0.02	0.5	24
Intradermal test[a]	0.1	–	48

Note: a: Intradermal test would not be taken into consideration in the permeation rate study as the substance is directly injected into the dermal layer; b: average of the value was used during the calculation; c: 48 hours would be used to calculate the minimum J_{expt} of respective allergens which would initiate an allergenic response as longer exposure has a greater chance of resulting in an allergenic response.

Fraction of absorption was introduced to the calculation to determine the true amount of allergens that have permeated into the skin to cause ACD. With all these parameters, the calculation could be simplified into Eq. 5.1 whereby *C* refers to minimum concentration, *V* refers to volume, *A* refers to area of skin, *T* refers to time of application, *J* refers to flux and *F* refers to fraction of absorption which would be assumed as 0.05 if there was no percutaneous study of the allergen. $F = 0.05$ was estimated by obtaining the average value across various compounds ranging from $0.01 < F < 0.1$ (Gilpin et al., 2010; Saghir et al., 2010; Pažoureková et al., 2011; Ross et al., 2011).

$$J(\mu g/cm^2/hr) = C(\mu g/\mu l) \times V(\mu l) \times \frac{1}{(A(cm^2) \times T(hr))} \times F \qquad [5.1]$$

5.2.5 *Analysis of EC3 and flux*

EC3 derived from murine LLNA is defined as the dermal application concentration (% w/v) of the test chemical required to provoke a three-fold increase in lymph node cell (LNC) proliferative activity (Kimber et al., 2002). It has been well documented by the European Centre for Ecotoxicology and Toxicology of Chemicals (ECETOC) in the determination of allergenic potency of compounds (Basketter et al., 2000). Regression analysis was conducted by Minitab® 16 Statistical Software (M16SS) while the correlation of EC3 and flux was expressed as a 2-dimensional graph in Microsoft Excel®. Values of EC3 and flux were converted to logarithm form to normalize the wide distribution. This mathematical relationship would be validated by cross-validation of the training set (24 allergens from the database) using the leave-one-out method while the applicability of this predictive model would be confirmed by the validation set (eight allergens from external sources).

5.3 Results

5.3.1 Prevalence of allergens

Out of the 514 cosmetic ingredients, 151 were known allergens, 150 were possible allergens and 213 were unknown. One hundred and fifty-one allergenic ingredients are most commonly found in anti-ageing, oil regulating, skin repairing, tanning, ultraviolet (UV) protection and whitening products, Table 5.3. Of the identified allergens, the top ten most frequently used ingredients were Methylparaben, Tocopheryl acetate, Citral, Eugenol, Amyl cinnamal, Farnesol, Geraniol, Propylparaben, Hexyl cinnamal and Lyral (Table 5.4). These ingredients

Table 5.3 Prevalence of cosmeceutics containing at least one allergen

Rank	Function	Prevalence (%)	Rank	Function	Prevalence (%)
1	Anti-ageing	100	7	Whitening	100
2	Oil regulating	100	8	Treatment for blemish/acne	95
3	Others*	100	9	Moisturizing	91
4	Skin repairing	100	10	Cleansing	83
5	Tanning	100	11	Soothing	69
6	UV protection	100			

* Consists of cosmetic products intended for firming, foundation, astringent, pore refining.

Table 5.4 **Top ten ingredients with allergenic property**

Rank	Allergenic cosmetic ingredients	Prevalence (%)
1	Methylparaben	51.1
2	Tocopheryl acetate	48.9
3	Citral	40.9
4	Eugenol	40.4
5	Amyl cinnamal	39.6
6	Farnesol	39.6
7	Geraniol	39.6
8	Propylparaben	39.6
9	Hexyl cinnamal	39.1
10	Lyral	39.1

have the intended function of mainly being preservatives and of fragrance. In addition to these alarming findings, up to 92.9% of the cosmeceutics from the local pharmacy could potentially cause ACD.

5.3.2 Analysis of ȩLog P and MW

Ingredients might acquire allergenic property if they had ȩLog P between values 1 to 3 and MW between 150 to 250 Daltons as illustrated in Figure 5.3. This showed that for the optimal amounts of allergens to induce the sensitization phase of ACD, the hydrophobic property had to be compatible to that of the *stratum corneum* (Roberts and Walters, 1998) for partitioning and the compound should be of a relatively low molecular weight to facilitate passive diffusion across the skin (Aptula et al., 2007).

5.3.3 Correlation of EC3 and flux

Out of 168 allergens, 24 had their EC3 reported in literature. Regression analysis revealed the correlation of Log EC3 and Log Flux as shown in Figure 5.4. Cross validation by leave-one-out method had derived $q^2 = 0.4874$ while predictivity of this model by the validation set had obtained $r^2_{ext} = 0.6384$.

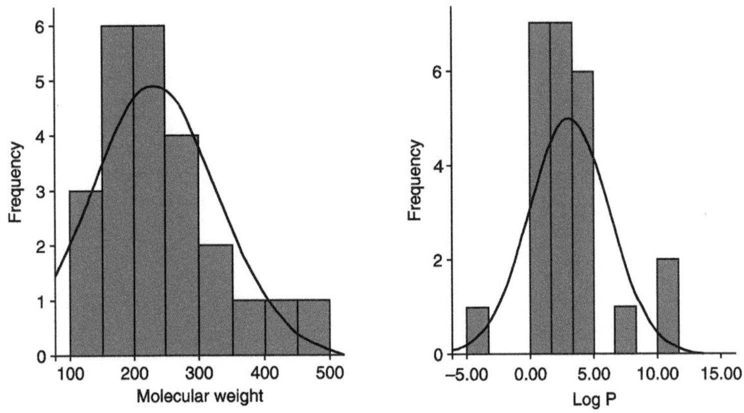

Figure 5.3 **Histograms of ęLog P and MW of the allergens (N = 24)**

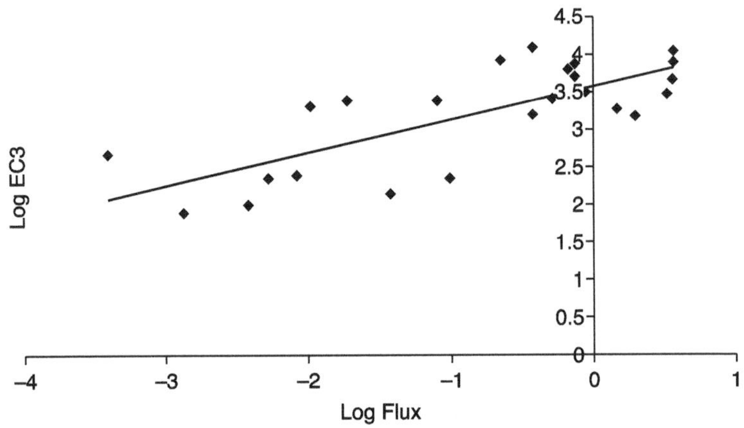

Figure 5.4 **Correlation of Log EC3 and Log Flux**

Log EC3 = 0.4281 (Flux) + 3.5699; $r^2 = 0.5551$; $q^2 = 0.4874$; r^2ext = 0.6384; $p < 0.001$

5.3.4 Predictive modelling for allergenic potency of existing sensitizers

By inferring a linear correlation ($r^2 = 0.5551$; $p < 0.001$) between the EC3 value and flux, allergenic potency may be determined by flux using the equation of Log EC3 = 0.4281 (Log Flux) + 3.5699. Based on the classification of the allergenic potency by EC3 as stated in ECETOC in Table 5.5, allergens with a low EC3 were considered strong sensitizers

Table 5.5 **Potency of the known allergens based on mathematically derived EC3 by flux (Gerberick et al., 2007)**

Flux (μg/cm²/hr)	EC3 values *(μg/cm²)	Potency
$<8.4\times10^{-6}$	<25	Very strong sensitizer
8.4×10^{-6}–1.8×10^{-3}	25–250	Strong sensitizer
1.8×10^{-3}–4.0×10^{-1}	250–2500	Moderate sensitizer
4.0×10^{-1}–8.6×10^{1}	2500–25 000	Weak sensitizer
$>8.6\times10^{1}$	>25 000	Very weak sensitizer

* The unit of EC3 is supposed to be %w/v stated in the protocol of ECETOC. However, for the standardization of unit with flux, a unit of %w/v is converted to μg/cm² by multiplying by a factor of 250 (Griem et al., 2003).

and vice versa. In other words, a potent allergen would require a low dose to evoke 3-fold increase in LNC activity while a weak allergen would require a higher dose to reach the same threshold.

5.4 Discussion

There is an immense breadth and diversity of approaches in the designing of new predictive sensitization risk assessments. This is often carried out by the derivation of the relationship between a physical chemical and a pharmacologic parameter (Basketter et al., 1992; Cronin and Dearden, 1997; Kostoryz et al., 2006). The positive correlation of human lowest observed effect level (LOEL) dose and EC3 (Griem et al., 2003; Basketter et al., 2005) is a crucial platform in the validation of EC3 with respect to human clinical data. Henceforth, it is possible to determine the allergenic potency by extrapolating EC3 with the corresponding human LOEL dose of sensitizing ingredient which evokes ACD on human subjects. This method will be of great significance as the prediction is based on human data. Hence, flux is proposed as an alternative parameter to predict EC3. According to the equation of Fick's first law, steady-state flux (J_{ss}) is calculated using the equation $J_{ss} = K_p.C$ which encompasses permeability coefficient (K_p) and concentration of the substance that has undergone dermal absorption (dose-related) (Korinth et al., 2005). It is a multidisciplinary parameter as it is governed by the properties of test substance (lipophilicity, molecular weight (MW), hydrogen bonding capacity charge of the compound) (Van De Waterbeemd et al., 1996) and the property of the skin (composition, thickness and surface area). With a linear correlation of EC3 and flux ($r^2=0.5551$), flux is appropriate to be the predictive parameter to estimate EC3 which determines allergenic potency of known cosmeceutic sensitizers on humans.

The significance deviation in cross-validation ($q^2=0.4874$) and external validation ($r^2_{ext}=0.6384$) could be the result of the assumption on fraction of absorption ($F=0.05$). This assumption is made due to the lack of percutaneous studies on cosmeceutics compared to drugs which pose greater adverse effect on humans. In addition, the value of *F* derived from percutaneous studies varies with the type of assays[1] employed (Brain et al., 1998; Kreilgaard, 2001), the vehicle in which the test substances are formulated, the type of skin and other factors. Therefore, flux of the allergens calculated from the assumed *F* may not be a good estimation as different substances have varying *F* dependent on their unique physical and chemical properties. For better prediction of *F* and flux on the risk assessment of cosmetic ingredients, *in vitro* percutaneous study by permeation cells (Bronaugh and Stewart, 1985) is recommended as it can derive steady state flux with close approximation under precisely controlled experimental conditions. This form of *in vitro* study enables the use of human skin models (Wagner et al., 2000) to simulate the actual condition of dermal absorption of substances on human subjects where a biological response is observed. Standardization of procedures and robustness of the experiment is necessary to achieve scientific recognition of such a model in the research field of cosmetics.

Ideally, flux should be incorporated into the guideline to advise manufacturers on the amount of allergens contained within the cosmetic products. In this regard, flux over a fixed period of time can be viewed as the maximum dose of the allergens to be added into the cosmetic products that will not evoke an allergic response. However, due to the skin inherent barrier property, *F* has to be factored in when calculating the flux. For instance, given that the applied dose is 1000 μg/cm²/hr, with *F* of 0.05, the flux of the allergen will be much lower at 20 μg/cm²/hr. With flux studies, *F* can be calculated and be used to calculate the ceiling dose which does not cause any allergic reaction.

Therefore, Eq. 5.1 is modified into Eq. 5.2 whereby *D* refers to the maximum applied dose, *C* refers to minimum concentration, *V* refers to volume, *A* refers to area of skin and *T* refers to time of application, with the assumption of 100% absorption ($F=1$) of the applied allergen into the skin. An advantage of such an assumption is that compliance within the maximum applied dose will most likely avoid allergic reactions if 100% absorption does not evoke an allergenic response. In other words, the flux of that particular allergen ($F<1$) will definitely not cause any sensitization as the magnitude of flux is lower than that of the maximum applied dose due to inherent barrier properties of the skin. In this way, cosmeceutical companies are able to calculate and comply within the maximum applied dose of allergens to be formulated in each individual product without the risk of any allergic response. Table 5.6 is a list of allergens which have the calculated maximum applied dose.

$$D(\mu g/cm^2/hr) < C\ (\mu g/\mu l) \times V(\mu l) \times \frac{1}{(A\ (cm^2) \times T\ (hr))} \qquad [5.2]$$

5.5 Conclusion

From this research, it is concluded that flux is a promising parameter for quantitative risk assessment on allergenic substances taken by the transdermal route. As such, allergenic prediction of known allergens may rely less on animal assays such as LLNA and can be substituted by convenient *in vitro* percutaneous studies to determine flux in predicting EC3. With regards to the proposed guideline, cosmeceuticals will be able to comply with the maximum tolerable dose of allergens so as to minimize the likelihood of undesired ACD events associated with the use of their products and ensure the safety of the consumers upon using cosmeceutics.

Table 5.6 **Recommended guidelines of the maximum allowable dose of allergens**

No.	Allergen	Minimum Concentr. (μg/μl)	Volume (μl)	Area (cm²)	Time (hr)	Maximum dose (μg/cm²/hr)	Reference
1	2-Bromo-2-nitropropane-1,3-diol	0.5	17.5	0.5	48	<0.365	Storrs and Bell, 1983
2	4-methylbenzylidene Camphor	100	17.5	0.5	48	<72.9	Buhrv, 1980
3	Allantoin	5	17.5	0.5	48	<3.65	Hansen, 1983
4	Alpha lipoic acid	0.25	17.5	0.5	48	<0.182	Neri et al., 2006
5	Aluminium hydroxide	100	17.5	0.5	48	<72.9	Lopez et al., 1994

(*continued*)

Table 5.6 **Recommended guidelines of the maximum allowable dose of allergens (*continued*)**

No.	Allergen	Minimum Concentr. (μg/μl)	Volume (μl)	Area (cm^2)	Time (hr)	Maximum dose (μg/ cm^2/hr)	Reference
6	Aluminium starch Octenylsuccinate	–	–	–	–	–	Vermaat et al., 2008
7	Ammonium hydroxide	300	17.5	0.5	48	<219	Lopez et al., 1994
8	Amyl cinnamal	10	85	1.75	48	<10.1	Goossens, 2011
9	Ascorbyl palmitate	10	17.5	0.5	48	<7.29	Travassos and Goossens, 2012
10	Asiatic acid	100	17.5	0.5	48	<72.9	Hausen, 1993
11	Avobenzone	100	17.5	0.5	48	<72.9	Hughes and Stone, 2007
12	Benzalkonium chloride	1	17.5	0.5	48	<0.729	Herbst et al., 2004
13	Benzoic acid	20	17.5	0.5	48	<14.6	Toxicology, 2001
14	Benzophenone-4	30	17.5	0.5	48	<21.9	Hughes and Stone, 2007
15	Benzoyl peroxide	1	17.5	0.5	48	<0.729	Hausten et al., 1985
16	Benzyl alcohol	10	17.5	0.5	48	<7.29	Van Oosten et al., 2009
17	Benzyl salicylate	20	17.5	0.5	48	<14.6	Van Oosten et al., 2009
18	Benzyladehyde	50	17.5	0.5	48	<36.5	Forsbeck and Skog, 1977
19	Beta carotene	20	17.5	0.5	48	<14.6	Buhrv, 1980
20	BHA	0.1	17.5	0.5	48	<0.0729	Toxicology, 1984b
21	Bisabolol	10	17.5	0.5	48	<7.29	Andersen, 1999a
22	Bisoctrizole	10	17.5	0.5	48	<7.29	Groot and Frosch, 2011
23	Butylated hydroxytoluene (BHT)	20	17.5	0.5	48	<14.6	Marks Jr et al., 1998

24	Butylene glycol	200	100	25	12	<66.7	Toxicology, 1985d
25	Butylparaben	30	17.5	0.5	24	<43.8	Menné and Hjorth, 1988
26	Butylphenyl methylpropional	100	17.5	0.5	24	<146	Groot and Frosch, 2011
27	C12-15 Alkyl Ethylhexanoate	–	–	–	–	–	Jírová et al., 2010
28	C20-40 Pareth-10	–	–	–	–	–	Bárány et al., 1999
29	C30-38 Olefin/isopropyl Maleate/MA copolymer	–	–	–	–	–	Kai et al., 2011
30	Ceresin	–	–	–	–	–	Schwartz, 1936
31	Ceteareth	–	–	–	–	–	Andersen, 1999b
32	Cetearyl glucoside	–	–	–	–	–	Travassos and Goossens, 2012
33	CetearylIsononanoate	–	–	–	–	–	Le Coz and Bressieux, 2003
34	Cetrimonium bromide	2.5	17.5	0.5	48	<1.82	Toxicology, 1997
35	Cetyl alcohol	10	17.5	0.5	48	<7.29	Toxicology, 1988c
36	Cetyl palmitate	25	17.5	0.5	48	<18.2	Toxicology, 1982c
37	Chlorhexidine acetate	5	17.5	0.5	48	<3.65	Toxicology, 1993a
38	Chlorhexidine digluconate	5	17.5	0.5	48	<3.65	Toxicology, 1993a
39	Chlorocresol	5	17.5	0.5	48	<3.65	Andersen and Hamann, 1984
40	Chlorphenesin	10	17.5	0.5	48	<7.29	Groot and Frosch, 2011
41	Citral	20	17.5	0.5	48	<14.6	Van Oosten et al., 2009
42	Coal tar	50	17.5	0.5	48	<36.5	Groot and Frosch, 2011

(*continued*)

Table 5.6 Recommended guidelines of the maximum allowable dose of allergens (*continued*)

No.	Allergen	Minimum Concentr. (μg/μl)	Volume (μl)	Area (cm^2)	Time (hr)	Maximum dose (μg/ cm^2/hr)	Reference
43	Coco-betaine	10	17.5	0.5	48	<7.29	Herbst et al., 2004
44	Colloidal silver	1	17.5	0.5	48	<0.729	Groot and Frosch, 2011
45	Copper sulphate	50	17.5	0.5	48	<36.5	Nordlind and Liden, 1992
46	Decyl glucoside	5	17.5	0.5	48	<3.65	Andersen and Goossens, 2006
47	Decyl oleate	–	–	–	–	–	Toxicology, 1982a
48	Di C12-15 Alkyl fumarate	–	–	–	–	–	Lammintausta et al., 2010
49	Diazolidinyl urea	4	17.5	0.5	48	<2.92	Toxicology, 1990
50	Dichlorobenzyl alcohol	10	17.5	0.5	48	<7.29	Perrenoud et al., 1994
51	Diisostearyl malate	150	17.5	0.5	48	<109	Hayakawa et al., 1987
52	DMDM hydantoin	2	17.5	0.5	48	<1.46	Toxicology, 1988a
53	Ethoxydiglycol	10	17.5	0.5	48	<7.29	Toxicology, 1985d
54	Ethylhexylglycerin	50	17.5	0.5	48	<36.5	Anonymous, 2012
55	Ethylparaben	30	17.5	0.5	48	<21.9	Toxicology, 1984c
56	Eugenol	20	17.5	0.5	48	<14.6	Addo et al., 1982
57	Farnesol	50	17.5	0.5	48	<36.5	Van Oosten et al., 2009
58	FD & C Yellow N6	–	–	–	–	–	Søsted et al., 2004
59	Fragrance mix	80	17.5	0.5	48	<58.3	Herbst et al., 2004
60	Geraniol	320	17.5	0.5	48	<233	Lapczynski et al., 2008

61	Glyceryl Isostearate	355	17.5	0.5	48	<259	Hayakawa et al., 1987
62	Glycolic acid	5	17.5	0.5	48	<3.65	Andersen, 1998
63	Glycyrrhetinic acid	1	17.5	0.5	48	<0.729	Toxicology, 2007
64	Hexyl cinnamal	100	17.5	0.5	48	<72.9	Groot and Frosch, 2011
65	Hexylene glycol	1.3	17.5	0.5	48	<0.948	Toxicology, 1985d
66	Homosalate	50	17.5	0.5	48	<36.5	Groot and Frosch, 2011
67	Hydrogenated lanolin	–	–	–	–	–	Sugai and Higashi, 1975
68	Hydrogenated polyisobutene	40	17.5	0.5	48	<29.2	Toxicology, 2008
69	Imidurea	20	17.5	0.5	48	<14.6	Marks Jr et al., 2000
70	Iodopropynyl butylcarbamate	1	17.5	0.5	48	<0.729	Groot and Frosch, 2011
71	Iron oxides (CI77492)	8	17.5	0.5	48	<5.83	Zugerman, 1985
72	Isobutylparaben	–	–	–	–	–	Yazar et al., 2011
73	Isononyl Isononanoate	200	17.5	0.5	48	<146	Goossens, 2009
74	Isopropyl alcohol	100	17.5	0.5	48	<72.9	Dromgoole and Maibach, 1990
75	Isopropyl lanolate	200	17.5	0.5	48	<146	Anonymous, 2009
76	Isopropyl myristate	100	17.5	0.5	48	<72.9	Groot and Frosch, 2011
77	Isopropyl stearate	10	17.5	0.5	48	<7.29	Toxicology, 1985c
78	Isopropylparaben	10	17.5	0.5	48	<7.29	Toxicology, 1995
79	Kojic acid	1	17.5	0.5	48	<0.729	Nakagawa et al., 1995
80	Lactic acid	20	17.5	0.5	48	<14.6	Andersen, 1998
81	Lanolin	300	17.5	0.5	48	<219	Groot and Frosch, 2011

(continued)

Table 5.6 Recommended guidelines of the maximum allowable dose of allergens (*continued*)

No.	Allergen	Minimum Concentr. (μg/μl)	Volume (μl)	Area (cm^2)	Time (hr)	Maximum dose (μg/ cm^2/hr)	Reference
82	Lanolin alcohol	300	17.5	0.5	48	<219	Herbst et al., 2004
83	Laureth-23	30	17.5	0.5	48	<21.9	Toxicology, 1983
84	Limonene	20	17.5	0.5	48	<14.6	Van Oosten et al., 2009
85	Linalool	100	17.5	0.5	48	<72.9	Van Oosten et al., 2009
86	Lyral	50	17.5	0.5	48	<36.5	Groot and Frosch, 2011
87	Menthyl anthranilate	10	17.5	0.5	48	<7.29	Marzulli and Maibach, 1975
88	Methoxycinnamate	20	17.5	0.5	48	<14.6	Ortiz and Yiannias, 2004
89	Methyl methacrylate crosspolymer	15	17.5	0.5	48	<10.9	Toxicology, 2002
90	Methylchloroisothiazolinone	0.1	17.5	0.5	48	<0.0729	Groot and Frosch, 2011
91	Methyldibromoglutaronitrile	0.1	85	1.75	48	<0.101	Toxicology, 1996
92	Methylene blue	–	–	–	–	–	Hölzle et al., 2009
93	Methylisothiazolinone	0.01	17.5	0.5	48	<0.00729	Toxicology, 1992
94	Methylparaben	30	17.5	0.5	48	<21.9	Toxicology, 1984b
95	Microcrystalline wax	–	–	–	–	–	Adams et al., 1985
96	Myristyl myristate	80	17.5	0.5	48	<58.3	Toxicology, 1982b
97	Octisalate	50	17.5	0.5	48	<36.5	Avenel-Audran, 2010
98	Octocrylene	100	17.5	0.5	48	<72.9	Karlsson et al., 2011

99	Octyl dimethyl PABA	50	17.5	0.5	48	<36.5	Fotiades et al., 1995
100	Octyldodecanol	300	17.5	0.5	48	<219	Toxicology, 1985a
101	Oxybenzone	30	17.5	0.5	48	<21.9	Marks et al., 2000
102	Palmitic acid	–	–	–	–	–	Toxicology, 1987b
103	Panthenol (Vit B5)	5	17.5	0.5	48	<3.65	Toxicology, 1987b
104	PCA	–	–	–	–	–	Goossens et al., 2002
105	PEG-22/dodecyl glycol copolymer	20	17.5	0.5	48	<14.6	Goossens et al., 2002
106	PEG-4	–	–	–	–	–	Fisher, 1978
107	PEG-4 dilaurate	–	–	–	–	–	Adams et al., 1985
108	PEG-6	–	–	–	–	–	Toxicology, 1993b
109	PEG-8	30	17.5	0.5	48	<21.9	Toxicology, 1993b
110	Phenoxyethanol	10	17.5	0.5	48	<7.29	Groot and Frosch, 2011
111	Phenylbenzimidozole sulfonic acid	50	17.5	0.5	48	<36.5	And and Ros, 1998
112	Polypropylene glycol-2	–	–	–	–	–	Johnson, 1999
113	Polyquaternium-10	–	–	–	–	–	Toxicology, 1988b
114	Polysorbate 20	50	17.5	0.5	48	<36.5	Toxicology, 1984a
115	Polysorbate 60	50	17.5	0.5	48	<36.5	Toxicology, 1984a
116	Polysorbate 80	50	17.5	0.5	48	<36.5	Toxicology, 1984a
117	Polysorbate blend	–	–	–	–	–	Toxicology, 1984a
118	Polyvinyl alcohol	130	17.5	0.5	48	<94.8	Bindu Nair, 1998
119	Polyvinylpyrrolidone	100	17.5	0.5	48	<72.9	Nair, 1998

(continued)

Table 5.6 **Recommended guidelines of the maximum allowable dose of allergens (*continued*)**

No.	Allergen	Minimum Concentr. (μg/μl)	Volume (μl)	Area (cm^2)	Time (hr)	Maximum dose (μg/ cm^2/hr)	Reference
120	Potassium sorbate	–	–	–	–	–	Travassos and Goossens, 2012
121	Propyl gallate	0.035	17.5	0.5	48	<0.0255	Toxicology, 1985b
122	Propylene carbonate	5.4	17.5	0.5	48	<3.94	Toxicology, 1987a
123	Propylene glycol	10	100	25	12	<3.33	Hannuksela and Salo, 1986
124	Propylene glycol dicaprylate	50	100	25	12	<16.7	Johnson, 1999
125	Propylparaben	30	17.5	0.5	48	<21.9	Toxicology, 1984c
126	Quatermium-15	10	17.5	0.5	48	<7.29	Groot and Frosch, 2011
127	Resorcinol	50	100	25	12	<16.7	Hannuksela and Salo, 1986
128	Retinal	0.05	17.5	0.5	48	<0.0365	Groot and Frosch, 2011
129	Silk protein	–	–	–	–	–	Hatch and Maibach, 1985
130	Sodium bisulfite	10	17.5	0.5	48	<7.29	Vena et al., 1994
131	Sodium cocoyl isethionate	2.9	100	25	12	<0.967	Tupker et al., 1999
132	Sodium hyaluronate	–	–	–	–	–	Kowalzick and Ziegler, 2006
133	Sodium lauryl sulphate	0.2	85	1.75	48	<0.202	Kawai et al., 1992
134	Sodium metabisulfite	10	17.5	0.5	48	<7.29	Vena et al., 1994
135	Sodium stearoyl/ isostearoyl lactylate	–	–	–	–	–	Jensen and Andersen, 2005

136	Sodium sulfite	10	17.5	0.5	48	<7.29	Vena et al., 1994
137	Sodium sulphate	–	–	–	–	–	Van Der Valk et al., 1985
138	Sorbic acid	25	100	25	12	<8.33	Hannuksela and Salo, 1986
139	Sorbitol	100	17.5	0.5	48	<72.9	De Waard-van der Spek and Oranje, 2009
140	Stearalkonium hectorite	–	–	–	–	–	Guillot et al., 1982
141	Stearic acid	130	17.5	0.5	48	<94.8	Toxicology, 1987b
142	Stearyl alcohol	300	17.5	0.5	48	<218.8	Giovinazzo et al., 1980
143	Styrene/acrylates copolymer	–	–	–	–	–	Quartier et al., 2006
144	Sulphur	100	17.5	0.5	48	<72.9	Groot and Frosch, 2011
145	T-butyl alcohol	–	–	–	–	–	Dromgoole and Maibach, 1990
146	Tocopheryl acetate (Vit E)	40	17.5	0.5	48	<29.2	De Groot et al., 1991
147	Triclosan	20	17.5	0.5	48	<14.6	Wetter et al., 2005
148	Tricontanyl PVP	–	–	–	–	–	Quartier et al., 2006
149	Triethanolamine	20	17.5	0.5	48	<14.6	Wetter et al., 2005
150	Vit B6	10	17.5	0.5	48	<7.29	Murata et al., 1998
151	VP/eicosene copolymer	–	–	–	–	–	Gallo et al., 2004

5.6 Note (to 'type of assays' on page 64)

1 *In vitro* assays such as horizontal skin diffusion cell, skin stripping, attenuated total reflectance fourier transform infrared (ATR-FTIR) spectroscopy, isolated perfused tissue models, autoradiography, laser scanning confocal microscopy (LSCM) and *in vivo* assays such as cutaneous micro-dialysis.

Essential monographs

DOI: 10.1533/9781908818713.75

This section of the book entails the detailed description of 502 ingredients commonly found in the cosmeceutical products. This includes the international nomenclature of cosmetic ingredients (INCI), other common names, chemical structure, chemical formulae, molecular weight, chemical abstracts service (CAS), intended function and partition coefficient (Log P) from SciFinder®, Cosmetic Ingredient Review (CIR), Specialchem4cosmetics®, Sigmaaldrich®, Cosmeticsinfo® and the *International Cosmetic Ingredient Dictionary*. Through our thorough evaluations of the published literature, we have suggested appropriate classification of carcinogenicity and allergenicity to better guide formulators, clinicians, academics, health care professionals working in the community and hospitals and students interested in the field of cosmeceutics and dermatology. We have also included a popularity ranking to allow manufacturers to know how widely the ingredients are used so as to allow industry players to understand the prevalence of the usage of the ingredient. The recommendations of the monograph are included to provide an easy guide on the intended safety levels of the ingredients.

Carcinogenicity (Please refer to Figure 4.1)

Category	Recommendations
1	Use within proposed limit
2	Safe to use
3	Use with caution

Allergenicity

Potency	Flux (μg/cm²/hr)
Very weak sensitizer	>8.6×10^{1}
Weak sensitizer	4.0×10^{-1} to 8.6×10^{1} (inclusive)
Moderate sensitizer	1.8×10^{-3} to 4.0×10^{-1} (inclusive)
Strong sensitizer	8.4×10^{-6} to 1.8×10^{-3} (inclusive)
Very strong sensitizer	<8.4×10^{-6}

Excipient function

Intended function	Function description
Abrasive	Ingredients used for abrading, smoothing or polishing, such as emery or pumice
Absorbent	Ingredients that have the capacity to absorb or soak up liquids
Adhesive	Ingredients that unite or bond surfaces together
Antiacne agent	Ingredients that reduce the number of acne blemishes, acne pimples, blackheads, and whiteheads
Anticaking agent	Ingredients or processing aids that prevent powdered or granular substances from forming clumps
Antidandruff agent	Ingredients that help to control dandruff, seborrheic dermatitis, and psoriasis
Antifoaming agent	Ingredients that reduce the tendency of finished products to generate foam when shaken
Antioxidant	Ingredients that prevent or slow deterioration due to chemical reaction with oxygen
Antiperspirant agent	Ingredients that are applied to the skin to reduce the production of perspiration at the site of application
Antistatic agent	Ingredients that prevent or inhibit the build-up of static electricity
Artificial nail builder	Ingredients that are used in nail enhancement products to build or lengthen the nail
Astringent	Ingredients that induce a tightening or tingling sensation of the skin
Binder	Ingredients that hold together the ingredients of a compressed tablet or cake
Buffering agent	Ingredients that minimize the change in the pH of a solution when an acid or a base is added to the solution

Bulking agent	Non-reactive, solid ingredients that are used to dilute other solids, or to increase the volume of a product
Chelating agent	Ingredients that inactivate metallic ions so as to prevent the deterioration of cosmetic products
Cleansing agent	Surfactants that clean skin and hair by helping water to mix with oil and dirt so that they can be rinsed away
Colourant	Ingredients that impart colour to cosmetic products
Corrosion inhibitor	Prevents corrosion of the packaging
Cosmetic biocide	Ingredients that help to cleanse the skin or to prevent odour by destroying or inhibiting the growth of micro-organisms
Demulcent	An agent that forms a soothing film when put onto the surface of a mucous membrane such as the inside of the mouth. A demulcent is meant to relieve the irritation of the inflamed mucous membrane
Denaturant	Ingredients added to ethyl alcohol (grain alcohol) to make it unsuitable for drinking, usually by imparting an intensely bitter taste
Deodorant	Ingredients that reduce or eliminate unpleasant odour and that protect against the formation of such odours on the skin
Depilating agent	Ingredients that chemically break down hair fibres so that unwanted hair can be removed by simply wiping it from the skin
Emollient	Ingredients that act as lubricants on the skin surface, which give the skin a soft and smooth appearance
Emulsifying agent	Surfactants that help to form emulsions by reducing the surface tension of the substances to be emulsified
Emulsion stabilizer	Ingredients that help to keep an emulsion from separating into its oil and liquid components
Epilating agent	Waxes or other substances that are heated, applied to the skin, and stripped off quickly to remove unwanted hair
Exfoliant	Ingredients that help to remove dead skin cells from the skin surface
Film former	Ingredients that dry to form a thin coating on the skin, hair or nails
Flavouring agent	Ingredients that impart a flavour or a taste to a product

Foam booster	Surfactants that increase foaming capacity or that stabilize foams
Fragrance	Substances that impart an odour to a product
Hair colourant	Ingredients that impart colour to hair
Hair conditioning	Ingredients that enhance the appearance and feel of hair, by increasing hair body, suppleness, or sheen, or by improving the texture of hair that has been damaged physically or by chemical treatment
Hair fixative	Ingredients that help hair hold its style by inhibiting the hair's ability to absorb moisture
Hairwaving and straightening agent	Substances that modify hair fibres to facilitate changes to the structure of the fibres, such as with permanent waves or with hair straightening
Humectant	Ingredients that increase the water content of the top layers of the skin by drawing moisture from the surrounding air
Hydrotrope	Surfactants that have the ability to enhance the water solubility of another surfactant
Nail conditioning agent	Ingredients that enhance the appearance and feel of nails, by moisturizing the nail, increasing nail sheen, or by reducing nail brittleness and flaking
Occlusive agent	Ingredients that slow the loss of water from the skin by forming a barrier on the skin's surface
Opacifying agent	Substances that reduce the clear or transparent appearance of cosmetic products. Some opacifying agents are used in skin make-up for hiding blemishes
Oral care agent	Ingredients that polish the teeth, reduce oral odour, or otherwise cleanse or deodorize the teeth and mouth
Oxidizing agent	Ingredients that restore hair or skin to its normal oxidized state after exposure to the reducing agent in permanent waving, or that aid in oxidative hair dyeing
pH adjuster	Ingredients that are used to control the pH of cosmetic products
Plasticizer	Materials that soften synthetic polymers by reducing brittleness and cracking
Preservative	Ingredients that prevent or retard bacterial growth, and thus protect cosmetic products from spoilage
Propellant	Compressed gases that are used to expel products from aerosols

Skin bleaching agent	Ingredients that bleach or lighten skin by suppressing melanin (pigment) formation within skin cells
Skin conditioning	Ingredients that enhance the appearance of dry or damaged skin by reducing flaking and restoring suppleness
Slip modifier	Ingredients that help other substances to flow more easily and more smoothly, without reacting chemically
Skin protectant	An ingredient that temporarily protects injured or exposed skin from harmful or annoying stimuli, and that may provide relief to such skin
Solubilizing agent	Surfactants that help another ingredient to dissolve in a solvent in which it would not normally dissolve
Solvent	Substances, usually liquids, that are used to dissolve other substances
Surface modifier	Substances that are added to other cosmetic ingredients to make those ingredients either attract or repel water
Surfactant	An ingredient that helps two substances that normally do not mix to become dissolved or dispersed in one another. Also called a surface active agent
Suspending agent	Suspending agents function by modifying a solid's surface characteristics by adsorption. Changing the surface properties of a solid, keeps the particles from coming together and falling out of solution
UV absorber	Ingredients that protect cosmetic products or packaging from deterioration by absorbing, reflecting, or scattering UV rays. These ingredients may also be used to protect the hair from UV rays
UV filter	UV filters are ingredients that filter certain UV rays that are found in sunlight and, to a lesser degree, artificial light. UV filter is a general term that is used for sunscreen agents, ingredients used to protect the skin from UV rays, and ultraviolet light absorbers (ingredients used to protect products, packaging and hair from UV rays)
Viscosity controlling agent	Materials used to alter the thickness of liquid cosmetic products
Viscosity decreasing agent	Substances that decrease the thickness of liquid cosmetic products
Viscosity increasing agent	Substances that increase the thickness of the liquid portion of cosmetic products

Care has been taken to ensure the accuracy of the information presented. However, the authors are not responsible for errors or omissions or for any consequences on application of the information in this monograph and make no warranty, expressed or implied, with respect to the current accuracy of the contents of the monograph. Application of this information in a particular situation remains the professional responsibility of the manufacturers, formulators, clinicians, health care professionals, academicians, or any other parties that use this monograph; the maximum limits and potentials described and recommended may not be considered absolute and universal recommendations. The authors have exerted every effort to ensure that the dosage and formulae written in this text are in accordance with the current published literature at the time of publication. However, in view of ongoing research, changes in government regulations and the constant flow of information relating to cosmeceutics, dermatology and permeability studies, the reader is urged to check the latest safety data sheet for any amendments and for any added warnings and precautions.

2-Bromo-2-Nitropropane-1,3-Diol

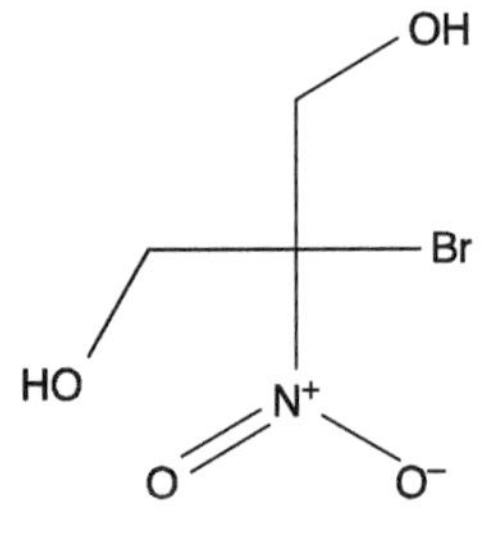

Other names: Bronopol, BNPD, BNPK
INCI: 2-Bromo-2-Nitropropane-1,3-Diol
CAS no: 52-51-7
Molecular formula: $C_3H_6BrNO_4$
Molecular weight: 199.99
Rank of popularity: 188/502
Intended function: Preservative
Log P: 1.15
Allergenic potential: Moderate sensitizer (max dose = 0.365 μg/cm^2/hr)

4-Methylbenzylidene Camphor

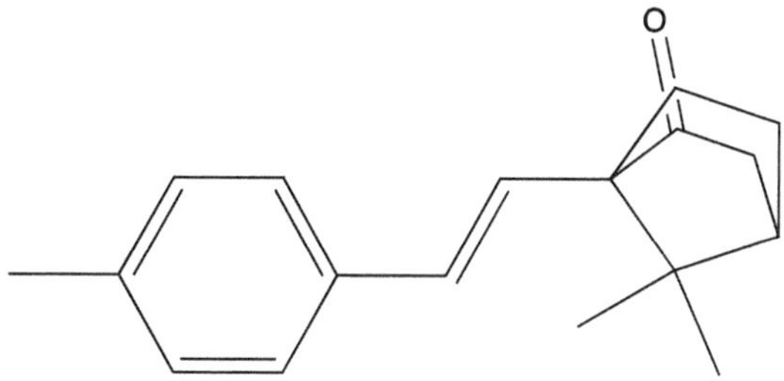

Other names: Enacamene, Enzacamene
INCI: 4-Methylbenzylidene Camphor
CAS no: 36861-47-9/ 38102-62-4
Molecular formula: $C_{18}H_{22}O$
Molecular weight: 254.37
Rank of popularity: 127/502
Intended function: UV absorber, UV filter
Log P: 3.39
Carcinogenic potential: Category 3 (use with precaution)
Allergenic potential: Weak sensitizer (max dose = 72.9 μg/cm^2/hr)

Acetylated Lanolin Alcohol

Other names: Lanolin, Alcohols, Acetates
INCI: Acetylated Lanolin Alcohol
CAS no: 61788-49-6
Rank of popularity: 129/502
Intended function: Emollient, Hair conditioning, Occlusive agent

Acrylamide/Sodium acryloyldimethyltaurate copolymer

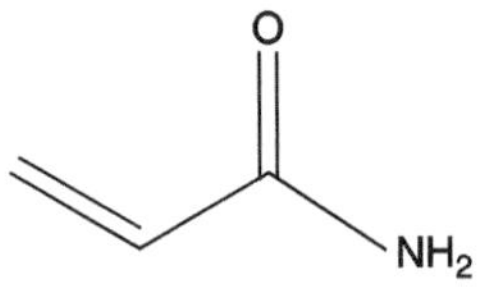

Acrylamide

Other names: Simulgel 600
INCI: Acrylamide/ Sodium acryloyldimethyltaurate copolymer
CAS no: 38193-60-1
Rank of popularity: 189/502
Intended function: Emulsion stabilizer, Viscosity increasing agent
Note: The structure does not represent the polymer. Only individual components are shown.

Acrylates Crosspolymer

INCI: Acrylates Crosspolymer
Rank of popularity: 115/502
Intended function: Absorbent

Acrylates/ C10-30 Alkyl Acrylate Crosspolymer

INCI: Acrylates/ C10-30 Alkyl Acrylate Crosspolymer
Rank of popularity: 30/502
Intended function: Emulsion stabilizer, Viscosity increasing agent

Acrylates/Octylacrylamide Copolymer

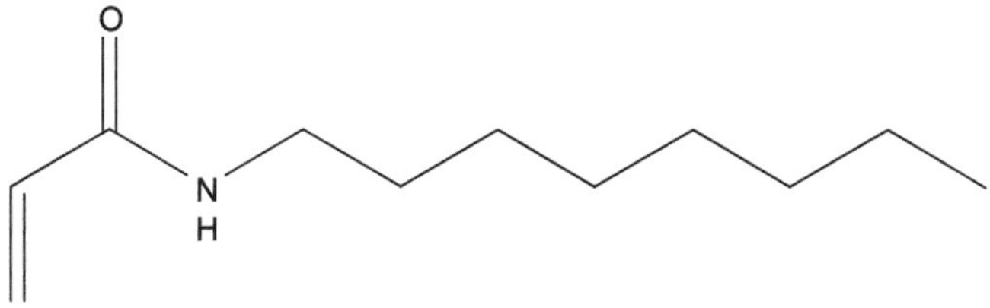

Octylacrylamide

INCI: Acrylates/Octylacrylamide Copolymer
CAS no: 129702-02-9
Rank of popularity: 331/502
Intended function: Film former, Hair fixative

Adipic Acid/ Diethylene Glycol/ Glycerin Crosspolymer

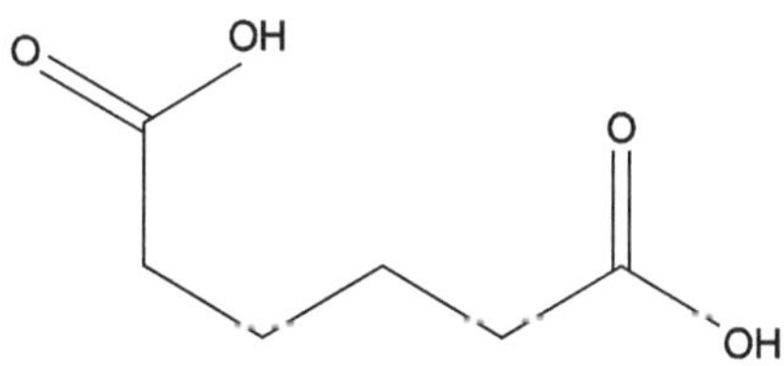

Adipic Acid

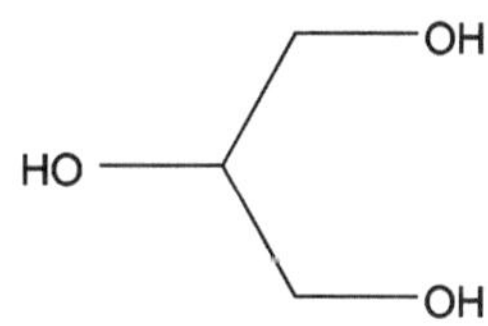

Glycerin

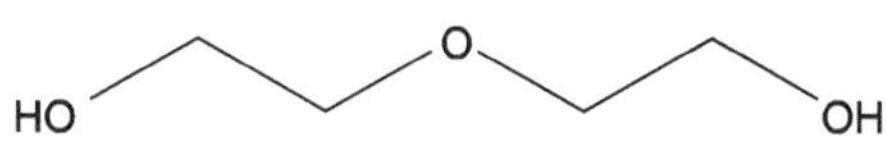

Diethylene Glycol

INCI: Adipic Acid/Diethylene Glycol/Glycerin Crosspolymer
CAS no: 26760-54-3
Rank of popularity: 155/502
Intended function: Film former
Note: The structure does not represent the polymer. Only individual components are shown.

Alanine

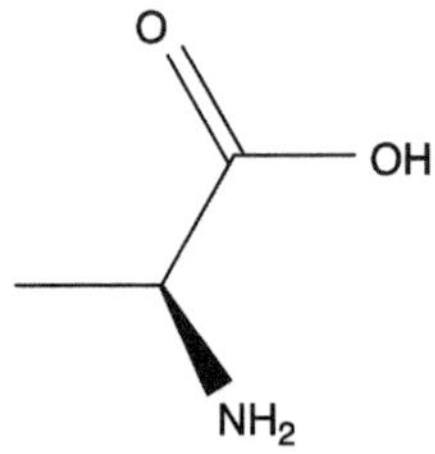

Other names: L-alanine, alaninum, 2-aminopropionic acid
INCI: Alanine
CAS no: 56-41-7 (L-form)
Molecular formula: $C_3H_7NO_2$
Molecular weight: 89.09
Rank of popularity: 239/502
Intended function: Antistatic agent, Hair conditioning, Skin conditioning
Log P: –0.57

Allantoin

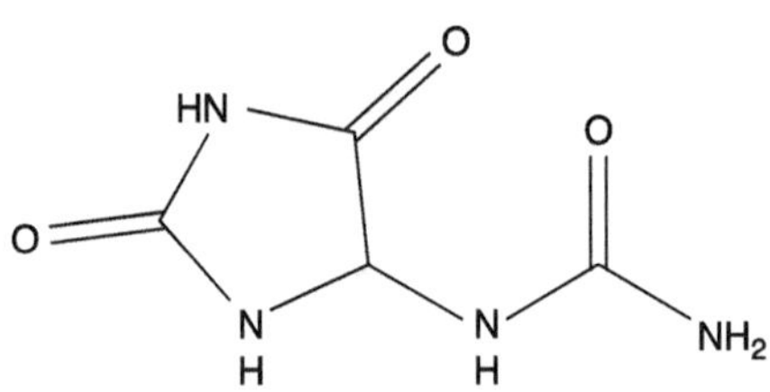

Other names: Glyoxyldiureid, Glyoxyldiureide, Glyoxylic diureide
INCI: Allantoin
CAS no: 97-59-6
Molecular formula: $C_4H_6N_4O_3$
Molecular weight: 158.12
Rank of popularity: 47/502
Intended function: Skin conditioning, Skin protectant
Log P: –1.52
Allergenic potential: Weak sensitizer (max dose = 3.65 $\mu g/cm^2/hr$)

Alpha Hydroxy Acid

Other names: AHA, Organic acids (glycolic acid, lactic acid, citric acid, a-hydroxyoctanoic acid, and α-hydroxydecanoic acid)
INCI: AHA
Rank of popularity: 332/502
Intended function: Exfoliant, pH adjuster, Humectant
Carcinogenic potential: Category 1 (use within limit on body = 10.0 %w/w)

Alpha Lipoic Acid

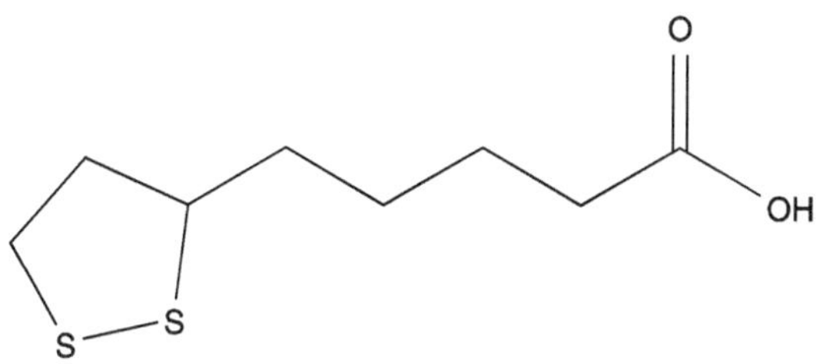

Thioctic acid

Other names: 1,2-Dithiolane-3-pentanoic acid
INCI: Thioctic acid
CAS no: 1077-28-7
Molecular formula: $C_8H_{14}O_2S_2$
Molecular weight: 206.32
Rank of popularity: 333/502
Intended function: Antioxidant
Log P: 2.87
Allergenic potential: Moderate sensitizer (max dose = 0.182 μg/cm²/hr)

Alpha-Isomethyl Ionone

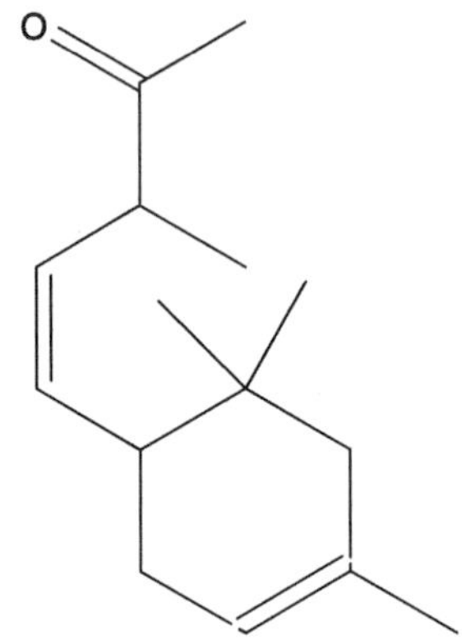

Other names: Isomethyl-alpha-ionone
INCI: Alpha-Isomethyl Ionone
CAS no: 127-51-5
Molecular formula: $C_{14} H_{22} O$
Molecular weight: 206.32
Rank of popularity: 240/502
Intended function: Fragrance, Skin conditioning
Log P: 4.08

Alumina

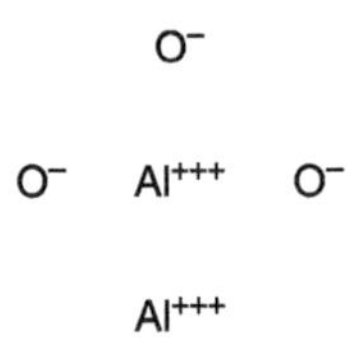

Aluminium oxide

Other names: Aluminum oxide, Aluminum sesquioxide, Aluminum trioxide
INCI: Alumina
CAS no: 1333-84-2(hydrated)/ 1344-28-1
Molecular formula: $Al(OH)_3$
Molecular weight: 77.97
Rank of popularity: 93/502
Intended function: Abrasive agent, Absorbent, Anticaking agent, Bulking agent, Opacifying agent, Viscosity increasing agent

Aluminium Chlorohydrate

$[Al_2(OH)_5]n.\ nCl$

Other names: Aluminum hydroxychloride, Aluminum chloride hydroxide, Aluminum chlorohydrol, Aluminum oxychloride, Aluminum chloride basic
INCI: Aluminium Chlorohydrate
CAS no: 1327-41-9/ 7784-13-6/ 12042-91-0
Molecular formula: $Al_2ClH_5O_5$
Molecular weight: 174.45
Rank of popularity: 334/502
Intended function: Antiperspirant agent, Astringent, Deodorant agent

Aluminium Hydroxide

OH^-

Al^{+++} OH^-

OH^-

Other names: Alumina hydrate, Aluminum trihydroxide, Trihydroxy aluminum
INCI: Aluminium Hydroxide
CAS no: 1333-84-2/ 21645-51-2
Molecular formula: AlH_3O_3
Molecular weight: 78.00
Rank of popularity: 65/502
Intended function: Opacifying agent, Skin protectant
Log P: 0.50
Allergenic potential: Weak sensitizer (max dose = 72.9 μg/cm²/hr)

Aluminium Starch Octenylsuccinate

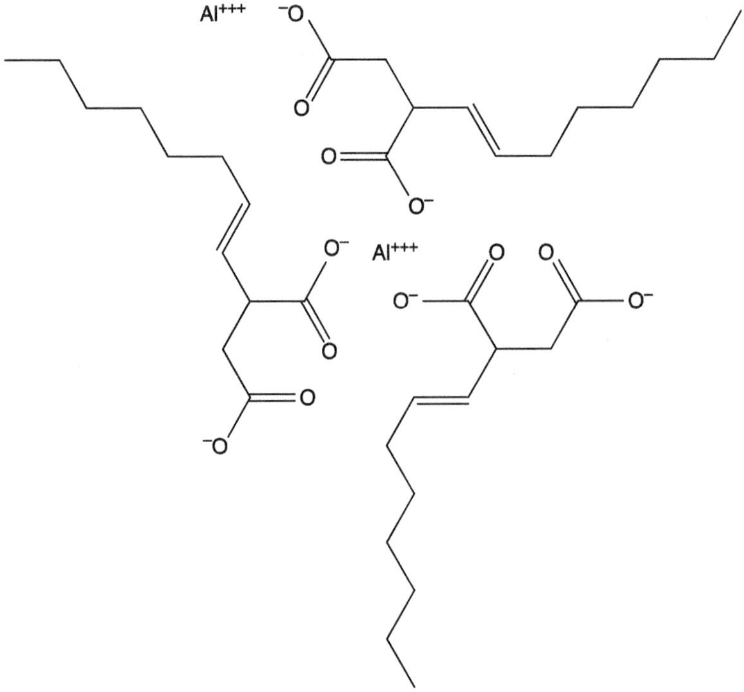

Aluminium Octenylsuccinate

Other names: Starch, Hydrogen octenylbutanedioate
INCI: Aluminium Starch Octenylsuccinate
CAS no: 9087-61-0
Molecular formula: $C_{21}H_{44}O_3$
Molecular weight: 344.57
Rank of popularity: 80/502
Intended function: Absorbent, Anticaking agent, Viscosity increasing agent
Allergenic potential: Maximum dose not stated
Note: The structure does not represent the polymer. Only individual components are shown.

Aluminium Stearate

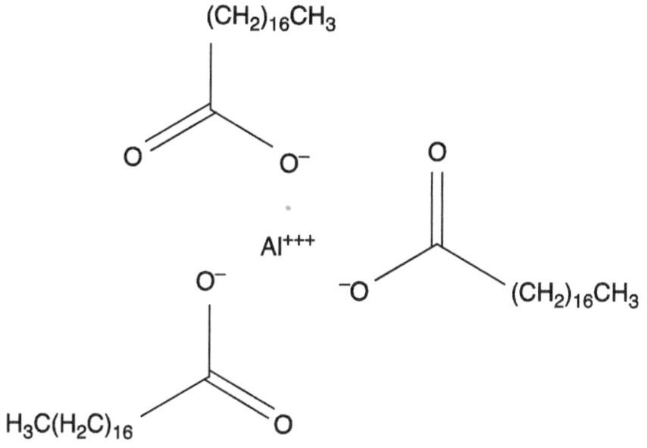

Other names: Aluminium stearate, Aluminum dihydroxide stearate, Aluminum monostearate, Dibasic aluminum stearate
INCI: Aluminium Stearate
CAS no: 7047-84-9
Molecular formula: $C_{18}H_{37}AlO_4$
Molecular weight: 296.46
Rank of popularity: 116/502
Intended function: Anticaking agent, Colourant, Emulsion stabilizer, Viscosity increasing agent

Aluminium Sucrose Octasulfate

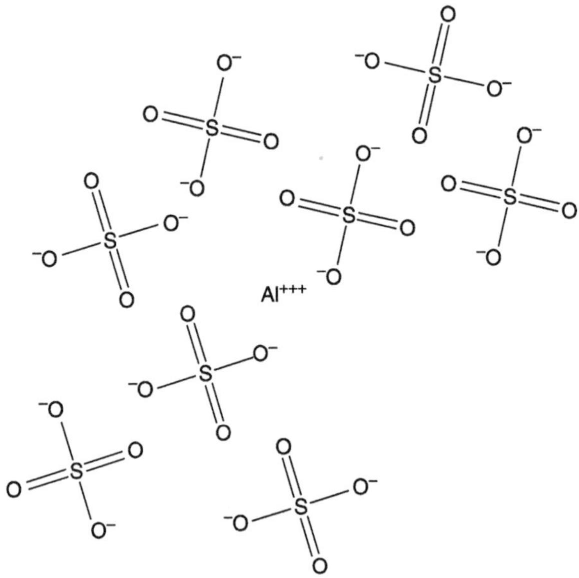

Aluminium Octasulfate

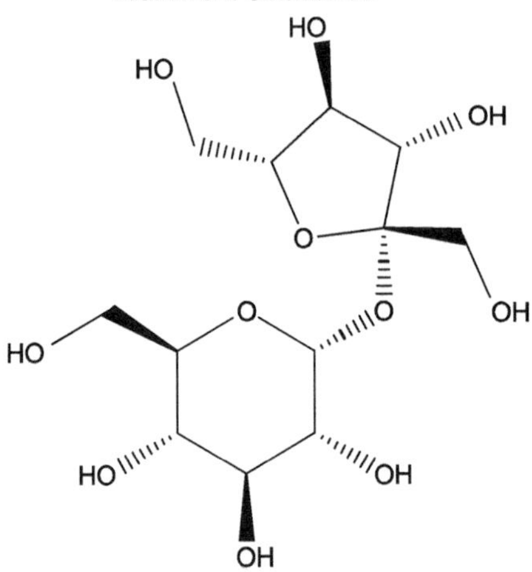

Sucrose

Other names: Sucralfate
INCI: Aluminium Sucrose Octasulfate
CAS no: 54182-58-0
Molecular formula: $C_{12} H_{54} Al_{16} O_{75} S_8$
Molecular weight: 2086.73

Rank of popularity: 335/502
Intended function: Skin conditioning
Note: The structure does not represent the polymer. Only individual components are shown.

Amaranth

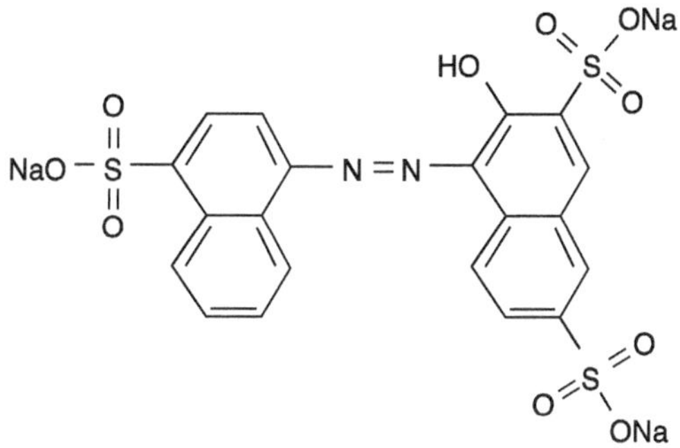

Other names: Amaranth, Cl 16185, Food red 9, Japan red 2, Red no. 2
INCI: Acid red 27
CAS no: 915-67-3
Molecular formula: $C_{20}H_{14}N_2O_{10}S_3 \cdot 3Na$
Molecular weight: 607.49
Rank of popularity: 336/502
Intended function: Colourant
Carcinogenic potential: Category 2 (safe to use)

Ammonium Acryloyldimethyltaurate/VP Copolymer

INCI: Ammonium Acryloyldimethyltaurate/VP Copolymer
Molecular formula: copolymer of ammonium acryloyldimethyltaurate and vinylpyrrolidone monomers
Rank of popularity: 241/502
Intended function: Viscosity increasing agent

Ammonium Chloride

$NH_4^+\ Cl^-$

Other names: Ammonii chloridum, Ammonium muriate, Sal ammoniac, Salmiac
INCI: Ammonium Chloride
CAS no: 12125-02-9
Molecular formula: NH_4Cl
Molecular weight: 53.49
Rank of popularity: 337/502
Intended function: Fragrance, Viscosity increasing agent
Log P: –0.09
Carcinogenic potential: Category 3 (use with precaution)

Ammonium Glycolate

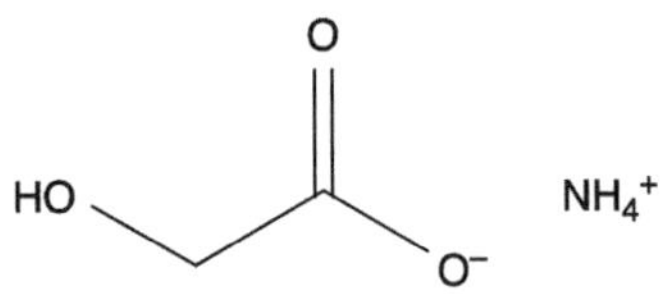

Other names: Ammonium hydroxyacetate
INCI: Ammonium Glycolate
CAS no: 35249-89-9
Molecular formula: $C_2H_7NO_3$
Molecular weight: 93.08
Rank of popularity: 156/502
Intended function: Exfoliant, ph adjuster

Ammonium Glycyrrhizate

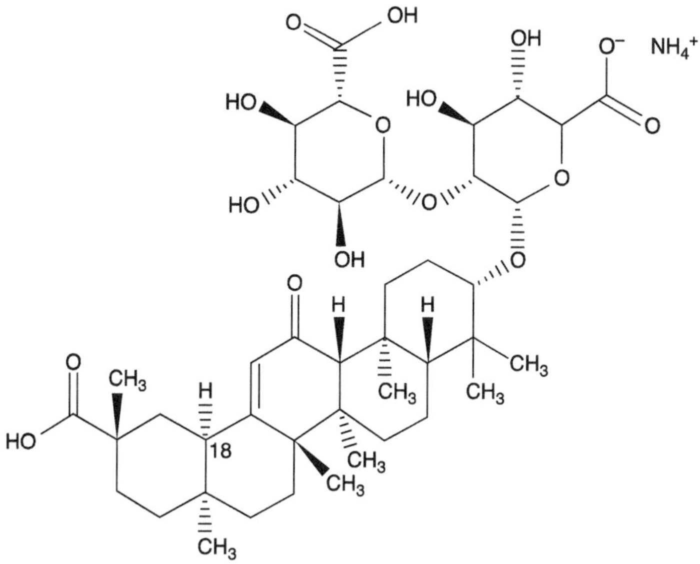

Other names: Glycyrrhizin ammonium salt, Glycyrrhizic acid ammonium salt, Monoammonium glycyrrhizinate
INCI: Ammonium Glycyrrhizate
CAS no: 53956-04-0
Molecular formula: $C_{42}H_{62}O_{16} \cdot H_3N$
Molecular weight: 83.99
Rank of popularity: 190/502
Intended function: Fragrance, Skin conditioning

Ammonium Hydroxide

$$NH_4^+ \quad OH^-$$

Other names: Ammonia water, Aqua ammonium, Spirit of hartshorn, Strong ammonia solution
INCI: Ammonium Hydroxide
CAS no: 1336-21-6
Molecular formula: H_5NO
Molecular weight: 35.05
Rank of popularity: 94/502
Intended function: Denaturant, ph adjuster
Log P: –0.76
Allergenic potential: Very weak sensitizer (max dose = 219 μg/cm²/hr)

Ammonium Polyacryloyldimethyl Taurate

INCI: Ammonium Polyacryloyldimethyl Taurate
CAS no: 62152-14-1
Rank of popularity: 130/502
Intended function: Emulsion stabilizer, Viscosity increasing agent

Amyl Cinnamal

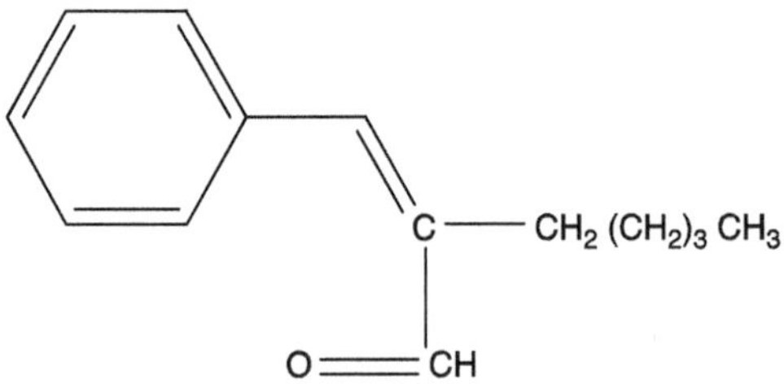

Other names: Alpha-amylcinnamaldehyde, Alpha-amyl cinnamic aldehyde
INCI: Amyl Cinnamal
CAS no: 122-40-7
Molecular formula: $C_{14}H_{20}O$
Molecular weight: 202.29
Rank of popularity: 242/502
Intended function: Fragrance
Log P: 4.36
Allergenic potential: Weak sensitizer (max dose = 10.1 μg/cm^2/hr)

Arachidyl Alcohol

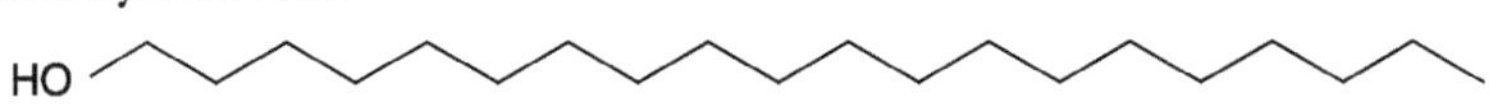

Other names: Arachic alcohol, Arachidic alcohol, 1-eicosanol, Eicosyl alcohol
INCI: Arachidyl Alcohol
CAS no: 629-96-9
Molecular formula: $C_{20}H_{42}O$
Molecular weight: 298.55
Rank of popularity: 338/502
Intended function: Emollient, Emulsion stabilizer, Viscosity increasing agent
Log P: 8.99

Arbutin

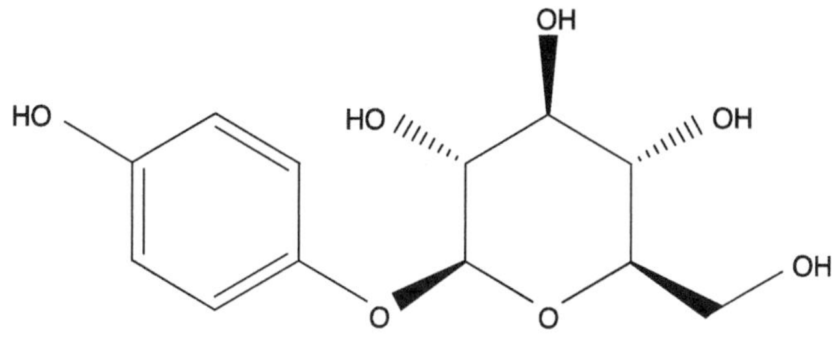

Other names: Arbutine, 4-hydroxyphenyl-beta-D-glucopyranoside, p-hydroxyphenyl beta-D-glucoside
INCI: Arbutin
CAS no: 497-76-7
Molecular formula: $C_{12}H_{16}O_7$
Molecular weight: 272.25
Rank of popularity: 243/502
Intended function: Antioxidant, Skin bleaching agent, Skin conditioning
Log P: –1.35
Carcinogenic potential: Category 3 (use with precaution)

Arginine

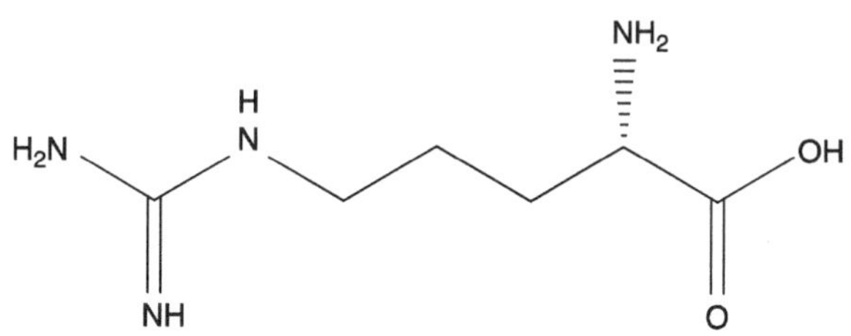

Other names: L-Arginine
INCI: Arginine
CAS no: 74-79-3(L form)/7200-25-1
Molecular formula: $C_6H_{14}N_4O_2$
Molecular weight: 174.20
Rank of popularity: 73/502
Intended function: Antistatic agent, Hair conditioning, Oral care agent, Skin conditioning
Log P: –1.65
Carcinogenic potential: Category 3 (use with precaution)

Argireline

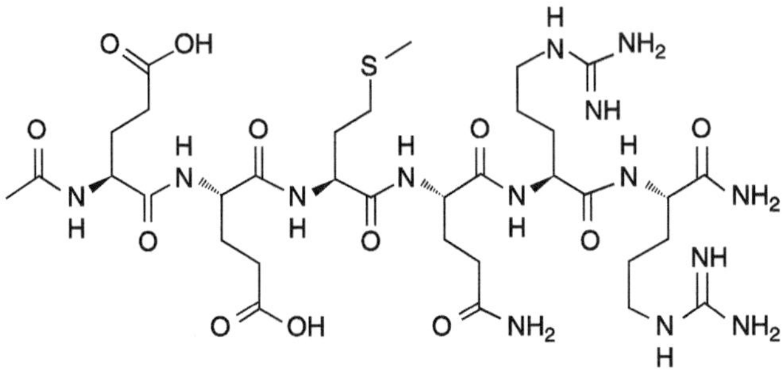

Other names: Acetyl hexapeptide-3
INCI: Acetyl hexapeptide-3
CAS no: 616204-22-9
Molecular formula: $C_{34}H_{60}N_{14}O_{12}S$
Molecular weight: 888.99
Rank of popularity: 340/502
Intended function: Humectant
Log P: –5.81

Ascorbyl Glucoside

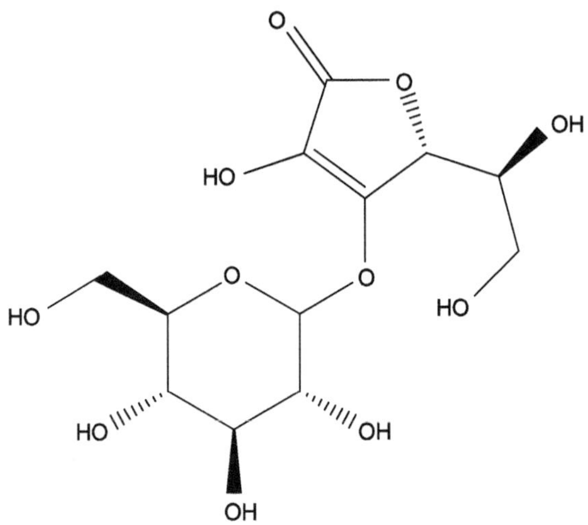

INCI: Ascorbyl Glucoside
CAS no: 129499-78-1
Molecular formula: $C_{12}H_{18}O_{11}$
Molecular weight: 338.26
Rank of popularity: 131/502
Intended function: Antioxidant
Log P: –4.66

Ascorbyl Methyslilanol Pectinate

INCI: Ascorbyl Methyslilanol Pectinate
CAS no: 227200-22-8
Rank of popularity: 244/502
Intended function: Antioxidant, Viscosity increasing agent

Ascorbyl Palmitate

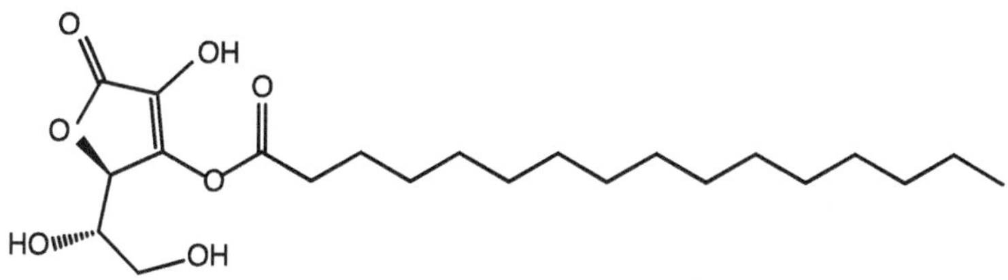

Other names: Ascorbic acid palmitate, Ascorylapalmitic acid
INCI: Ascorbyl Palmitate
CAS no: 137-66-6
Molecular formula: $C_{22}H_{38}O_7$
Molecular weight: 414.53
Rank of popularity: 110/502
Intended function: Antioxidant, Fragrance
Log P: 4.97
Allergenic potential: Weak sensitizer (max dose = 7.29 μg/cm^2/hr)

Asiatic Acid

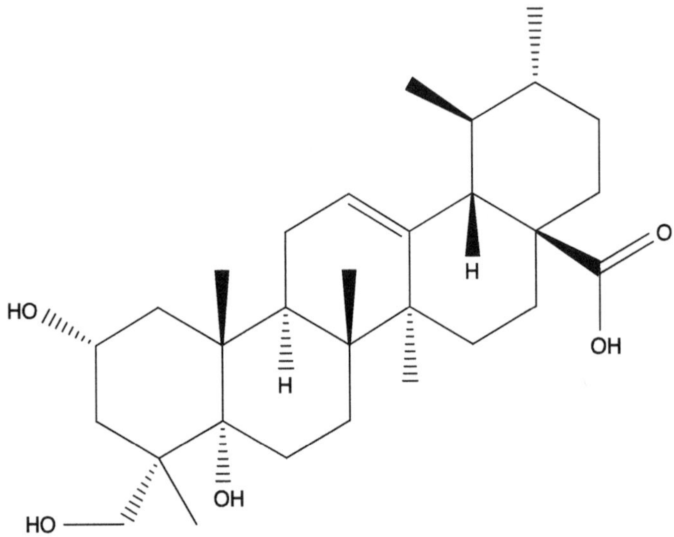

Other names: 2α,23-Dihydroxyursolic acid, Dammarolic acid
INCI: Asiatic Acid
CAS no: 464-92-6
Molecular formula: $C_{30}H_{48}O_5$
Molecular weight: 488.70
Rank of popularity: 341/502
Intended function: Skin conditioning
Log P: 5.75
Allergenic potential: Weak sensitizer (max dose = 72.9 μg/cm²/hr)

Avobenzone

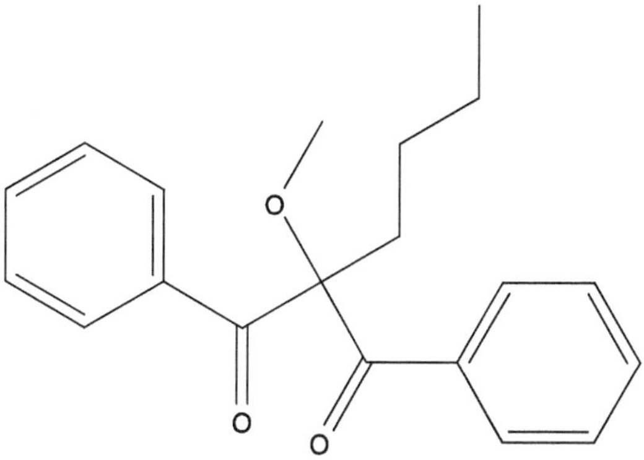

Other names: Butyl methoxydibenzoylmethane
INCI: Butyl methoxydibenzoylmethane
CAS no: 70356-09-1
Molecular formula: $C_{20}H_{22}O_3$
Molecular weight: 310.39
Rank of popularity: 34/502
Intended function: UV absorber, UV filter
Log P: 4.19
Allergenic potential: Weak sensitizer (max dose = 72.9 μg/cm²/hr)

Barium Sulphate

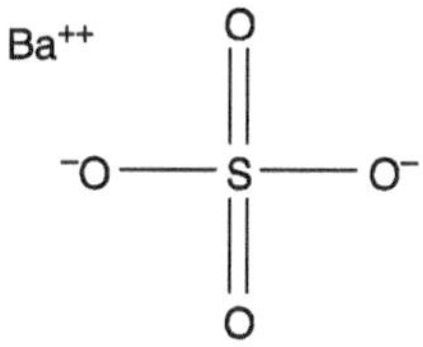

Barium Sulfate

Other names: Blanc fixe, Cl 77120, Pigment white 21, Pigment white 22
INCI: Barium Sulfate
CAS no: 7727-43-7
Molecular formula: Ba. H_2O_4S
Molecular weight: 235.41
Rank of popularity: 245/502
Intended function: Colourant, Opacifying agent
Carcinogenic potential: Category 2 (safe to use)

Behentrimonium Methosulphate

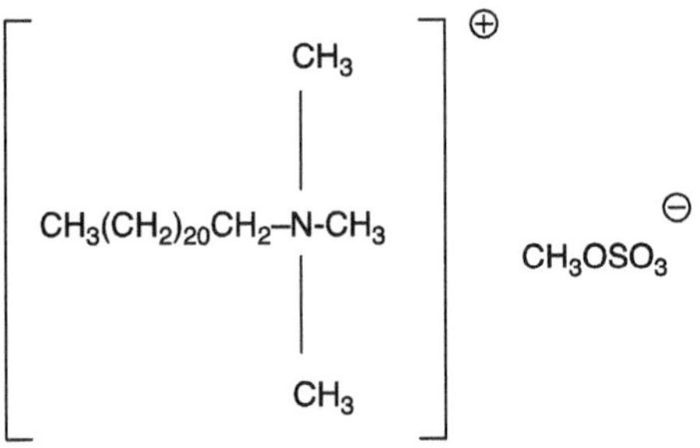

Other names: Behenyl trimethyl ammonium methosulfate
INCI: Behentrimonium Methosulfate
CAS no: 81646-13-1/ 241148-21-0
Molecular formula: $C_{25}H_{54}N \cdot CH_3O_4S$
Molecular weight: 479.80
Rank of popularity: 342/502
Intended function: Antistatic agent, Hair conditioning

Behenyl Alcohol

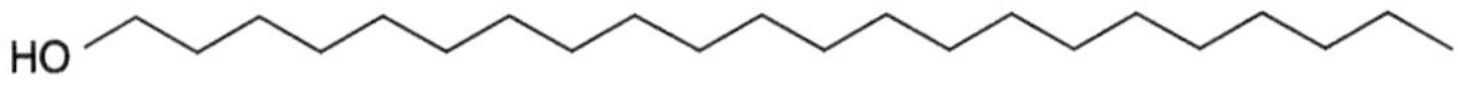

Other names: 1-docosanol
INCI: Behenyl Alcohol
CAS no: 661-19-8
Molecular formula: $C_{22}H_{46}O$
Molecular weight: 326.60
Rank of popularity: 157/502
Intended function: Binder, Emollient, Emulsion stabilizer, Viscosity increasing agent
Log P: 10.01

Bemotrizinol

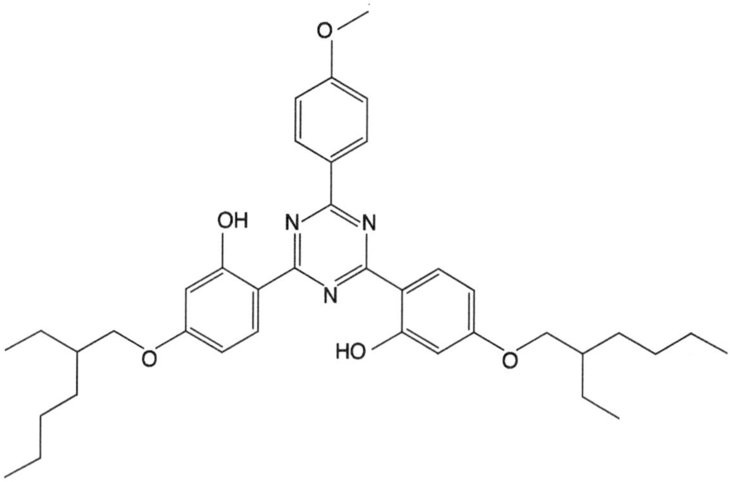

Other names: Bis-ethylhexyloxyphenol methoxyphenyl triazine
INCI: Bis-ethylhexyloxyphenol methoxyphenyl triazine
CAS no: 187393-00-6
Molecular formula: $C_{38}H_{49}N_3O_5$
Molecular weight: 627.81
Rank of popularity: 95/502
Intended function: Skin conditioning, UV absorber, UV filter
Log P: 12.93

Bentonite

Other names: Bentonitum, CI77004, Soap clay
INCI: Bentonite
CAS no: 1302-78-9
Molecular formula: $Al_2O_3 \cdot 4SiO_2 \cdot H_2O$
Rank of popularity: 246/502
Intended function: Absorbent, Bulking agent, Emulsion stabilizer, Opacifying agent, Suspending agent, Viscosity increasing agent
Carcinogenic potential: Category 2 (safe to use)

Benzalkonium Chloride

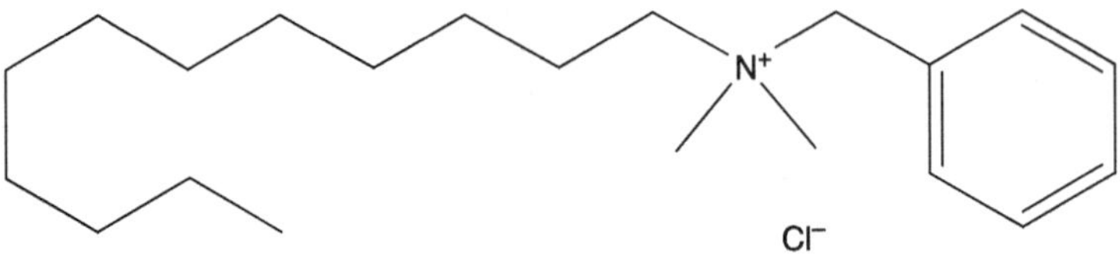

Other names: Alkylbenzyldimethylammonium chloride
INCI: Benzalkonium Chloride
CAS no: 8001-54-5/ 61789-71-7/ 68391-01-5/ 68424-85-1/ 85409-22-9
Molecular weight: 424.15
Rank of popularity: 191/502
Intended function: Antistatic agent, Deodorant, Preservative, Surfactant
Log P: 10.05
Allergenic potential: Weak sensitizer (max dose = 0.729 μg/cm²/hr)

Benzoic Acid

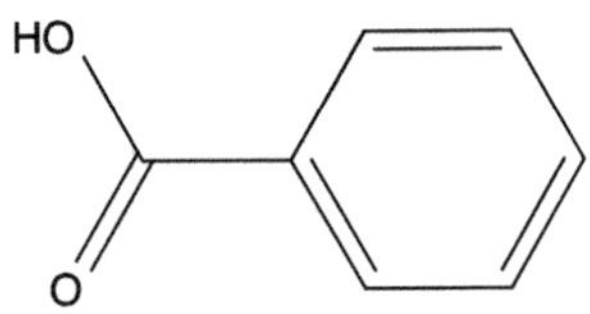

Other names: Acidum benzoicum, Benzenecarboxylic acid, Benzeneformic acid, Carboxybenzene, Dracyclic acid, Phenylcarboxylic acid, Phenylformic acid
INCI: Benzoic Acid
CAS no: 65-85-0
Molecular formula: $C_7H_6O_2$
Molecular weight: 122.12
Rank of popularity: 132/502
Intended function: Fragrance, pH adjuster, Preservative
Log P: 1.56
Carcinogenic potential: Category 3 (use with precaution)
Allergenic potential: Weak sensitizer (max dose = 14.6 μg/cm²/hr)

Benzophenone-4

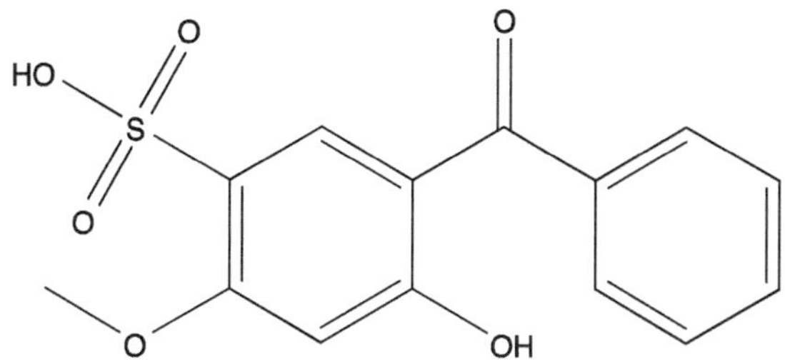

Other names: Sulisobenzone
INCI: Benzophenone-4
CAS no: 4065-45-6
Molecular formula: $C_{14}H_{12}O_6S$
Molecular weight: 308.31
Rank of popularity: 247/502
Intended function: UV absorber, UV filter
Log P: 0.99
Allergenic potential: Weak sensitizer (max dose = 21.9 μg/cm^2/hr)

Benzoyl Peroxide

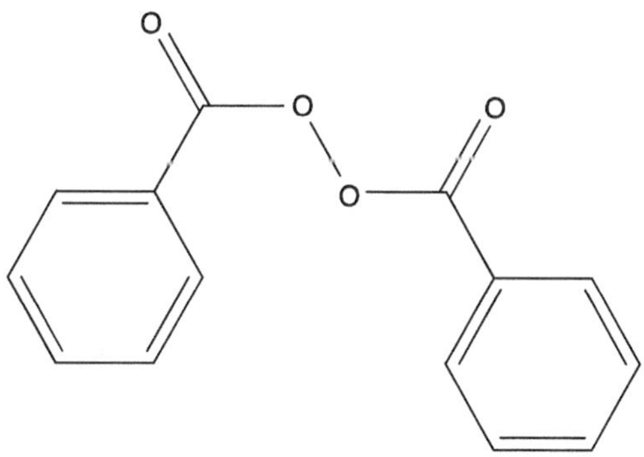

Other names: Dibenzoyl peroxide
INCI: Benzoyl Peroxide
CAS no: 94-36-0
Molecular formula: $C_{14}H_{10}O_4$
Molecular weight: 242.20
Rank of popularity: 158/502
Intended function: Antiacne agent, Oxidizing agent
Log P: 3.46
Carcinogenic potential: Category 2 (safe to use)
Allergenic potential: Weak sensitizer (max dose = 0.729 μg/cm^2/hr)

Benzyl alcohol

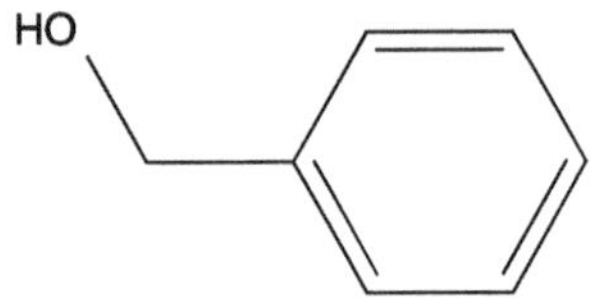

Other names: Benzenemethanol, Benzylic alcohol, Phenylcarbinol, Phenylmethanol, Phenylmethyl alcohol, Alpha-toluenol
INCI: Benzyl alcohol
CAS no: 100-51-6
Molecular formula: C_7H_8O
Molecular weight: 108.14
Rank of popularity: 81/502
Intended function: Fragrance, Preservative, Solvent, Viscosity decreasing agent
Log P: 1.06
Carcinogenic potential: Category 3 (use with precaution)
Allergenic potential: Weak sensitizer (max dose = 7.29 $\mu g/cm^2/hr$)

Benzyl Salicylate

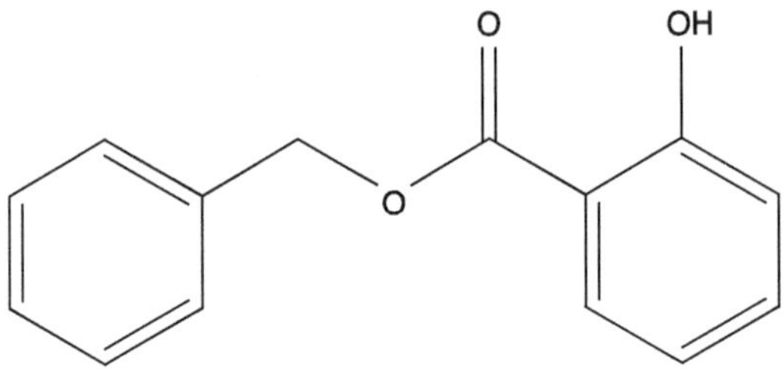

Other names: Benzyl 2-hydroxybenzoate, Phenylmethyl 2-hydroxybenzoate
INCI: Benzyl Salicylate
CAS no: 118-58-1
Molecular formula: $C_{14}H_{12}O_3$
Molecular weight: 228.24
Rank of popularity: 343/502
Intended function: Fragrance, UV absorber
Log P: 4.21
Carcinogenic potential: Category 3 (use with precaution)
Allergenic potential: Weak sensitizer (max dose = 14.6 $\mu g/cm^2/hr$)

Benzyladehyde

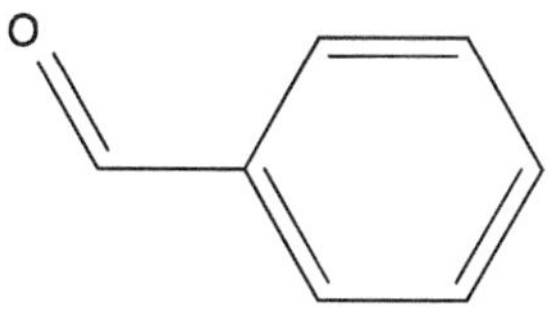

Other names: Artificial almond oil, Benzoic aldehyde, Phenylformaldehyde
INCI: Benzyladehyde
CAS no: 100-52-7
Molecular formula: C_7H_6O
Molecular weight: 106.12
Rank of popularity: 344/502
Intended function: Denaturant, Flavouring agent, Fragrance
Log P: 1.45
Carcinogenic potential: Category 3 (use with precaution)
Allergenic potential: Weak sensitizer (max dose = 36.5 μg/cm²/hr)

Beta Carotene

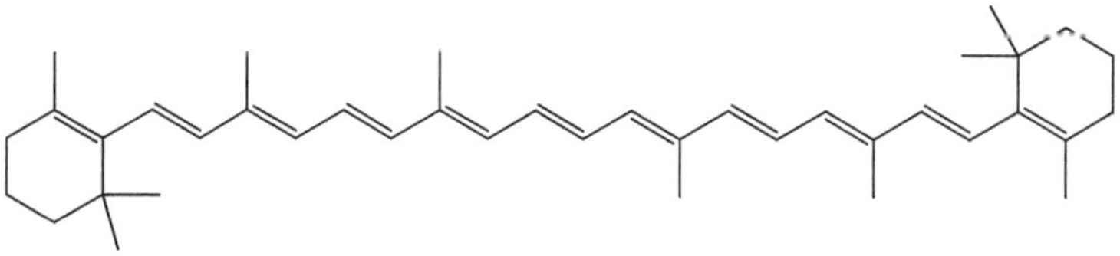

Other names: Cl75130, Food orange 5, Natural yellow 26
INCI: Beta-Carotene
CAS no: 7235-40-7/ 116-32-5/ 31797-85-0
Molecular formula: $C_{40}H_{56}$
Molecular weight: 536.87
Rank of popularity: 345/502
Intended function: Colourant, Skin conditioning
Log P: 14.76
Carcinogenic potential: Category 2 (safe to use)
Allergenic potential: Weak sensitizer (max dose = 14.6 μg/cm²/hr)

Betasitosterol

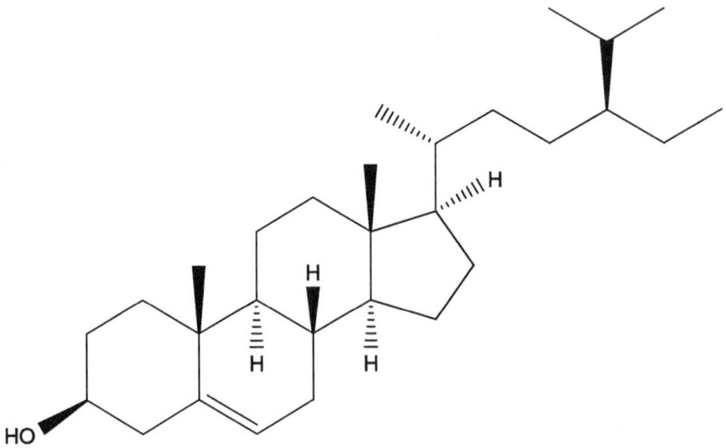

Other names: α-Dihydrofucosterol, 22, 23-Dihydrostigmasterol, 24β-Ethylcholesterol, 5-Stigmasten-3β-ol
INCI: Beta-Sitosterol
CAS no: 83-46-5
Molecular formula: $C_{29}H_{50}O$
Molecular weight: 414.71
Rank of popularity: 133/502
Intended function: Emulsion stabilizer, Fragrance, Skin conditioning
Log P: 10.48

Butylated hydroxyanisole

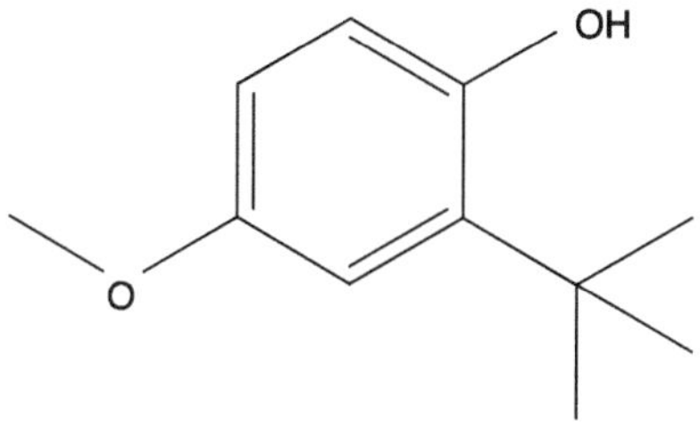

Other names: Butylated hydroxyanisole, Butylhydroxyanisol, Tert-butyl-4-methoxyphenol
INCI: BHA
CAS no: 25013-16-5
Molecular formula: $C_{11}H_{16}O_2$
Molecular weight: 180.11
Rank of popularity: 346/502
Intended function: Antioxidant, Fragrance
Log P: 3.78
Carcinogenic potential: Category 1 (use within limit on body = 5.2 % w/w; face >100% w/w; hands >100 % w/w)
Allergenic potential: Moderate sensitizer (max dose = 0.0729 μg/cm^2/hr)

Biosaccharide Gum-1

INCI: Biosaccharide Gum-1
Molecular formula: Polysaccharides derived from the fermentation of sorbitol
Molecular weight: >1 000 000
Rank of popularity: 248/502
Intended function: Skin conditioning

Biotin

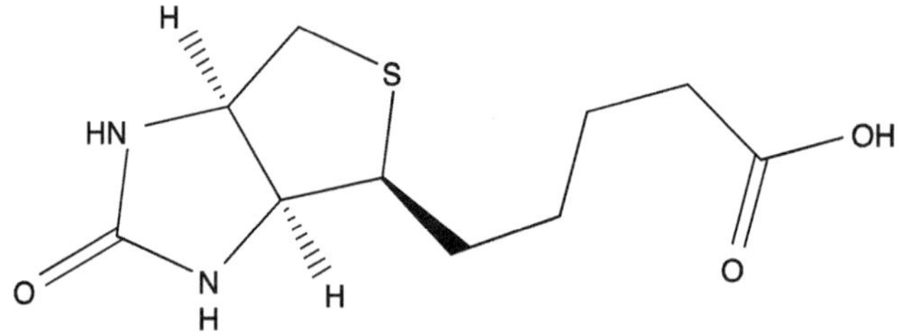

Other names: Biotinum, Coenzyme R, Vitamin B7, Vitamin H
INCI: Biotin
CAS no: 58-85-5
Molecular formula: $C_{10}H_{16}N_2O_3S$
Molecular weight: 244.31
Rank of popularity: 249/502
Intended function: Hair conditioning, Skin conditioning
Log P: 0.86
Carcinogenic potential: Category 3 (use with precaution)

Bisabolol

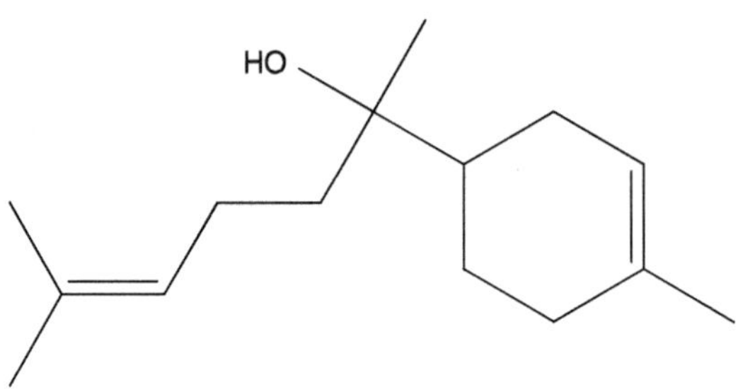

Other names: Levomenol
INCI: Bisabolol
CAS no: 515-69-5 / 23089-26-1
Molecular formula: $C_{15}H_{26}O$
Molecular weight: 222.37
Rank of popularity: 82/502
Intended function: Fragrance, Skin conditioning
Log P: 4.59
Allergenic potential: Weak sensitizer (max dose = 7.29 μg/cm^2/hr)

Bisoctrizole

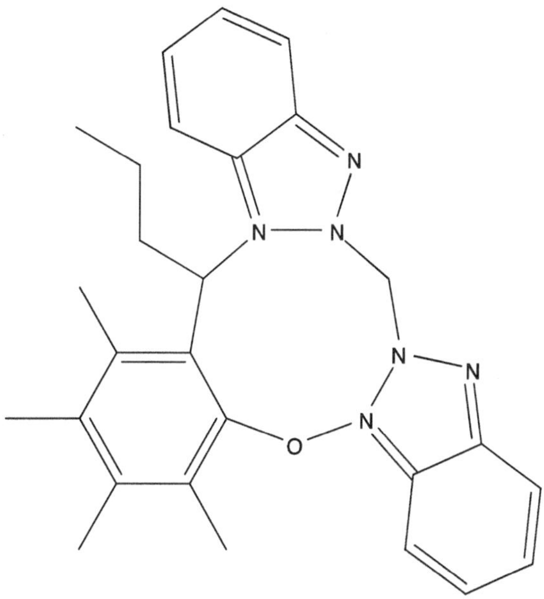

Other names: Methylene bis-benzotriazolyl tetramethylbutylphenol
INCI: Methylene bis-benzotriazolyl tetramethylbutylphenol
CAS no: 103597-45-1
Molecular formula: $C_{41}H_{50}N_6O_2$
Molecular weight: 658.87
Rank of popularity: 134/502
Intended function: UV filter
Log P: 14.48
Allergenic potential: Weak sensitizer (max dose = 7.29 μg/cm²/hr)

BIS-PEG/PPG-16/16PEG/PPG-16/16 Dimethicone

INCI: BIS-PEG/PPG-16/16PEG/PPG-16/16 Dimethicone
Rank of popularity: 347/502
Intended function: Emulsifying agent, Occlusive agent

Bis-Stearyl Ethylenediamine/Neopentyl Glycol/Stearyl Hydrogenated Dimer Dilinoleate Copolymer

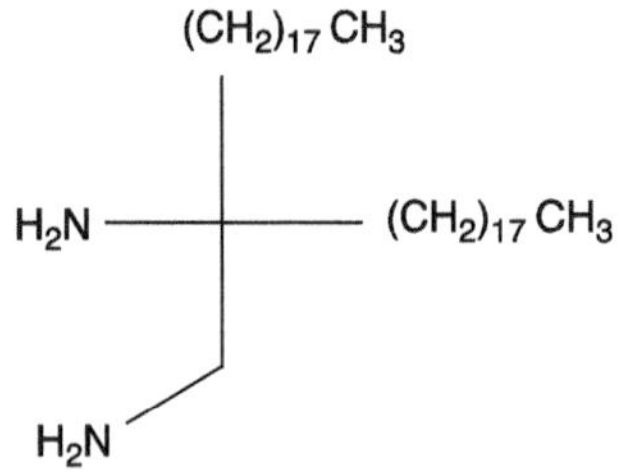

Bis-Stearyl Ethylenediamine

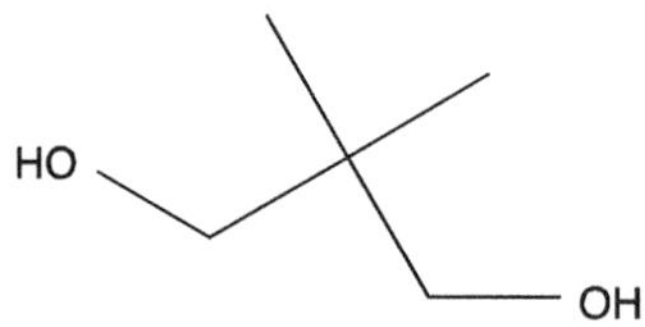

Neopentyl Glycol

INCI: Bis-Stearyl Ethylenediamine/Neopentyl Glycol/Stearyl Hydrogenated Dimer Dilinoleate Copolymer
Rank of popularity: 348/502
Intended function: Emollient, Occlusive agent, Skin protectant, Viscosity increasing agent
Note: The structure does not represent the polymer. Only individual components are shown.

Butylated Hydroxytoluene

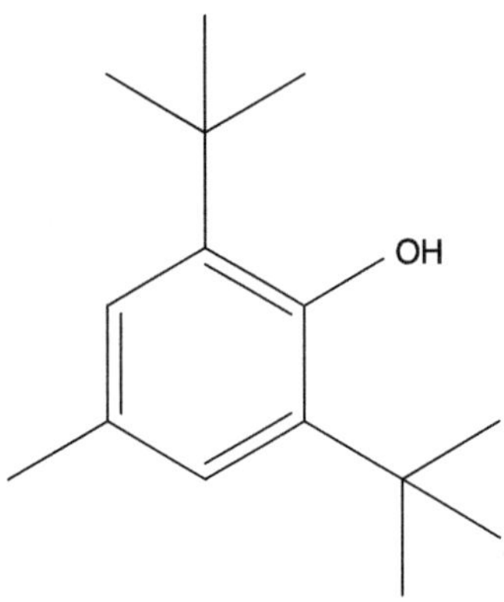

Other names: Butylated Hydroxytoluene, DBPC, Butylhydroxytoluenum, 2,6-di-t-butyl-p-cresol
INCI: BHT
CAS no: 128-37-0
Molecular formula: $C_{15}H_{24}O$
Molecular weight: 220.35
Rank of popularity: 33/502
Intended function: Antioxidant, Fragrance
Log P: 5.17
Allergenic potential: Weak sensitizer (max dose = 14.6 μg/cm^2/hr)

Butylene Glycol

Other names: 1,3-butanediol, 1,3-dihydroxybutane
INCI: Butylene Glycol
CAS no: 107-88-0
Molecular formula: $C_4H_{10}O_2$
Molecular weight: 90.12
Rank of popularity: 29/502
Intended function: Fragrance, Humectant, Skin conditioning, Solvent, Viscosity decreasing agent
Log P: –0.74
Allergenic potential: Weak sensitizer (max dose = 66.7 μg/cm^2/hr)

Butylparaben

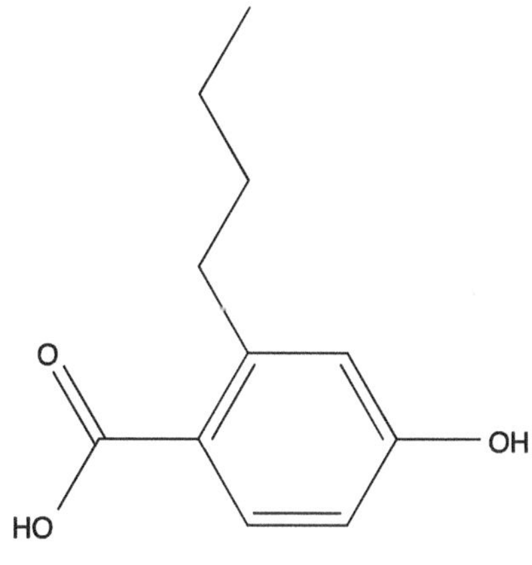

Other names: Butyl parasept, Chemynol B, CoSept B, Isocide BP, Microcare BHB, Nipabutyl, OriStar BPB, Paratexin B, Parido B, Unisept B
INCI: Butylparaben
CAS no: 94-26-8
Molecular formula: $C_{11}H_{14}O_3$
Molecular weight: 194.23
Rank of popularity: 16/502
Intended function: Fragrance, Preservative
Log P: 3.41
Carcinogenic potential: Category 2 (safe to use)
Allergenic potential: Weak sensitizer (max dose = 43.8 μg/cm^2/hr)

Butylphenyl Methylpropional

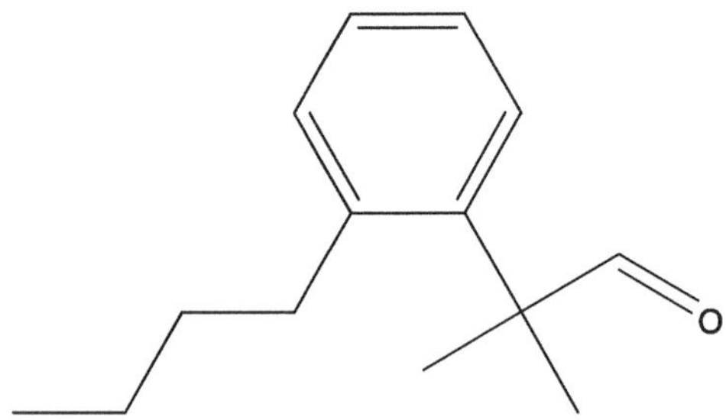

Other names: 2-(4-tert-Butylbenzyl)Propionaldehyde
INCI: Butylphenyl Methylpropional
CAS no: 80-54-6
Molecular formula: $C_{14}H_{20}O$
Molecular weight: 204.31
Rank of popularity: 349/502
Intended function: Fragrance
Log P: 3.84
Carcinogenic potential: Category 3 (use with precaution)
Allergenic potential: Very weak sensitizer (max dose = 146 μg/cm^2/hr)

C10-30 Cholesterol/Lanosterol Esters

Rank of popularity: 350/502
Intended function: Emulsifying agent, Skin conditioning

C12-14 Alkyl Benzoate

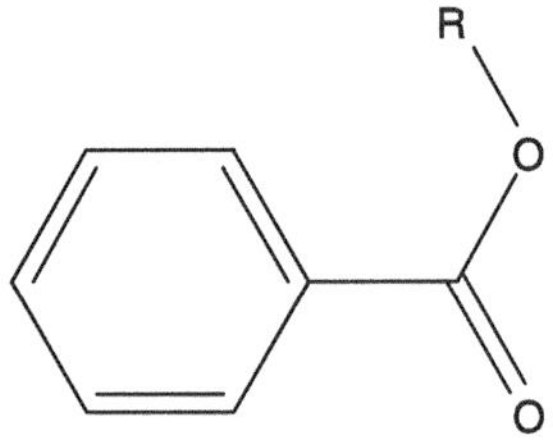

Alkyl Benzoate

Rank of popularity: 250/502
Intended function: Emollient

C12-15 Alkyl Benzoate

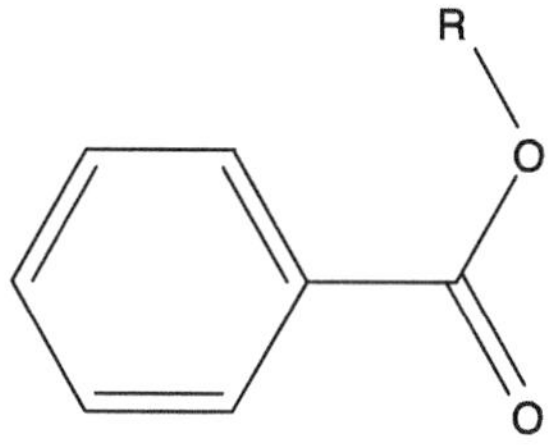

Alkyl Benzoate

Other names: Alkyl benzoate, C12-15 alcohols benzoate
INCI: C12-15 Alkyl Benzoate
CAS no: 68411-27-8
Rank of popularity: 28/502
Intended function: Emollient, Skin conditioning

C12-15 Alkyl Ethylhexanoate

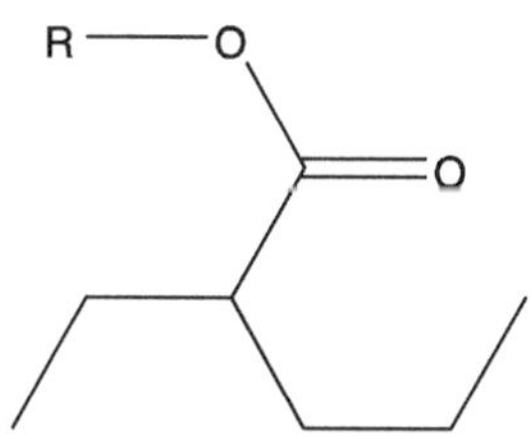

Alkyl Ethylhexanoate

Other names: C12-15 alcohols octanoate, C12-15 alkyl 2-ethylhexanoate, C12-15 alkyl octanoate
INCI: C12-15 Alkyl Ethylhexanoate
CAS no: 90411-66-8
Rank of popularity: 351/502
Intended function: Emollient
Allergenic potential: Maximum dose not stated

C12-15 Alkyl Octanoate

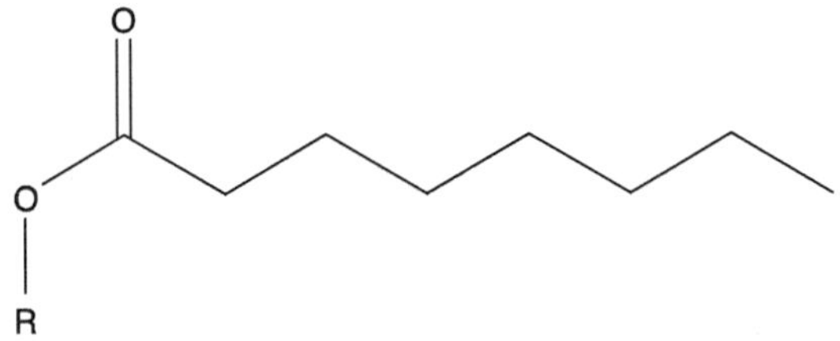

Alkyl Octanoate

Other names: Hexanoic acid, 2-ethyl-, C12-15-alkyl esters
INCI: C12-15 Alkyl Octanoate
CAS no: 90411-66-8
Rank of popularity: 192/502
Intended function: Emollient, Skin conditioning

C12-16 Alcohols

INCI: C12-16 Alcohols
CAS no: 68855-56-1
Rank of popularity: 354/502
Intended function: Antistatic agent, Emollient, Emulsion stabilizer, Hair conditioning, Viscosity increasing agent

C12-20 Alkyl Glucoside

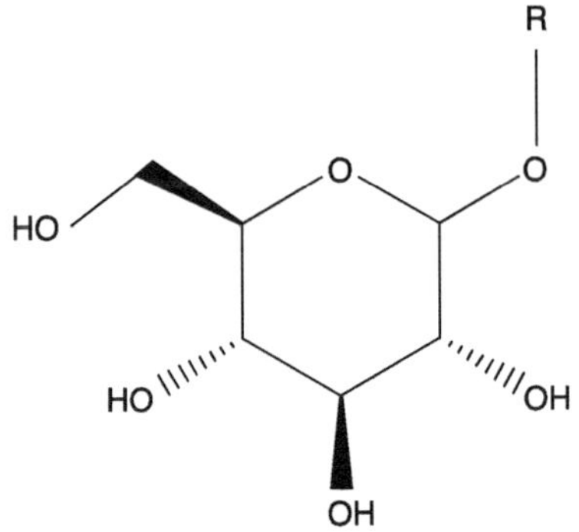

Alkyl Glucoside

INCI: C12-20 Alkyl Glucoside
Rank of popularity: 355/502
Intended function: Emulsifying agent

C13-14 Isoparaffin

INCI: C13-14 Isoparaffin
CAS no: 246538-79-4
Molecular formula: Mixture of branched-chain aliphatic hydrocarbons with 13 or 14 carbons in the chain
Rank of popularity: 49/502
Intended function: Emollient, Solvent

C14-22 Alcohols

Rank of popularity: 356/502
Intended function: Emulsion stabilizer

C20-40 Pareth-10

Other names: Performathox 450 ethoxylate
INCI: C20-40 Pareth-10
CAS no: 246538-83-0
Rank of popularity: 357/502
Intended function: Emulsifying agent
Allergenic potential: Max dose not stated

C30-38 olefin/Isopropyl Maleate/MA copolymer

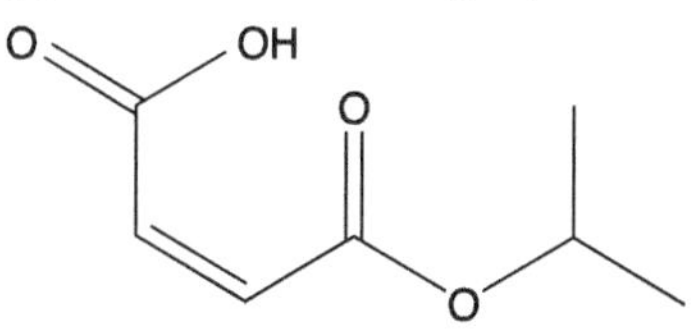

Isopropyl Maleate

INCI: C30-38 olefin/Isopropyl Maleate/MA copolymer
CAS no: 75535-27-2
Rank of popularity: 358/502
Intended function: Emulsifying agent, Viscosity increasing agent
Allergenic potential: Maximum dose not stated
Note: The structure does not represent the polymer. Only individual components are shown.

C30-45 Alkyl Methicone

INCI: C30-45 Alkyl Methicone
CAS no: 246864-88-0
Rank of popularity: 359/502
Intended function: Occlusive agent, Viscosity increasing agent

Caffeine

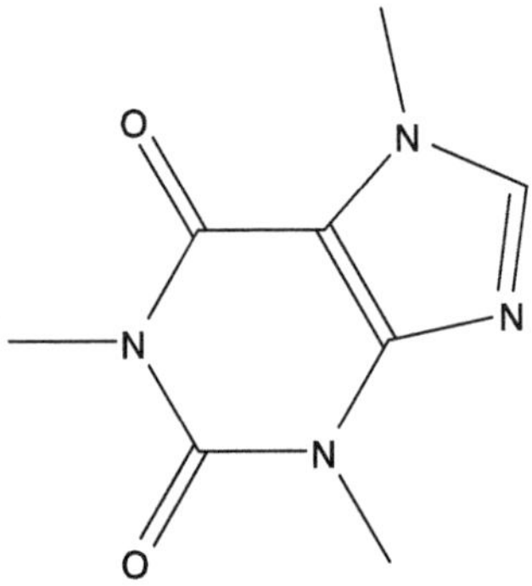

Other names: Anhydrous caffeine, Coffeinum, Methyltheobromine, 7-methyltheophylline
INCI: Caffeine
CAS no: 58-08-2
Molecular formula: $C_8H_{10}N_4O_2$
Molecular weight: 194.19
Rank of popularity: 135/502
Intended function: Fragrance, Skin conditioning
Log P: –0.63

Calamine

INCI: Calamine
CAS no: 8011-96-9
Molecular formula: Mixture of zinc oxide and iron oxide
Rank of popularity: 360/502
Intended function: Absorbent, Opacifying agent, Skin protectant

Calcium Pantetheine Sulfonate

INCI: Calcium Pantetheine Sulfonate
CAS no: 9007-03-8
Molecular formula: $C_{11}H_{22}N_2O_7S_2 \cdot 1/2Ca$
Molecular weight: 378.29
Rank of popularity: 159/502
Intended function: Hair conditioning, Skin conditioning
Log P: -6.11

Calcium Pantothenate

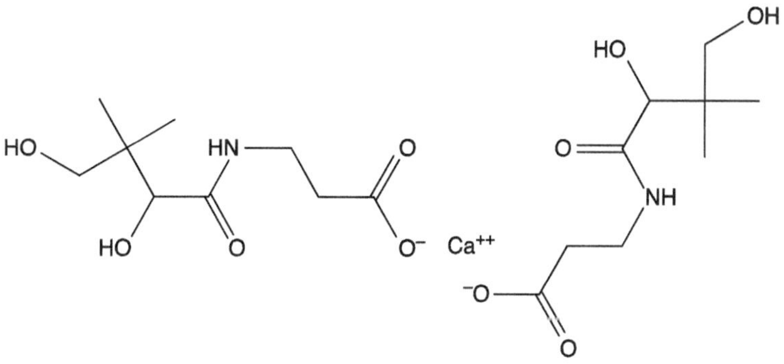

Other names: Vitamin B5 calcium salt
INCI: Calcium Pantothenate
CAS no: 137-08-6(D-form)
Molecular formula: $C_9H_{17}NO_5 \cdot 1/2Ca$
Molecular weight: 478.55
Rank of popularity: 361/502
Intended function: Antistatic agent, Hair conditioning
Log P of monomer: –0.86 (Pantothenic acid)
Carcinogenic potential: Category 3 (use with precaution)

Capryloyl Glycine

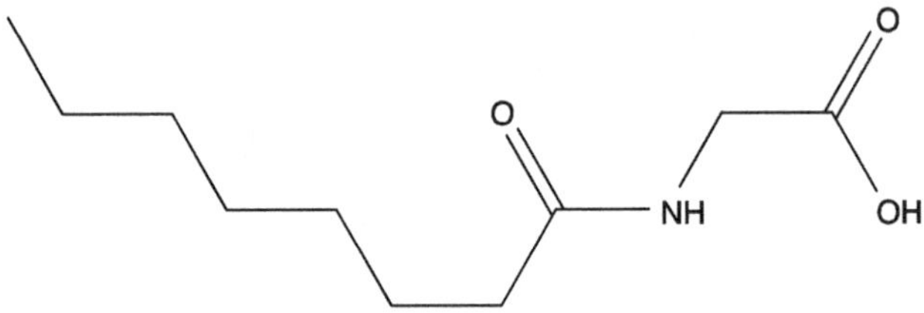

Other names: N-octanoyl-glycine, N-(1-oxooctyl) glycine
INCI: Capryloyl Glycine
CAS no: 14246-53-8
Molecular formula: $C_{10}H_{19}NO_3$
Molecular weight: 201.26
Rank of popularity: 251/502
Intended function: Cleansing agent, Hair conditioning
Log P: 1.07

Capryloyl Salicylic Acid

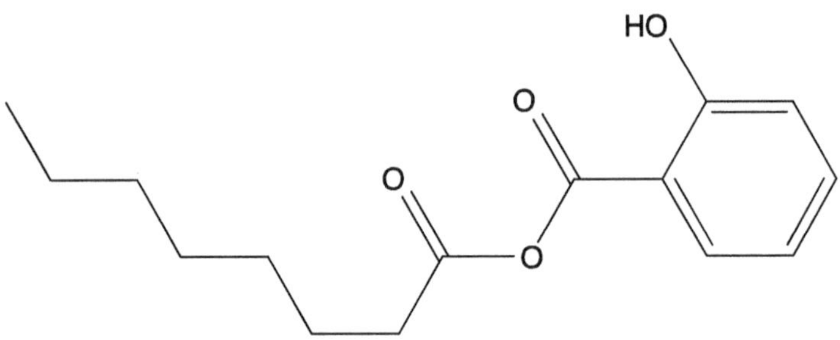

INCI: Capryloyl Salicylic Acid
CAS no: 70424-62-3
Molecular formula: $C_{19}H_{20}O_4$
Molecular weight: 264.32
Rank of popularity: 252/502
Intended function: Skin conditioning
Log P: 4.46

Caprylyl glycol

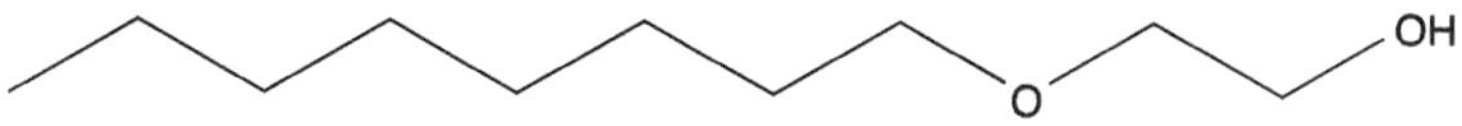

Other names: Capryl glycol, 1, 2-dihydroxyoctane, 1,2-octanediol, 1,2-octylene glycol
INCI: Caprylyl glycol
CAS no: 1117-86-8
Molecular formula: C8H18O2
Molecular weight: 146.23
Rank of popularity: 96/502
Intended function: Cleansing agent, Emollient, Foam booster, Hair conditioning, Humectant
Log P: 2.63

Caramel

Other names: Caramel colour, Natural brown 10
INCI: Caramel
CAS no: 8028-89-5
Rank of popularity: 362/502
Intended function: Colourant, Fragrance
Carcinogenic potential: Category 3 (use with precaution)

Carbomer

Other names: Carbomer 910, 934, 940,941, Carbopol 910, Carboxyvinylpolymer
INCI: Carbomer
CAS no: 9003-01-4/ 9007-16-3/ 9007-17-4/ 9062-04-8/ 76050-42-5
Molecular formula: Polymer of acrylic acid and polyalkenyl polyethers
Rank of popularity: 14/502
Intended function: Emulsion stabilizer, Viscosity increasing agent

Cellulose Acetate Butyrate

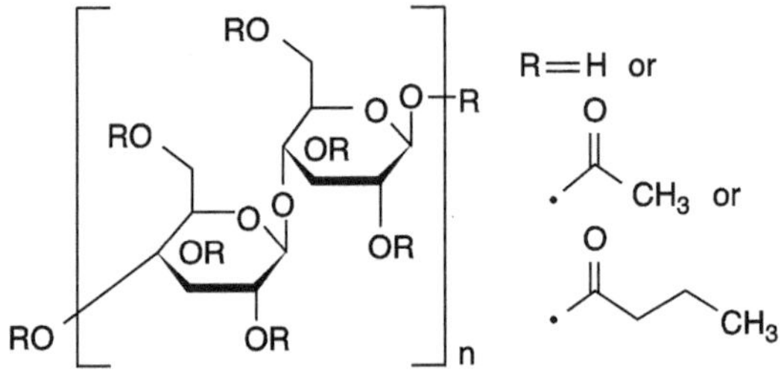

Other names: Acetobutyrate cellulose, Acetylpropionylcellulose, Cellaburate
INCI: Cellulose Acetate Butyrate
CAS no: 9004-36-8
Rank of popularity: 363/502
Intended function: Film former

Ceramide 3

Other names: Steroyl-C18-phytosphingosine, Steroyl-4-hydroxysphinganine
INCI: Ceramide 3
CAS no: 100403-19-8
Molecular formula: $C_{36}H_{73}NO_4$
Molecular weight: 583.97
Rank of popularity: 352/502
Intended function: Hair conditioning, Skin conditioning, Skin protectant

Ceresin

Other names: Cirine wax, Mineral wax, White ceresin wax, White ozokerite wax
INCI: Ceresin
CAS no: 8001-75-0
Molecular formula: Mixture of hydrocarbons obtained by purification of Ozokerite
Rank of popularity: 253/502
Intended function: Antistatic agent, Binder, Emulsion stabilizer, Hair conditioning, Epilating agent, Opacifying agent, Viscosity increasing agent
Allergenic potential: Maximum dose not stated

Ceteareth-20

Other names: PEG-20 cetostearyl alcohol, Polyethylene glycol 1000 cetyl/stearyl ether
INCI: Ceteareth-20
CAS no: 68439-49-6
Molecular formula: $R(OCH_2CH_2)_{20}OH$: R represents a blend of alkyl groups derived from cetyl and stearyl alcohol and ethoxylated (20 mol EO average molar ratio)
Rank of popularity: 69/502
Intended function: Solvent

Ceteareth-25

Other names: PEG-25 cetyl/stearyl ether, Polyethylene glycol (25) cetyl/stearyl ether
INCI: Ceteareth-25
CAS no: 68439-49-6
Molecular formula: $R(OCH_2CH_2)_{25}OH$: R represents a blend of alkyl groups derived from cetyl and stearyl alcohol and ethoxylated (25 mol EO average molar ratio)
Rank of popularity: 364/502
Intended function: Cleansing agent, Emulsifying agent, Solubilizing agent

Ceteareth-33

Other names: PEG-33 cetyl/stearyl ether, Polyethylene glycol (33) cetyl/stearyl ether
INCI: Ceteareth-33
CAS no: 68439-49-6
Molecular formula: $R(OCH_2CH_2)_{33}OH$: R represents a blend of alkyl groups derived from cetyl and stearyl alcohol and ethoxylated (33 mol EO average molar ratio)
Rank of popularity: 254/502
Intended function: Cleansing agent, Solubilizing agent

Ceteareth-6

Other names: PEG-6 cetyl/stearyl ether, Polyethylene glycol 300 cetyl/stearyl ether
INCI: Ceteareth-6
CAS no: 68439-49-6
Molecular formula: $R(OCH_2CH_2)_6OH$: R represents a blend of alkyl groups derived from cetyl and stearyl alcohol and ethoxylated (6 mol EO average molar ratio)
Rank of popularity: 255/502
Intended function: Emulsifying agent

Cetearyl Alcohol

Other names: Alcohol cetylicus et stearylicus, hexadecan-1-ol, octadecan-1-ol
INCI: Cetearyl Alcohol
CAS no: 8005-44-5/ 67762-27-0
Molecular formula: $(C_{16}H_{34}O)_n \cdot (C_{18}H_{38}O)_n$ (mixture of mostly cetyl (hexadecanol) and stearyl (octodecanol) alcohols)
Rank of popularity: 27/502
Intended function: Emollient, Emulsifying agent, Emulsion stabilizer, Foam booster, Opacifying agent, Viscosity increasing agent

Cetearyl Glucoside

Other names: OriStar CTG, Tego Care CG 90
INCI: Cetearyl Glucoside
CAS no: 246159-33-1
Molecular formula: C16-18 alkyl glycosides
Rank of popularity: 365/502
Intended function: Emulsifying agent
Allergenic potential: Maximum dose not stated

Cetearyl Isononanoate

Other names: Isononanoic acid cetyl/stearyl ether
INCI: Cetearyl Isononanoate
CAS no: 111937-03-2
Molecular formula: C16-18-alkyl esters
Rank of popularity: 256/502
Intended function: Emollient, Hair conditioning
Allergenic potential: Maximum dose not stated

Cetearyl Octanoate

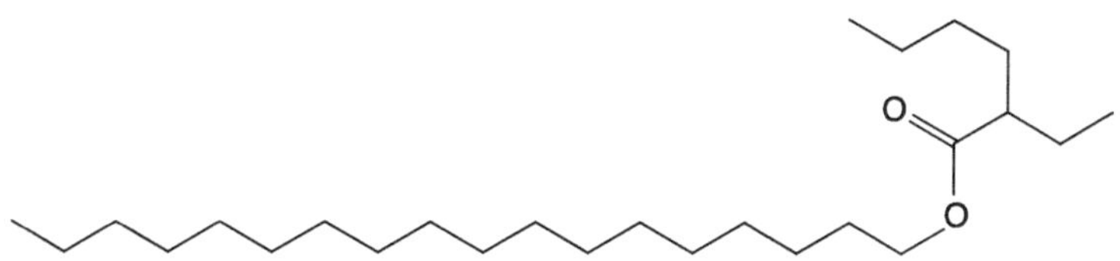

Other names: Cetyl 2-ethylhexanoate
INCI: Cetyl ethylhexanoate
CAS no: 59130-69-7
Molecular formula: $C_{24}H_{48}O_2$
Molecular weight: 368.64
Rank of popularity: 257/502
Intended function: Emollient
Log P: 10.82

Ceteth-10 Phosphate

INCI: Ceteth-10 Phosphate
CAS no: 50643-20-4
Molecular formula: Cetyl alcohol, phosphate and ethoxylated (10 mol EO average molar ratio)
Rank of popularity: 366/502
Intended function: Cleansing agent

Ceteth-20

Other names: Cetomacrogol 1000 BPC, PEG-20 cetyl ether, PEG-20 hexadecyl ether, Polyethylene glycol 1000 cetyl ether
INCI: Ceteth-20
CAS no: 9004-95-9
Molecular formula: Cetyl alcohol, ethyoxylated (20 mol EO average molar ratio)
Rank of popularity: 136/502
Intended function: Cleansing agent, Emulsifying agent, Solubilizing agent

Ceteth-24

Other names: Cetomacrogol 1000, PEG-24 cetyl ether, Polyethylene glycol (24) cetyl ether
INCI: Ceteth-24
CAS no: 9004-95-9
Molecular formula: Cetyl alcohol, ethyoxylated (24 mol EO average molar ratio)
Rank of popularity: 367/502
Intended function: Cleansing agent, Solubilizing agent

Cetomacrogol 1000

Other names: Cetomacrogolum 1000, Polyethylene glycol monohexadecyl ether; α-hexadecyl-ω-hydroxypoly(oxy-1,2-ethanediyl)
INCI: Cetomacrogol 1000
CAS no: 9004-95-9
Molecular formula: $(C_2H_4O)_n.C_{16}H_{34}O$
Rank of popularity: 368/502
Intended function: Surfactant

Cetrimonium Bromide

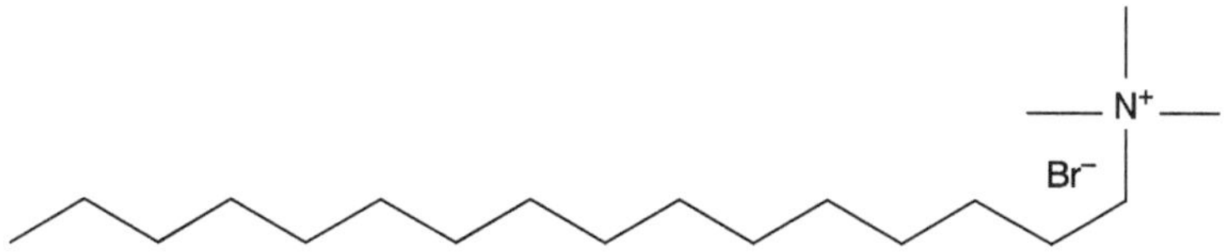

Other names: Cetab, Cetrimidum, Cetyl trimethyl ammonium bromide, Cetyltrimethylammonium bromide powder
INCI: Cetrimonium Bromide
CAS no: 57-09-0
Molecular formula: $C_{19}H_{42}N.\ Br$
Molecular weight: 364.45
Rank of popularity: 193/502
Intended function: Antistatic agent, Cosmetic biocide, Emulsifying agent
Log P: 7.76
Allergenic potential: Weak sensitizer (max dose = 1.82 μg/cm²/hr)

Cetyl Alcohol

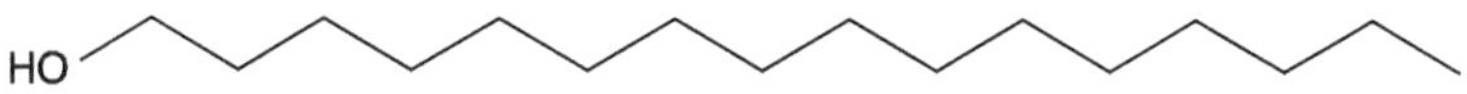

Other names: Alcohol cetylicus, cetanol, 1-hexadecanol, palmityl alcohol
INCI: Cetyl Alcohol
CAS no: 36653-82-4
Molecular formula: $C_{16}H_{34}O$
Molecular weight: 242.44
Rank of popularity: 13/502
Intended function: Emulsifying agent, Emulsion stabilizer, Foam booster, Fragrance, Opacifying agent, Viscosity increasing agent
Log P: 6.95
Allergenic potential: Weak sensitizer (max dose = 7.29 μg/cm²/hr)

Cetyl Dimethicone

INCI: Cetyl Dimethicone
CAS no: 191044-49-2
Rank of popularity: 97/502
Intended function: Antifoaming agent, Emollient, Occlusive agent

Cetyl Dimethicone Copolyol

INCI: Cetyl Dimethicone Copolyol
CAS no: 145686-34-6/ 251320-26-0
Rank of popularity: 194/502
Intended function: Emulsifying agent

Cetyl Esters

Other names: Synthetic spermaceti wax
INCI: Cetyl Esters
Rank of popularity: 258/502
Intended function: Emollient

Cetyl Hydroxyethylcellulose

Other names: Hexadecyl hydroxyethyl cellulose
INCI: Cetyl Hydroxyethylcellulose
Rank of popularity: 369/502
Intended function: Emulsion stabilizer, Viscosity increasing agent

Cetyl Palmitate

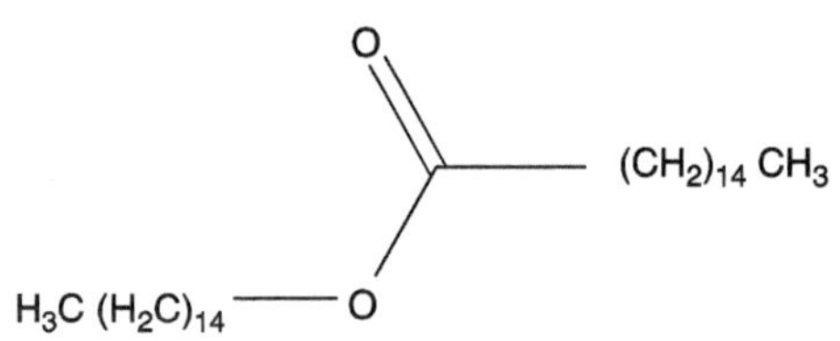

Other names: Hexadecyl palmitate, Palmityl palmitate
INCI: Cetyl Palmitate
CAS no: 540-10-3
Molecular formula: $C_{32}H_{64}O2$
Molecular weight: 480.85
Rank of popularity: 87/502
Intended function: Fragrance, Occlusive agent
Log P: 15.05
Allergenic potential: Weak sensitizer (max dose = 18.2 μg/cm²/hr)

Cetyl Phosphate

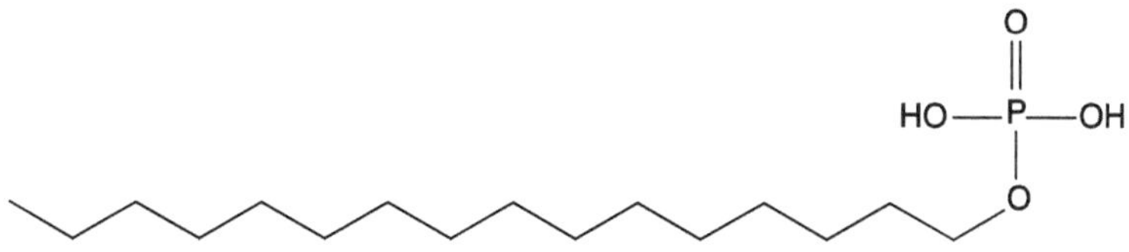

Other names: Cetyl dihydrogen phosphate, Monocetyl phosphate, Phosphoric acid monohexadecyl ester
INCI: Cetyl Phosphate
CAS no: 3539-43-3
Molecular formula: $C_{16}H_{35}O_4P$
Molecular weight: 322.42
Rank of popularity: 259/502
Intended function: Emulsifying agent
Log P: 5.06

Cetyl Ricinoleate

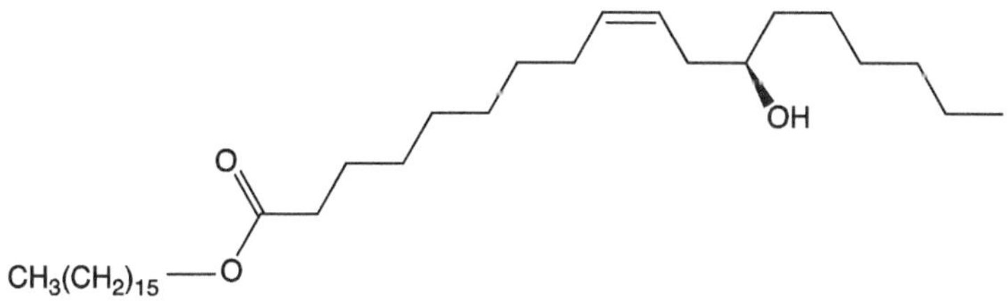

Other names: Hexadecyl 12-hydroxy-9-octadecenoate
INCI: Cetyl Ricinoleate
CAS no: 10401-55-5
Molecular formula: $C_{34}H_{66}O_3$
Molecular weight: 522.89
Rank of popularity: 370/502
Intended function: Occlusive agent
Log P: 13.85

Chlorhexidine Diacetate

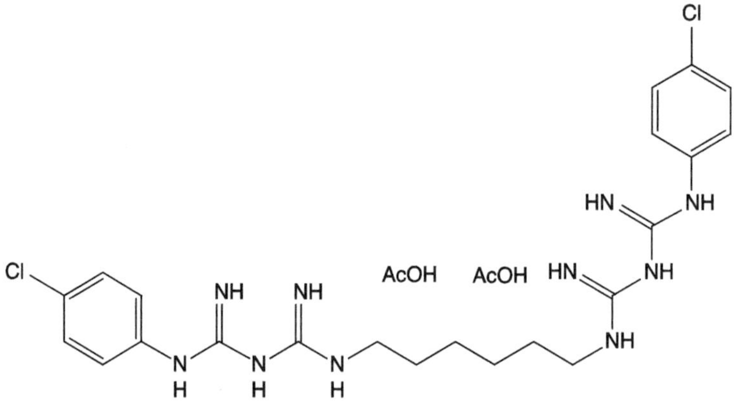

INCI: Chlorhexidine Diacetate
CAS no: 56-95-1
Molecular formula: $C_{22}H_{30}Cl_2N_{10} \cdot 2C_2H_4O_2$
Molecular weight: 625.55
Rank of popularity: 260/502
Intended function: Cosmetic biocide, Oral care agent, Preservative
Allergenic potential: Weak sensitizer (max dose = 3.65 μg/cm²/hr)

Chlorhexidine Digluconate

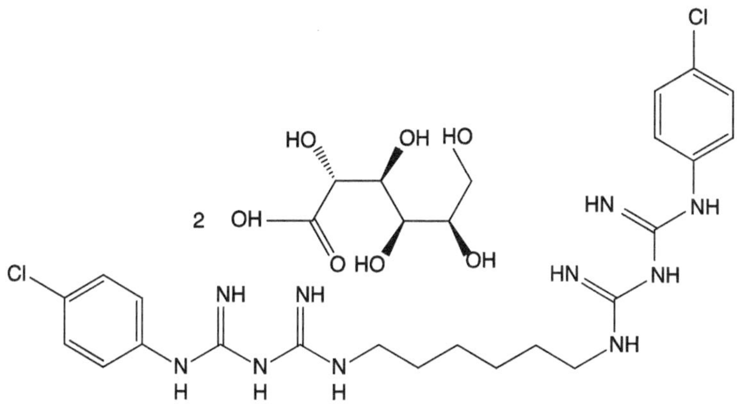

INCI: Chlorhexidine Digluconate
CAS no: 18472-51-0
Molecular formula: $C_{22}H_{30}Cl_2N_{10} \cdot 2C_6H_{12}O_7$
Molecular weight: 897.41
Rank of popularity: 195/502
Intended function: Cosmetic biocide, Oral care agent, Preservative
Log P: –4.70
Carcinogenic potential: Category 1 (use within limit on body = 5.0×10^{-2} % w/w; face = 3.0 % w/w; hands = 1.0 % w/w)
Allergenic potential: Weak sensitizer (max dose = 3.65 μg/cm^2/hr)

Chlorocresol

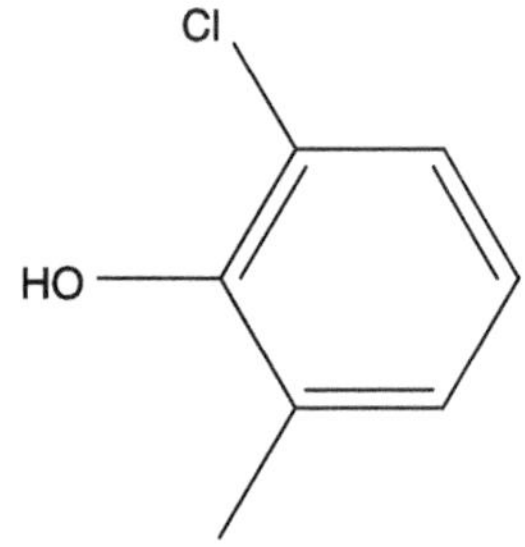

Other names: Chlorocresol, 4-Chloro-m-cresol, Chlorocresolum, Chloromethylphenol, Parachlorometacresol
INCI: p-Chloro-m-Cresol
CAS no: 59-50-7
Molecular formula: C_7H_7ClO
Molecular weight: 142.58
Rank of popularity: 160/502
Intended function: Cosmetic biocide, Preservative
Log P: 2.89
Allergenic potential: Weak sensitizer (max dose = 3.65 $\mu g/cm^2/hr$)

Chloroxylenol

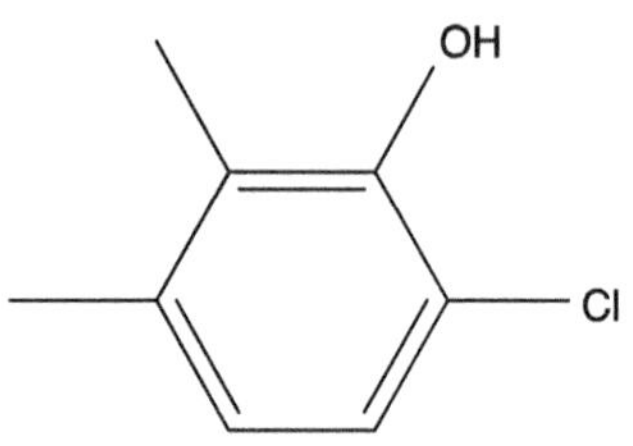

Other names: Chlorodimethylhydroxybenzene, PCMX, 4-Chloro-3,5-Xylenol
INCI: Chloroxylenol
CAS no: 88-04-0/ 1321-23-9
Molecular formula: C_8H_9ClO
Molecular weight: 156.61
Rank of popularity: 371/502
Intended function: Cosmetic biocide, Deodorant, Preservative
Log P: 3.38
Carcinogenic potential: Category 3 (use with precaution)

Chlorphenesin

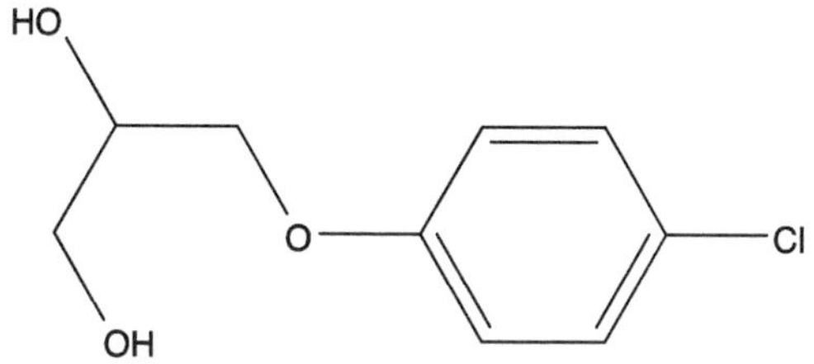

Other names: p-Chlorophenyl glyceryl ether
INCI: Chlorphenesin
CAS no: 104-29-0
Molecular formula: $C_9H_{11}ClO_3$
Molecular weight: 202.63
Rank of popularity: 52/502
Intended function: Cosmetic biocide
Log P: 1.71
Allergenic potential: Weak sensitizer (max dose = 7.29 μg/cm^2/hr)

Cholecalciferol

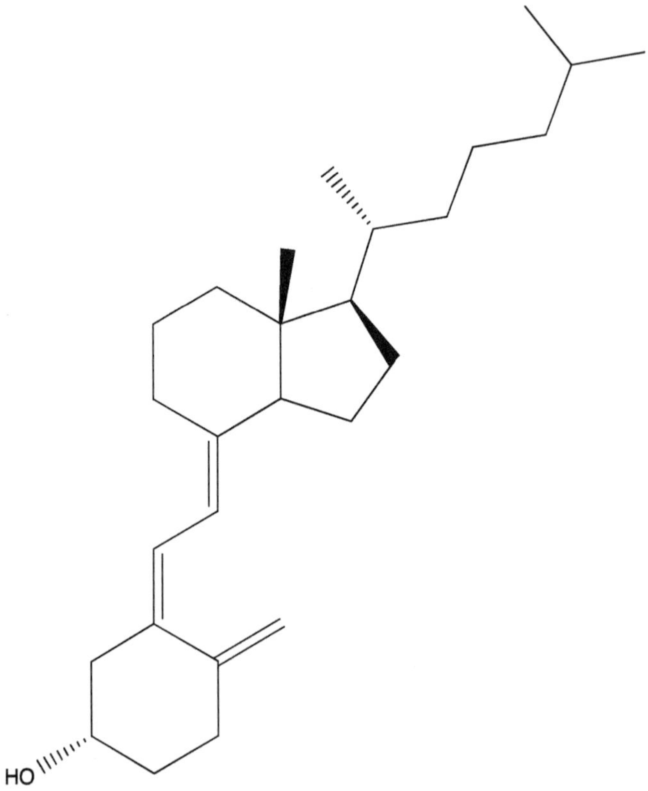

Other names: Arachitol, Colecalciferol, Vitamin D3
INCI: Cholecalciferol
CAS no: 67-97-0
Molecular formula: $C_{27}H_{44}O$
Molecular weight: 384.64
Rank of popularity: 261/502
Intended function: Skin conditioning
Log P: 9.09

Cholesterol

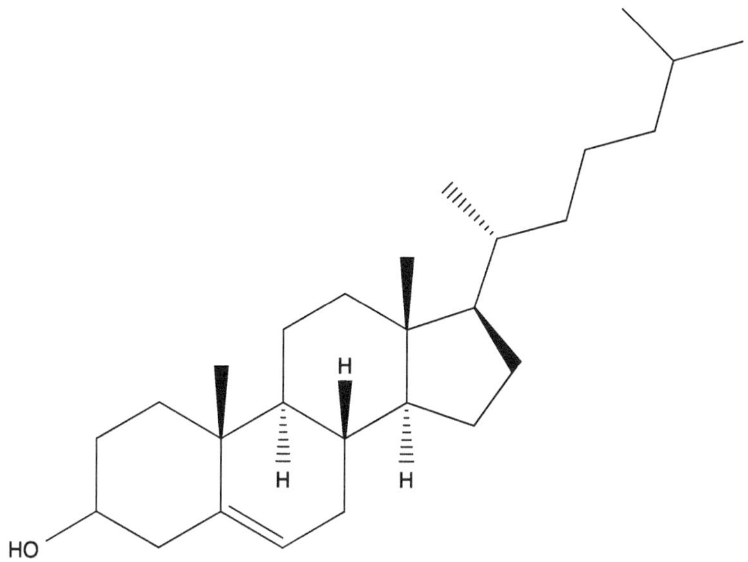

Other names: Cholesterin, Cholesteryl alcohol, Provitamin D3
INCI: Cholesterol
CAS no: 57-88-5
Molecular formula: $C_{27}H_{46}O$
Molecular weight: 386.65
Rank of popularity: 196/502
Intended function: Emulsion stabilizer, Skin conditioning, Viscosity increasing agent
Log P: 9.62
Carcinogenic potential: Category 2 (safe to use)

Choleth-24

Other names: PEG-24 cholesteryl ether, Polyethylene glycol (24) cholesteryl ether, Polyoxyethylene (24) cholesteryl ether
INCI: Choleth-24
CAS no: 27321-96-6
Molecular formula: $(C_2 H_4 O)_n C_{27} H_{46} O$
Rank of popularity: 372/502
Intended function: Emulsifying agent

Citral

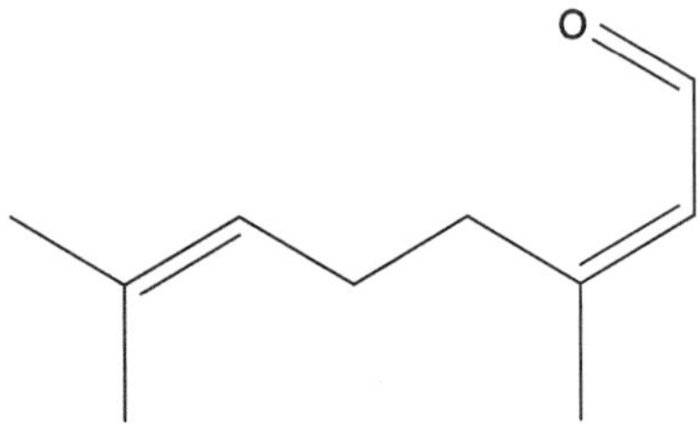

Other names: 3,7-dimethyl-2,6-octadienal, lemarome
INCI: Citral
CAS no: 5392-40-5
Molecular formula: $C_{10}H_{16}O$
Molecular weight: 152.23
Rank of popularity: 161/502
Intended function: Flavouring agent, Fragrance
Log P: 3.13
Allergenic potential: Weak sensitizer (max dose = 14.6 μg/cm^2/hr)

Citric Acid

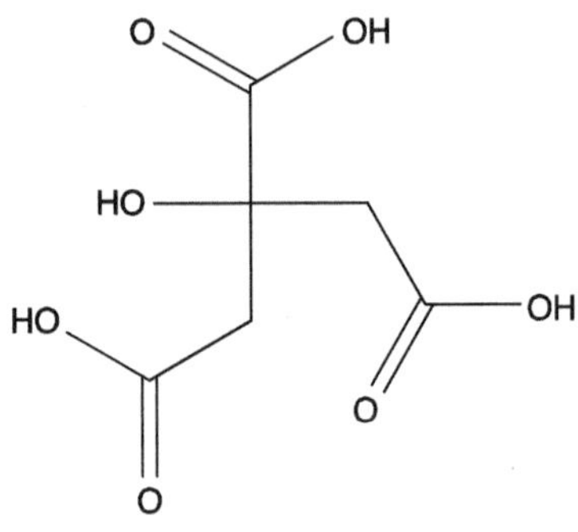

Other names: Acidum citricum, anhydrous citric acid
INCI: Citric Acid
CAS no: 77-92-9/ 5949-29-1
Molecular formula: $C_6H_8O_7$
Molecular weight: 192.12
Rank of popularity: 20/502
Intended function: Chelating agent, Fragrance, pH adjuster
Log P: –1.20

Coal Tar

INCI: Coal Tar
CAS no: 8007-45-2
Rank of popularity: 197/502
Intended function: Antidandruff agent, Cosmetic biocide, Denaturant
Carcinogenic potential: Category 2 (safe to use)
Allergenic potential: Weak sensitizer (max dose = 36.5 $\mu g/cm^2/hr$)

Coco-betaine

Other names: Coco dimethyl glycine, Coconut betaine
INCI: Coco-betaine
CAS no: 68424-94-2
Rank of popularity: 199/502
Intended function: Cleansing agent, Antistatic agent, Foam booster, Hair conditioning, Skin conditioning, Viscosity increasing agent
Allergenic potential: Weak sensitizer (max dose = 7.29 $\mu g/cm^2/hr$)

Collagen

Other names: Collagen fibre, Collagen sheet, Freeze-dried collagen sheet
INCI: Collagen
CAS no: 9007-34-5
Rank of popularity: 160/502
Intended function: Hair conditioning, Skin conditioning

Colloidal Silver

Other names: Suspension of silver particles in water prepared by electrolysis
INCI: Colloidal Silver
CAS no: 7440-22-4
Molecular formula: Ag
Molecular weight: 107.87
Rank of popularity: 353/502
Intended function: Cosmetic biocide, Slip modifier
Allergenic potential: Weak sensitizer (max dose = 0.729 $\mu g/cm^2/hr$)

Copper Gluconate

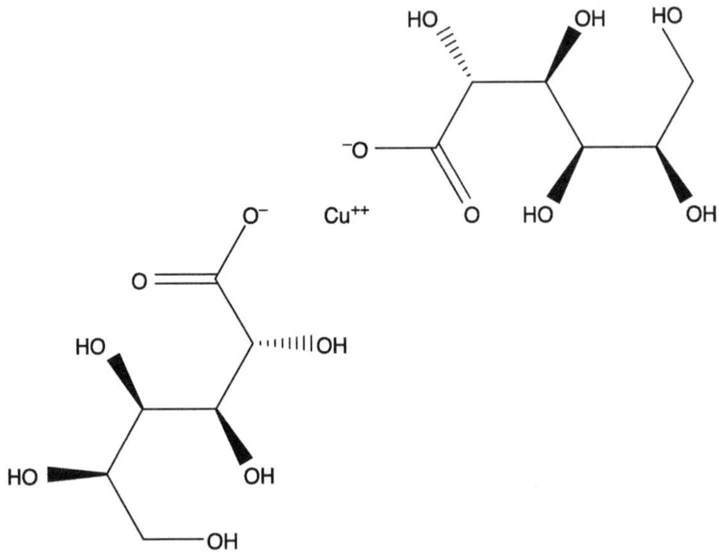

Other names: Bis (D-gluconato) copper, Cupric gluconate
INCI: Copper Gluconate
CAS no: 527-09-3
Molecular formula: $C_6H_{12}O_7 \cdot 1/2Cu$
Molecular weight: 453.84
Rank of popularity: 262/502
Intented function: Chelating agent, Skin conditioning
Carcinogenic potential: Category 2 (safe to use)

Copper Sulphate

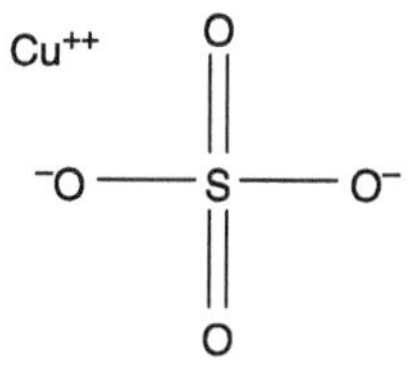

Other names: Copper (II) sulfate, Cupric sulfate, Sulfuric acid copper salt
INCI: Sopper sulfate
CAS no: 7758-98-7
Molecular formula: Cu · H_2O_4S
Molecular weight: 161.61
Rank of popularity: 263/502
Intended function: Skin conditioning
Log P: –3.45
Carcinogenic potential: Category 3 (use with precaution)
Allergenic potential: Weak sensitizer (max dose = 36.5 μg/cm^2/hr)

Cyclohexasiloxane

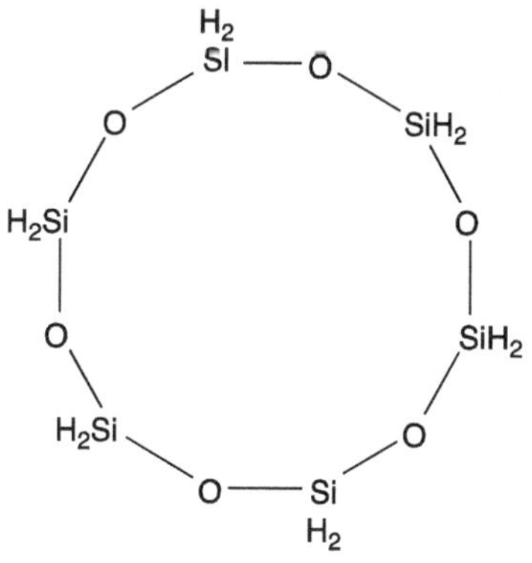

Other names: Cyclomethicone, Dodecamethylcyclohexasiloxane
INCI: Cyclohexasiloxane
CAS no: 540-97-6
Molecular formula: C_{12} H_{36} O_6 Si_6
Molecular weight: 444.92
Rank of popularity: 74/502
Intended function: Emollient, Hair conditioning, Solvent

Cyclomethicone

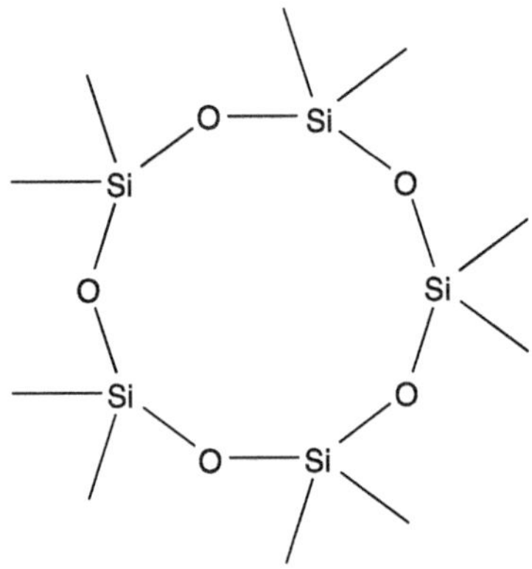

Other names: Generic name for several cyclic dimethyl polysiloxane compounds; cyclotetrasiloxane, cyclotrisiloxane, cyclopentasiloxane, cyclohexasiloxane, and cycloheptasiloxane
INCI: Cyclomethicone
CAS no: 69430-24-6
Molecular formula: $(C_2H_6OSi)_n$ where n = 3–7
Rank of popularity: 24/502
Intended function: Antistatic agent, Emollient, Hair conditioning, Humectant, Solvent, Viscosity controlling agent
Note: The structure is only an example of cyclomethicone.

Cyclopentasiloxane

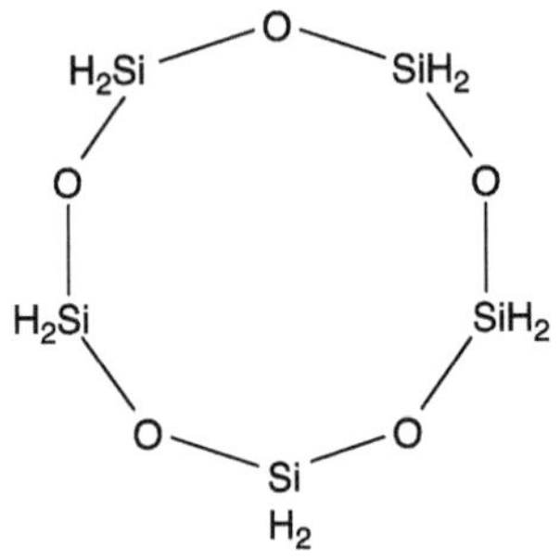

Other names: Cyclomethicone, Decamethylcyclopentasiloxane
INCI: Cyclopentasiloxane
CAS no: 541-02-6
Molecular formula: $C_{10}H_{30}O_5Si_5$
Molecular weight: 370.76
Rank of popularity: 31/502
Intended function: Emollient, Hair conditioning, Solvent

D & C Green N5

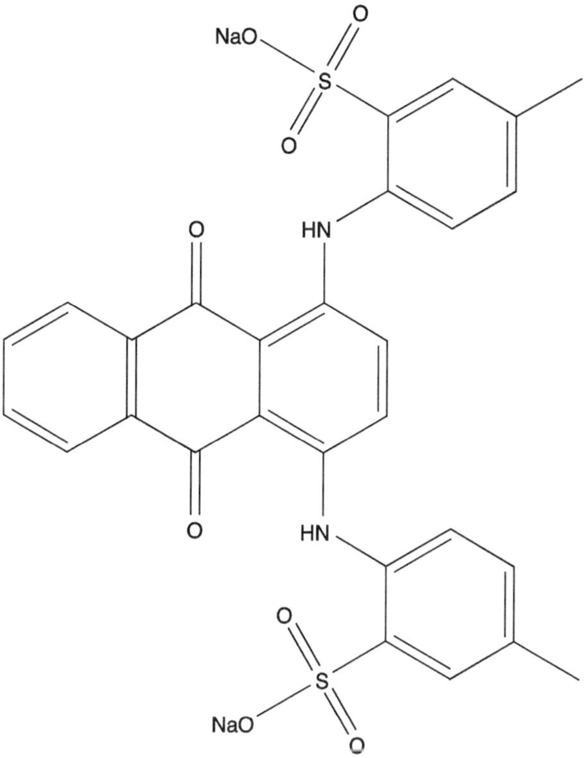

Other names: Cl61570, Acid green anthraquinone, Alizarincyanine green G, Green no.201, Japan green no.201, 2,2′-(9,10-dihydro-9,10 dioxo-1,4-anthracenediyl), diamino bis-(5-methyl-benzenesulfonic acid)
INCI: Acid green 25
CAS no: 4403-91-0
Molecular formula: $C_{28}H_{22}N_2O_8S_2 \cdot 2Na$
Molecular weight: 624.58
Rank of popularity: 373/502
Intended function: Colourant

D & C Red N33

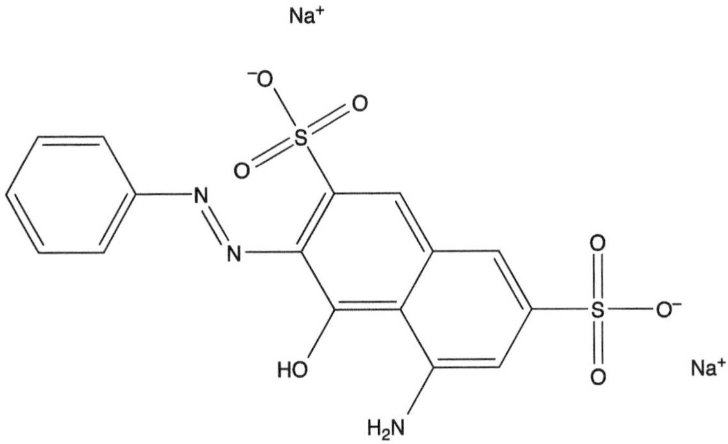

Other names: Cl17200, Fast acid fuchsine B, Food red 12, Red no. 227, Disodium 5-amino-4-hydroxy-3-(phenylazo)-naphthalene-2,7-disulfonate
INCI: Acid red 33
CAS no: 3567-66-6
Molecular formula: $C_{16}H_{13}N_3O_7S_2 \cdot 2Na$
Molecular weight: 469.39
Rank of popularity: 98/502
Intended function: Colourant

Diethanolamine cetyl phosphate

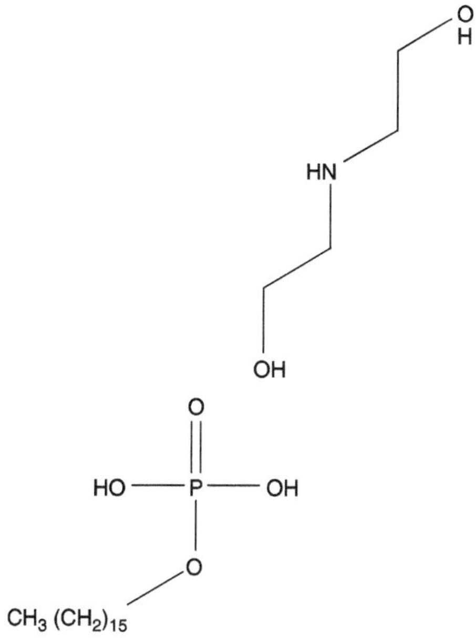

Other names: Diethanolamine cetyl phosphate
INCI: DEA-Cetyl Phosphate
CAS no: 61693-41-2/ 69331-39-1
Molecular formula: $C_{16}H_{35}O_4P \cdot xC_4H_{11}NO_2$
Rank of popularity: 137/502
Intended function: Emulsifying agent

Decyl Glucoside

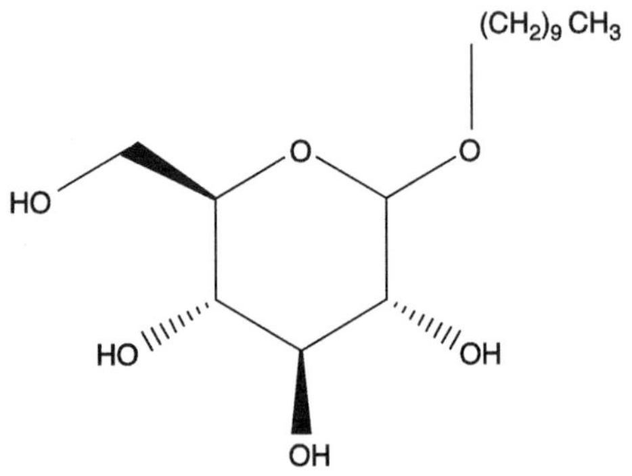

Other names: Decyl-beta-D- glucopyranoside
INCI: Decyl Glucoside
CAS no: 58846-77-8/ 68515-73-1/ 141464-42-8
Molecular formula: $C_{16}H_{32}O_6$
Molecular weight: 320.42
Rank of popularity: 138/502
Intended function: Cleansing agent, Emulsion stabilizer
Log P: 1.91
Allergenic potential: Weak sensitizer (max dose = 3.65 μg/cm²/hr)

Decyl Oleate

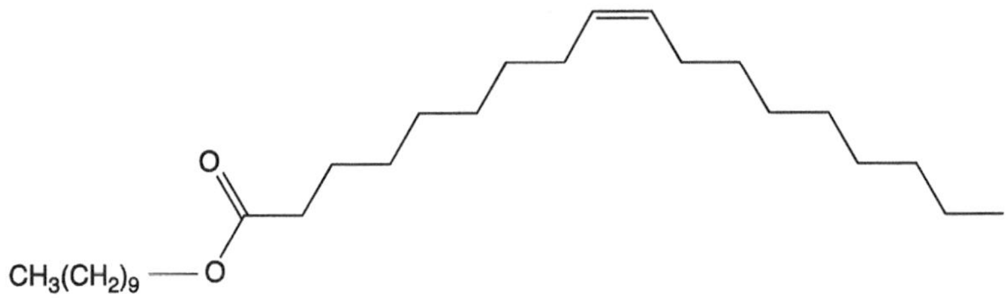

Other names: Decyl-9-octadecenoate
INCI: Decyl Oleate
CAS no: 3687-46-5
Molecular formula: $C_{28}H_{54}O_2$
Molecular weight: 422.73
Rank of popularity: 139/502
Intended function: Emollient
Log P: 12.60
Allergenic potential: Maximum dose not stated

Denatured Alcohol

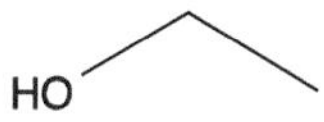

Other names: Denatured alcohol, Ethyl alcohol
INCI: Alcohol Denat.
CAS no: 64-17-5
Molecular formula: C_2H_6O
Molecular weight: 46.07
Rank of popularity: 25/502
Intended function: Antifoaming agent, Astringent, Solvent, Viscosity decreasing agent
Log P: –0.18
Carcinogenic potential: Category 2 (safe to use)

Di-C12-15 Alkyl Fumarate

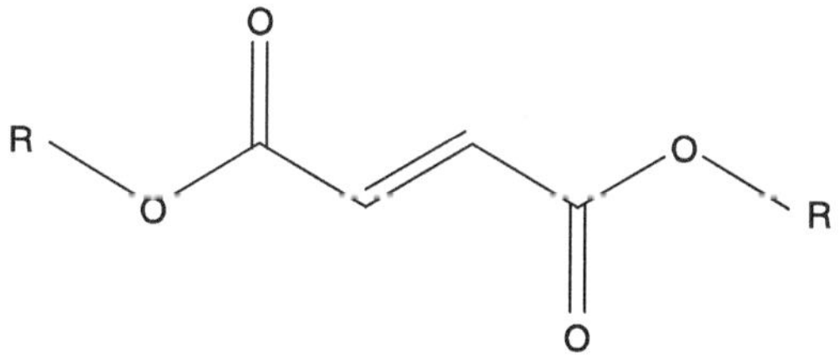

Dialkyl fumarate

Other names: Butenedioic acid (E), bis (C12-15-alkyl) esters
INCI: Di C12-15 Alkyl Fumarate
Rank of popularity: 374/502
Intended function: Emollient
Allergenic potential: Maximum dose not stated

Diazolidinyl urea

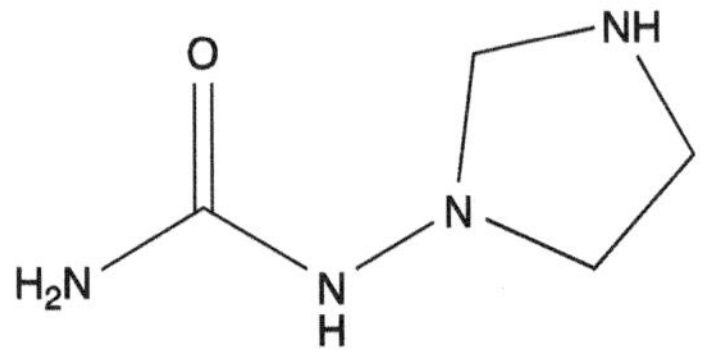

INCI: Diazolidinyl urea
CAS no: 78491-02-8
Molecular formula: $C_8H_{14}N_4O_7$
Molecular weight: 278.22
Rank of popularity: 26/502
Intended function: Preservative
Log P: –5.40
Carcinogenic potential: Category 2 (safe to use)
Allergenic potential: Weak sensitizer (max dose = 2.92 μg/cm^2/hr)

Di-C12-13 Alkyl Malate

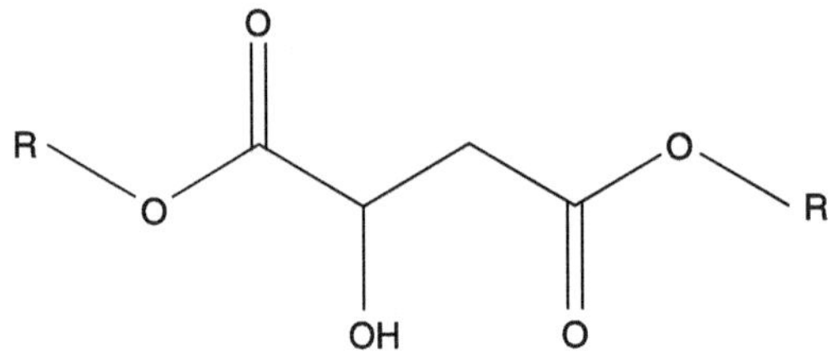

Dialkyl malate

Other names: Di-C12-13 alkyl hydroxybutandioate, Butandioic acid, hydroxy-, bis-(C12-13-alkyl) esters
INCI: Di-C12-13 Alkyl Malate
Rank of popularity: 375/502
Intended function: Emollient, Solvent

Dicaprylyl carbonate

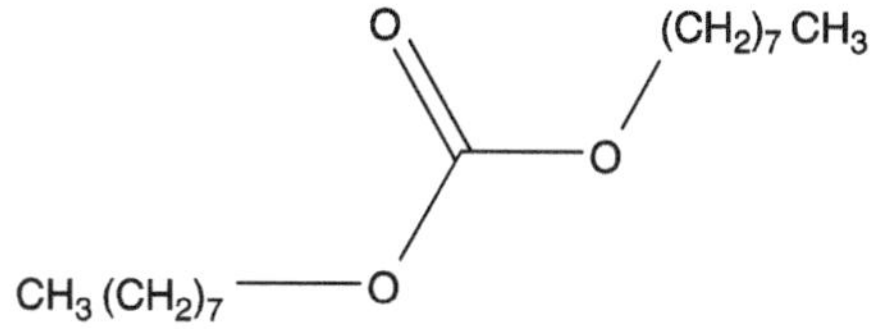

Other names: Carbonic acid dicaprylyl ester
INCI: Dicaprylyl carbonate
CAS no: 1680-31-5
Molecular formula: $C_{17}H_{34}O_3$
Molecular weight: 286.45
Rank of popularity: 264/502
Intended function: Emollient
Log P: 7.20

Dicetyl Phosphate

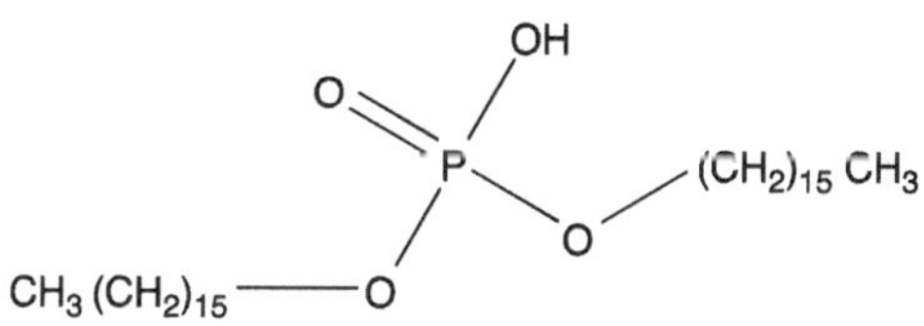

Other names: 1-hexadecanol hydrogen phosphate
INCI: Dicetyl Phosphate
CAS no: 2197-63-9
Molecular formula: $C_{32}H_{67}O_4P$
Molecular weight: 546.85
Rank of popularity: 376/502
Intended function: Emulsifying agent
Log P: 14.68

Dichlorobenzyl Alcohol

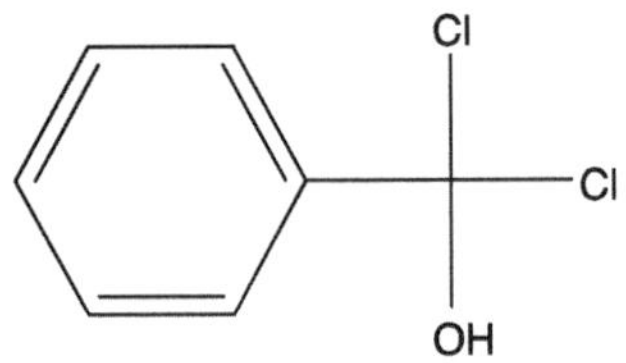

Other names: 2,4-dichlorobenzenemethanol
INCI: Dichlorobenzyl Alcohol
CAS no: 1777-82-8 / 12041-76-8
Molecular formula: $C_7H_6Cl_2O$
Molecular weight: 177.03
Rank of popularity: 200/502
Intended function: Cosmetic biocide, Preservative
Log P: 2.28
Allergenic potential: Weak sensitizer (max dose = 7.29 μg/cm²/hr)

Diglycol/CHDM (1,4-cyclohexanedimethanol)/Isophthalates/SIP Copolymer

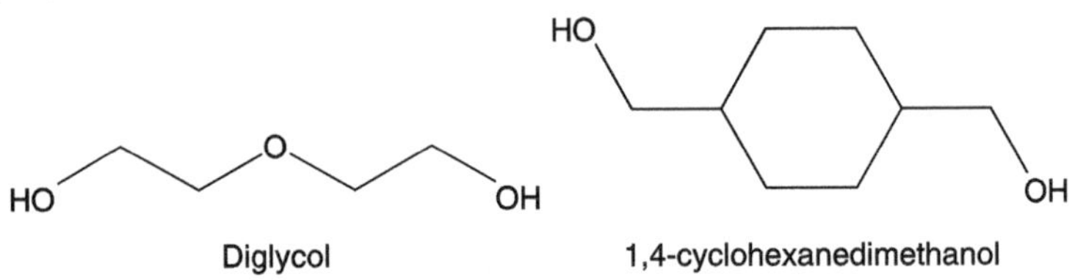

INCI: Diglycol/isophthalates/SIP copolymer
Rank of popularity: 377/502
Intended function: Film former
Note: The structure does not represent the polymer. Only individual components are shown.

Diiron Trioxide (CI77491)

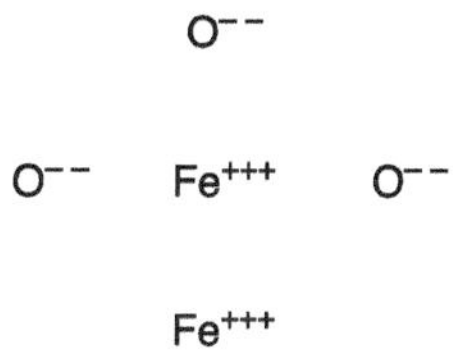

Other names: Ferric oxide, Iron oxides, Pigment brown 6 and 7, Pigment red 101
INCI: Cl77491
CAS no: 1317-61-9/ 1309-37-1/ 1345-25-1/ 1345-27-3/ 52357-70-7
Molecular formula: Fe_3O_4
Molecular weight: 231.53
Rank of popularity: 198/502
Intended function: Colourant

Diisopropyl Adipate

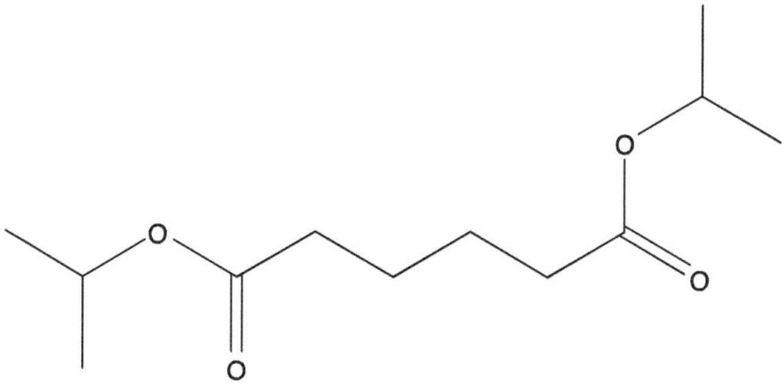

Other names: Bis (1-methylethyl) Hexanediate
INCI: Diisopropyl Adipate
CAS no: 6938-94-9
Molecular formula: $C_{12}H_{22}O_4$
Molecular weight: 230.30
Rank of popularity: 265/502
Intended function: Emollient, Fragrance, Plasticizer, Solvent
Log P: 2.68

Diisopropyl Sebacate

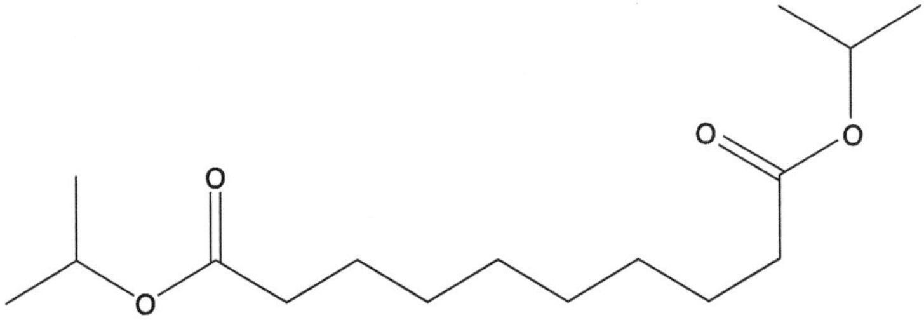

Other names: Bis (1-methylethyl) decanedioate
INCI: Diisopropyl Sebacate
CAS no: 7491-02-3
Molecular formula: $C_{16}H_{30}O_4$
Molecular weight: 286.41
Rank of popularity: 266/502
Intended function: Emollient, Plasticizer, Solvent
Log P: 4.63

Diisostearoyl polyglyceryl-3 Dimer Dilinoleate

INCI: Diisostearoyl polyglyceryl-3 Dimer
Rank of popularity: 378/502
Intended function: Emollient

Diisostearyl Malate

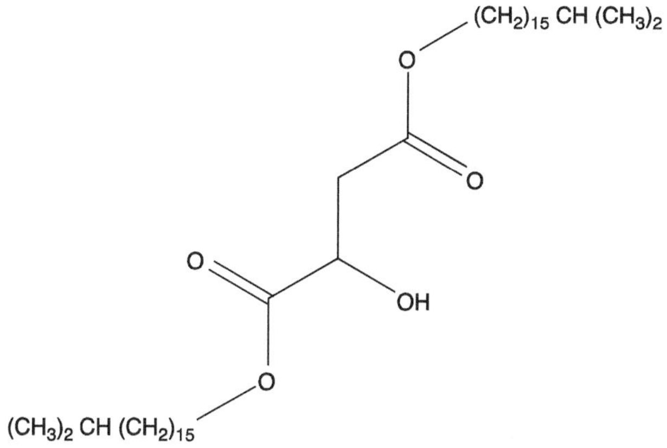

Other names: Bis (16-methyheptadecyl) hydroxybutanedioate
INCI: Diisostearyl Malate
CAS no: 67763-18-2/ 81230-05-9
Molecular formula: $C_{40}H_{78}O_5$
Molecular weight: 639.04
Rank of popularity: 379/502
Intended function: Emollient
Log P: 16.29
Allergenic potential: Very weak sensitizer (max dose = 109 μg/cm²/hr)

Diisostearoyl polyglyceryl-3 diisostearate

Rank of popularity: 380/502
Intended function: Emulsifying agent

Dilauryl Thiodipropionate

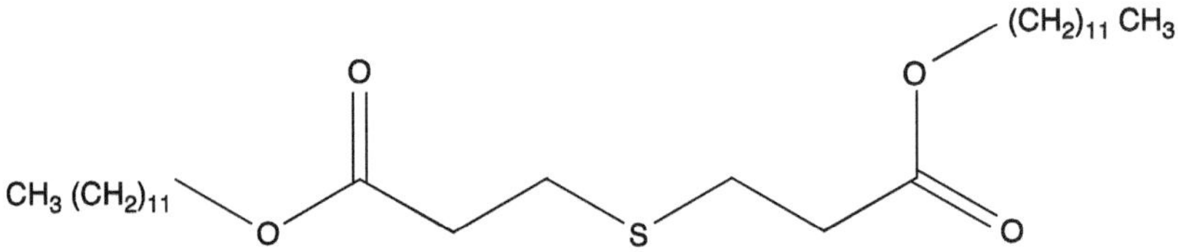

Other names: Didodecyl 3,3′-thiodipropionate
INCI: Dilauryl Thiodipropionate
CAS no: 123-28-4
Molecular formula: $C_{30}H_{58}O_4S$
Molecular weight: 502.84
Rank of popularity: 381/502
Intended function: Antioxidant
Log P: 11.92

Dimethiconol

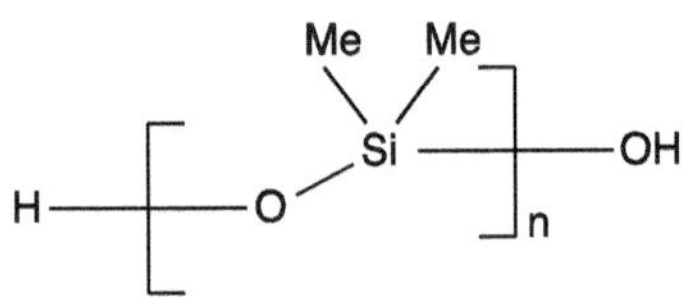

Other names: Dihydroxypolydimethylsiloxane
INCI: Dimethiconol
CAS no: 31692-79-2/ 70131-67-8
Molecular formula: $(C_2H_6OSi)_n\ H_2O$
Rank of popularity: 66/502
Intended function: Antifoaming agent, Emollient

Dimethicone

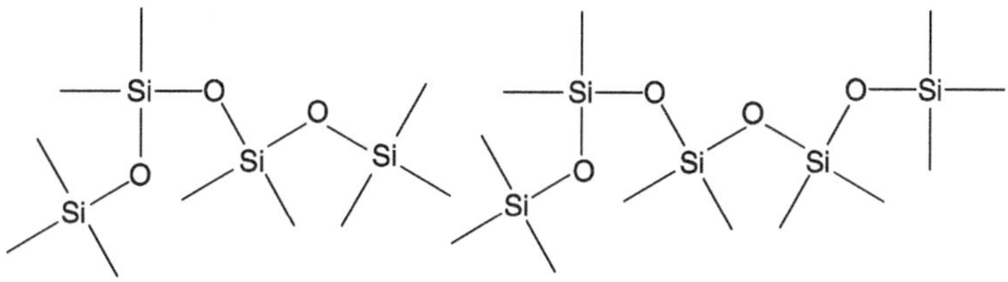

Decamethyltetrasiloxane Dodecamethylpentasiloxane

Other names: Decamethyltetrasiloxane, Dimethylpolysiloxane, Dimeticone, Dimeticonum, Dodecamethylpentasiloxane
INCI: Dimethicone
CAS no: 141-62-8/ 141-63-9/ 9006-65-9/ 9016-00-6/ 63148-62-9
Molecular formula: $(C_2H_6OSi)_x\ C_4H_{12}Si$
Rank of popularity: 8/502
Intended function: Antifoaming agent, Occlusive agent, Skin protectant

Dimethicone/Vinyl Dimethicone Crosspolymer

INCI: Dimethicone/Vinyl Dimethicone Crosspolymer
Rank of popularity: 267/502
Intended function: Viscosity increasing agent

Dimethiconol Behenate

Other names: Dimethicone propylethylenediamine behenate
INCI: Dimethicone propylethylenediamine behenate
CAS no: 132207-30-8
Rank of popularity: 382/502
Intended function: Occlusive agent

Dimethyl Capramide

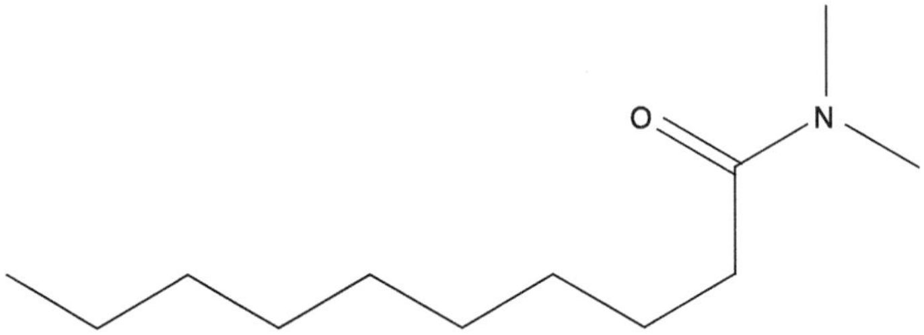

Other names: N,N-dimethyl decanamide
INCI: Dimethyl Capramide
CAS no: 14433-76-2
Molecular formula: $C_{12}H_{25}NO$
Molecular weight: 199.33
Rank of popularity: 383/502
Intended function: Emulsion stabilizer, Solvent
Log P: 3.82

Dimethyl Isosorbide

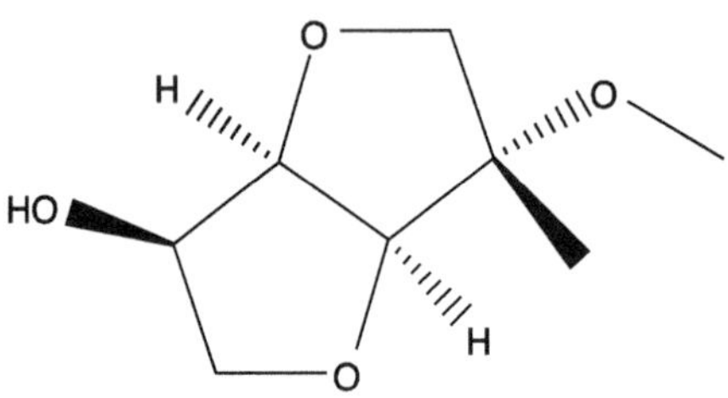

Other names: 1,4:3,6-Dianhydro-2,5-di-O-methyl-D-glucitol
INCI: Dimethyl Isosorbide
CAS no: 5306-85-4
Molecular formula: $C_8H_{14}O_4$
Molecular weight: 174.19
Rank of popularity: 268/502
Intended function: Solvent, Viscosity decreasing agent
Log P: –0.42

Dioctyl Ether

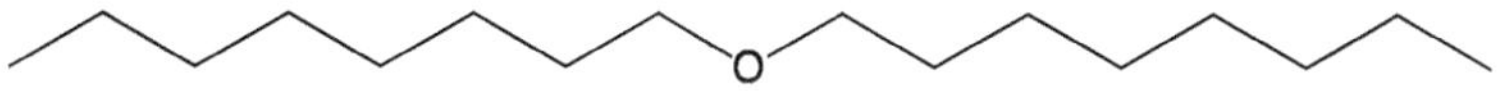

Other names: Dicaprylyl ether
INCI: Dicaprylyl ether
CAS no: 629-82-3
Molecular formula: $C_{16}H_{34}O$
Molecular weight: 242.44
Rank of popularity: 384/502
Intended function: Emollient, Solvent
Log P: 7.16

Dioctyl Succinate

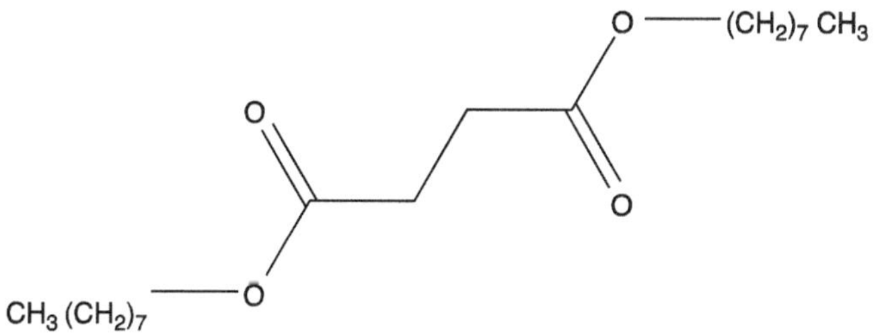

Other names: Diethylhexyl succinate
INCI: Diethylhexyl succinate
CAS no: 2915-57-3
Molecular formula: $C_{20}H_{38}O_4$
Molecular weight: 342.51
Rank of popularity: 385/502
Intended function: Emollient, Film former, Plasticizer, Solvent
Log P: 7.08

Dipalmitoyl Hydroxyproline

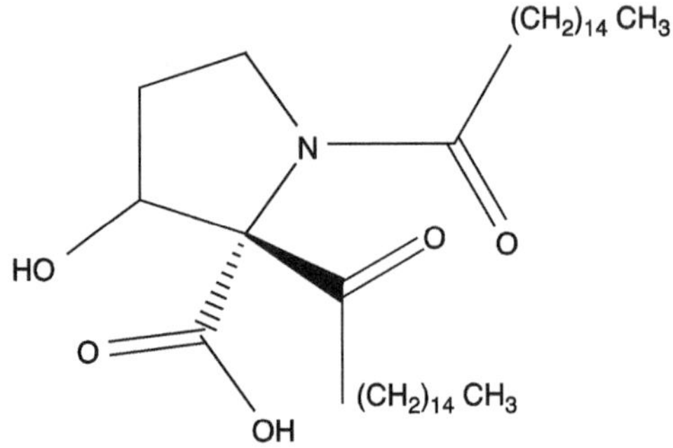

INCI: Dipalmitoyl Hydroxyproline
CAS no: 41672-81-5
Molecular formula: $C_{37}H_{69}NO_5$
Molecular weight: 607.95
Rank of popularity: 269/502
Intended function: Antistatic agent, Hair conditioning, Skin conditioning
Log P: 14.69

Diphenyl Dimethicone

INCI: Diphenyl dimethicone
Rank of popularity: 386/502
Intended function: Antifoaming agent, Occlusive agent
Log P: 14.69

Dipropylene Glycol

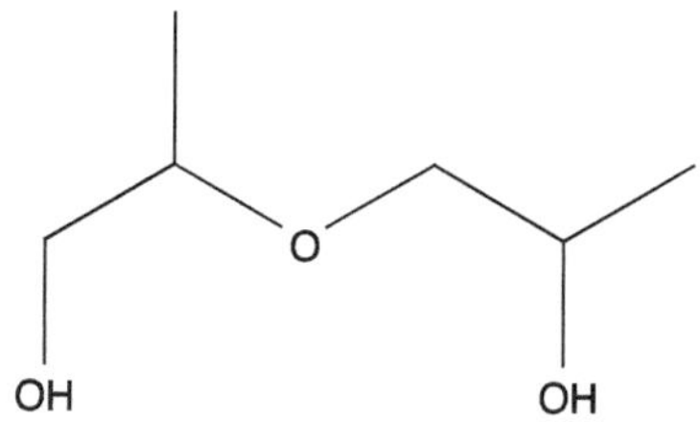

Other names: Hydroxypropyloxypropanol
INCI: Dipropylene Glycol
CAS no: 110-98-5/25265-71-8
Molecular formula: $C_6H_{14}O_3$
Molecular weight: 134.17
Rank of popularity: 201/502
Intended function: Fragrance, Solvent, Viscosity decreasing agent
Log P: -0.71

Dipropylene Glycol Dibenzoate

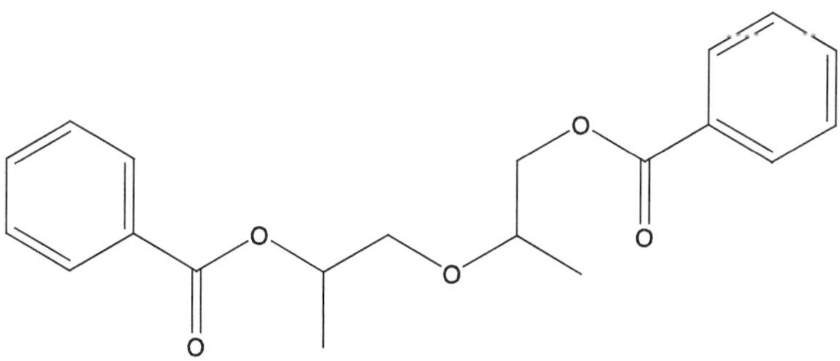

Other names: Polyoxypropylene (2) dibenzoate, PPG-2 dibenzoate
INCI: Dipropylene Glycol Dibenzoate
CAS no: 94-51-9/ 27138-31-4
Molecular formula: $C_{20}H_{22}O_5$
Molecular weight: 342.39
Rank of popularity: 387/502
Intended function: Emollient
Log P: 4.49

Disodium Cocoamphodiacetate

Other names: Cocoamphocarboxyglycinate,
INCI: Disodium Cocoamphodiacetate
CAS no: 68650-39-5
Rank of popularity: 388/502
Intended function: Cleansing agent, Foam booster, Hydrotrope, Hair conditioning

Disodium EDTA

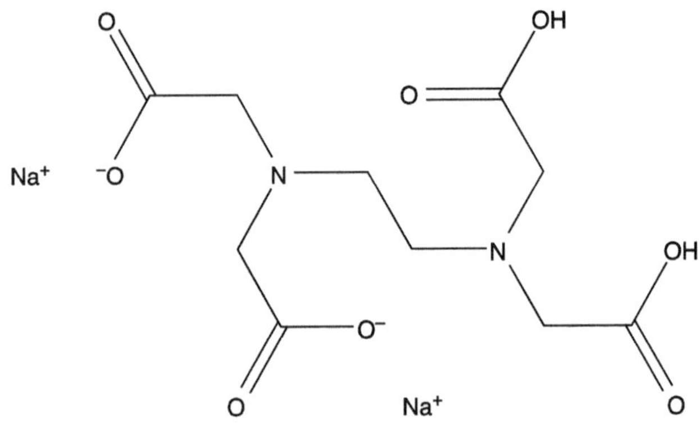

Other names: Disodium edetate
INCI: Disodium EDTA
CAS no: 139-33-3
Molecular formula: $C_{10}H_{16}N_2O_8 \cdot 2Na$
Molecular weight: 338.21
Rank of popularity: 11/502
Intended function: Chelating agent

Disodium Laureth Sulfosuccinate

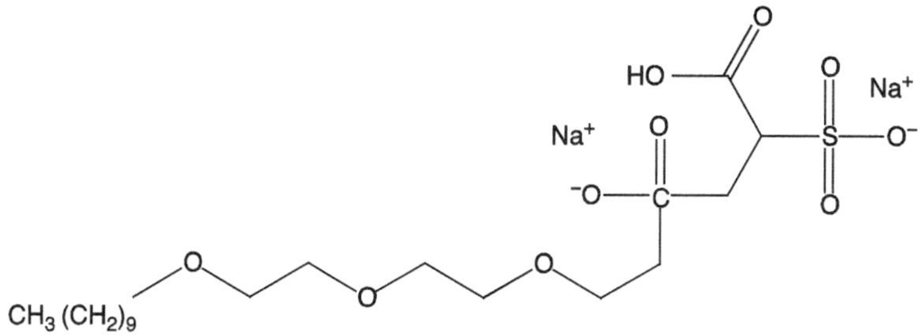

Other names: Disodium monolaureth sulfosuccinate
INCI: Disodium Laureth Sulfosuccinate
CAS no: 39354-45-5/ 40754-59-4/ 42016-08-0/ 58450-52-5/ 68815-56-5
Molecular formula: $(C_2H_4O)_x$ $C_{16}H_{30}O_7S$ ·2Na
Rank of popularity: 389/502
Intended function: Cleansing agent, Foam booster, Hydrotrope

Disodium Phosphate

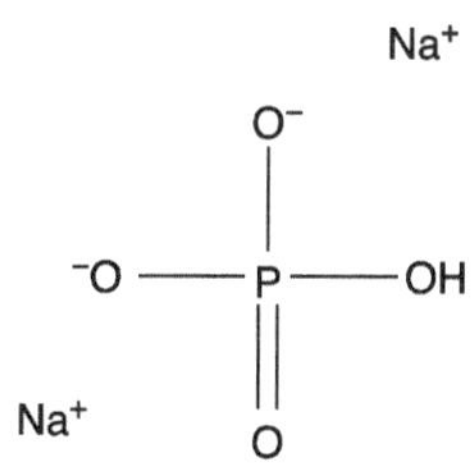

Other names: Dibasic sodium phosphate, Disodium hydrogen phosphate, Disodium orthophosphate
INCI: Disodium Phospate
CAS no: 7558-79-4/ 7782-85-6
Molecular formula: H_3O_4P ·2Na
Molecular weight: 143.97
Rank of popularity: 270/502
Intended function: Buffering agent, Corrosion inhibitor, Fragrance, pH adjuster

DMDM Hydantoin

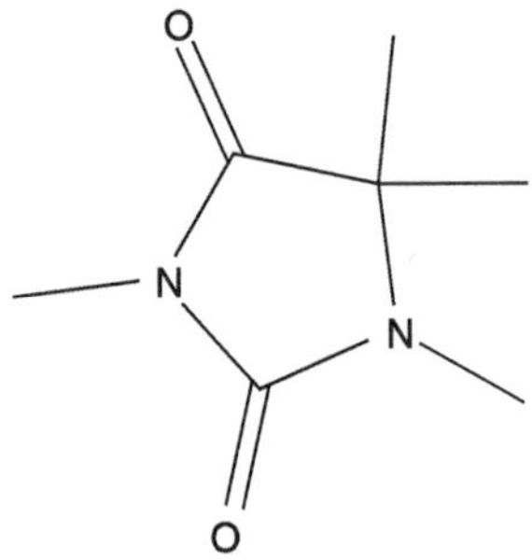

Other names: 1,3-dimethyl-5,5-dimethyl hydantoin
INCI: DMDM Hydantoin
CAS no: 6440-58-0
Molecular formula: $C_7H_{12}N_2O_4$
Molecular weight: 188.18
Rank of popularity: 117/502
Intended function: Preservative
Log P: –1.08
Allergenic potential: Weak sensitizer (max dose = 1.46 μg/cm^2/hr)

DNA

Other names: Deoxyribonucleic acid
INCI: DNA
CAS no: 9007-49-2
Rank of popularity: 390/502
Intended function: Skin conditioning

Drometriazole Trisiloxane

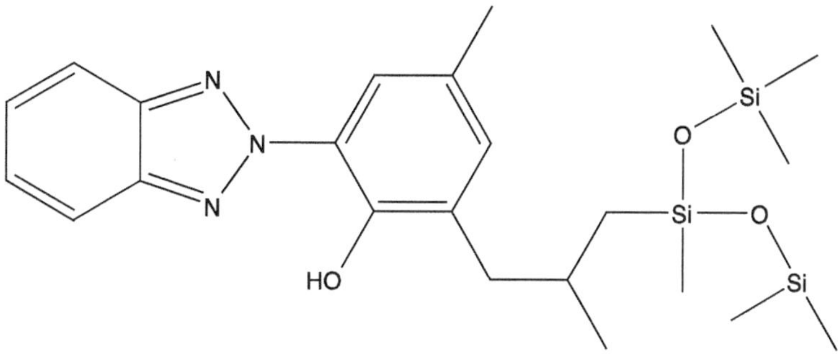

Other names: Dromiceius, emu oil
INCI: Drometriazole trisiloxane
CAS no: 155633-54-8
Molecular formula: $C_{24}H_{39}N_3O_3Si_3$
Molecular weight: 501.84
Rank of popularity: 56/502
Intended function: UV absorber, UV filter
Log P: 8.34

Ecamsule

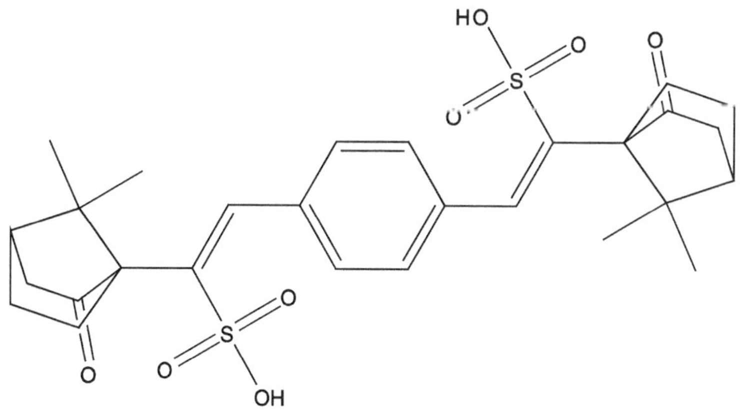

Other names: Terephthalylidene dicamphor sulfonic acid
INCI: Terephthalylidene dicamphor sulfonic acid
CAS no: 92761-26-7
Molecular formula: $C_{28}H_{34}O_8S_2$
Molecular weight: 52.69
Rank of popularity: 57/502
Intended function: UV absorber, UV filter
Log P: –1.82

EDTA

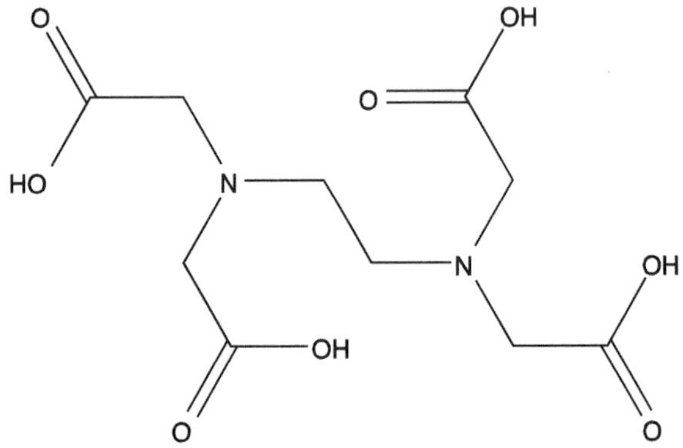

Other names: Edetic acid, Ethylene diamine tetre acetic acid
INCI: EDTA
CAS no: 60-00-4
Molecular formula: $C_{10}H_{16}N_2O_8$
Molecular weight: 292.23
Rank of popularity: 162/502
Intended function: Chelating agent
Log P: –0.84

Elastin

INCI: Elastin
CAS no: 9007-58-3
Rank of popularity: 391/502
Intended function: Hair conditioning, Skin conditioning
Carcinogenic potential: Category 2 (safe to use)

Emulsifying Wax

Other names: Emulsifying Wax N.F.
Rank of popularity: 99/502
Intended function: Emulsifying agent

Ethoxydiglycol

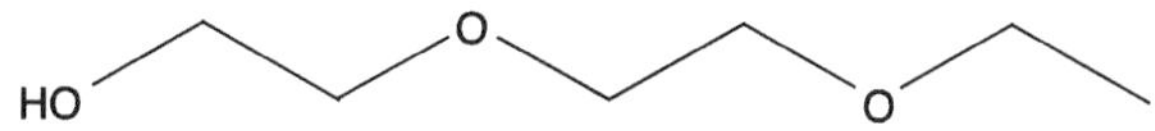

Other names: Diethylene glycol monoethyl ether
INCI: Ethoxydiglycol
CAS no: 111-90-0
Molecular formula: $C_6H_{14}O_3$
Molecular weight: 134.17
Rank of popularity: 111/502
Intended function: Fragrance, Solvent, Viscosity decreasing agent
Log P: -0.42
Allergenic potential: Weak sensitizer (max dose= 7.29 $\mu g/cm^2/hr$)

Ethylene/Acrylic Copolymer

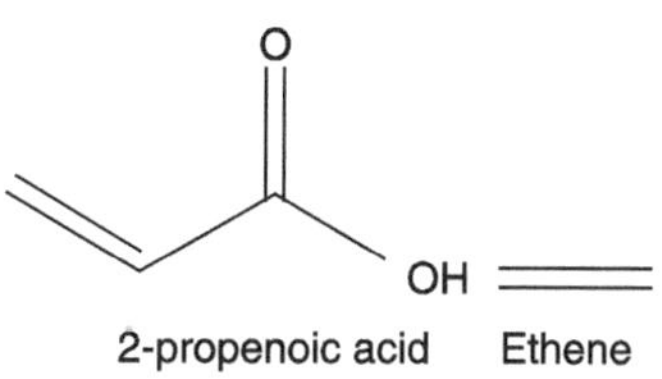

Other names: 2-propenoic acid with ethene
INCI: Ethylene/acrylic acid copolymer
CAS no: 9010-77-9
Rank of popularity: 392/502
Intended function: Binder, Film former, Viscosity increasing agent
Note: The structure does not represent the polymer. Only individual components are shown.

Ethylhexyl Palmitate

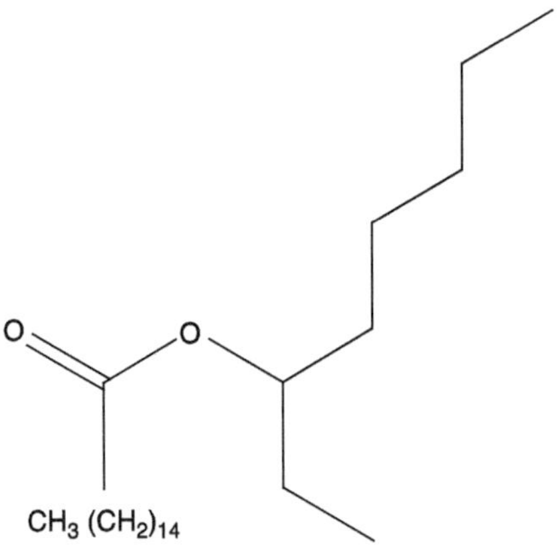

Other names: Elfacos EHP, 2-ethyl hexadecanoate, 2-ethylhexyl palmitate
INCI: Ethylhexyl Palmitate
CAS no: 29806-73-3
Molecular formula: $C_{24}H_{48}O_2$
Molecular weight: 368.64
Rank of popularity: 100/502
Intended function: Emollient, Fragrance
Log P: 11.15

Ethylhexyl Stearate

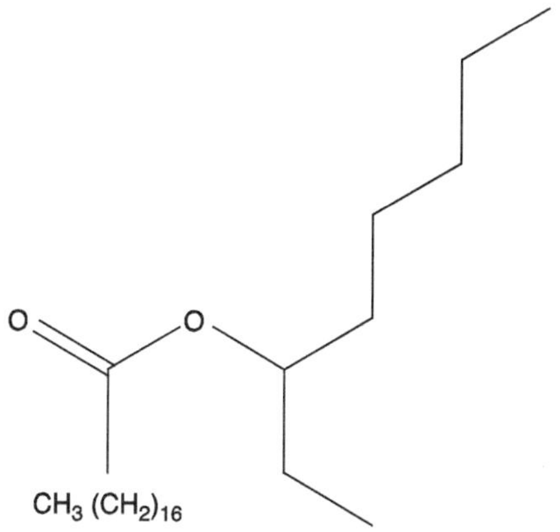

Other names: 2-ethylhexyl octadecanoate, 2-ethylhexyl stearate, Octyl Stearate
INCI: Ethylhexyl Stearate
CAS no: 22047-49-0
Molecular formula: $C_{26}H_{52}O_2$
Molecular weight: 396.69
Rank of popularity: 393/502
Intended function: Emollient
Log P: 11.84

Ethylhexyl Triazone

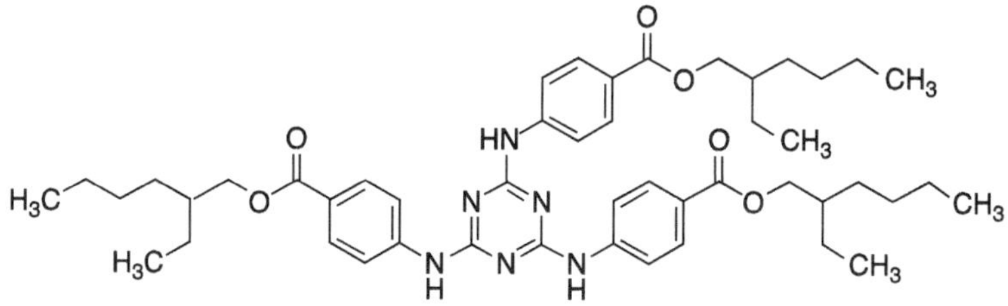

Other names: Octyl triazone
INCI: Ethylhexyl triazone
CAS no: 88122-99-0
Molecular formula: $C_{48}H_{66}N_6O_6$
Molecular weight: 823.07
Rank of popularity: 101/502
Intended function: UV filter
Log P: 16.13

Ethylhexylglycerin

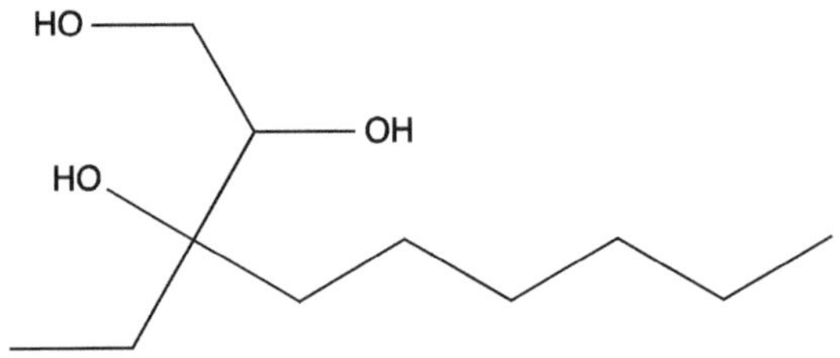

Other names: Octoxyglycerin
INCI: Ethylhexylglycerin
CAS no: 70445-33-9
Molecular formula: $C_{11}H_{24}O_3$
Molecular weight: 204.31
Rank of popularity: 118/502
Intended function: Deodorant, Skin conditioning
Log P: 2.47
Allergenic potential: Weak sensitizer (max dose = 36.5 μg/cm^2/hr)

Ethylparaben

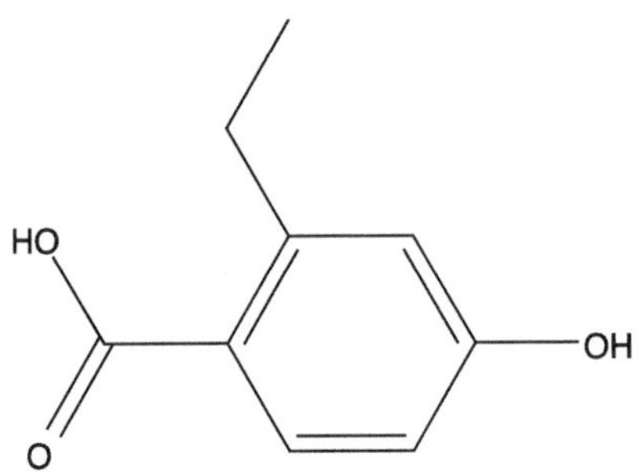

Other names: Ethyl 4-hydroxybenzoate, Ethyl parahydroxbenzoate
INCI: Ethylparaben
CAS no: 120-47-8
Molecular formula: $C_9H_{10}O_3$
Molecular weight: 166.17
Rank of popularity: 23/502
Intended function: Fragrance, Preservative
Log P: 2.39
Carcinogenic potential: Category 3 (use with precaution)
Allergenic potential: Weak sensitizer (max dose = 21.9 μg/cm^2/hr)

Eugenol

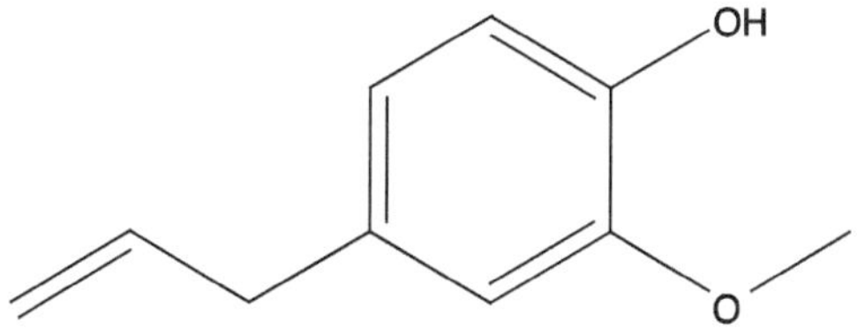

Other names: Allylguaiacol, Caryophyllic acid, Eugenic acid, Eugenolum, 2-hydroxy-5-allylanisole
INCI: Eugenol
CAS no: 97-53-0
Molecular formula: $C_{10}H_{12}O_2$
Molecular weight: 164.20
Rank of popularity: 394/502
Intended function: Denaturant, Fragrance
Log P: 2.40
Carcinogenic potential: Category 3 (use with precaution)
Allergenic potential: Weak sensitizer (max dose = 14.6 μg/cm²/hr)

Farnesol

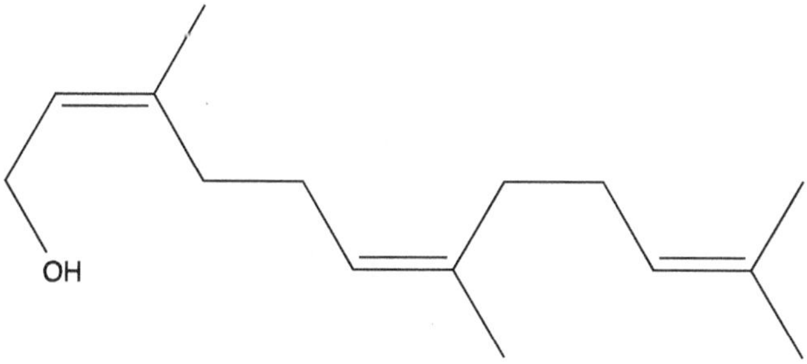

Other names: Trimethyl dodecatrienol
INCI: Farnesol
CAS no: 4602-84-0
Molecular formula: $C_{15}H_{26}O$
Molecular weight: 222.37
Rank of popularity: 271/502
Intended function: Fragrance
Log P: 4.83
Allergenic potential: Weak sensitizer (max dose = 36.5 μg/cm²/hr)

Fatty Alcohol

Other names: mixture of Cetearyl, Cetyl, Myristyl, Behenyl and Isostearyl Alcohol
Rank of popularity: 395/502
Intended function: Emollient, Emulsifying agent

FD & C Blue N1

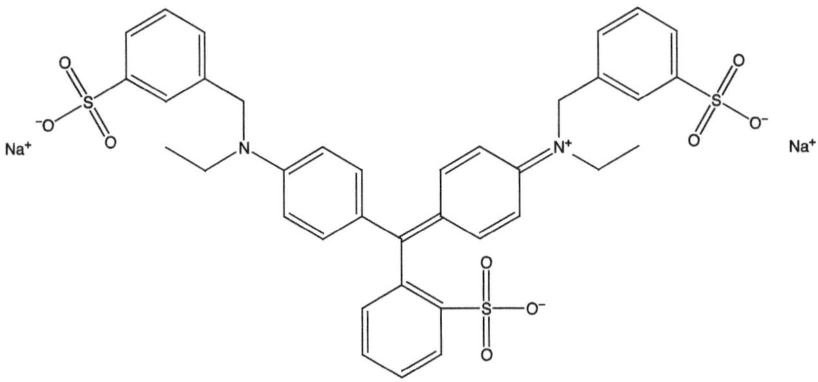

Other names: Acid blue 9, Blue no 1, Blue no 205, Brilliant blue FCF, Food blue 2, Japan blue 1 and 205
INCI: Cl42090
CAS no: 2650-18-2
Molecular formula: $C_{37}H_{36}N_2O_9S_3 \cdot 2Na$
Molecular weight: 794.86
Rank of popularity: 88/502
Intended function: Colourant

FD & C Green N3

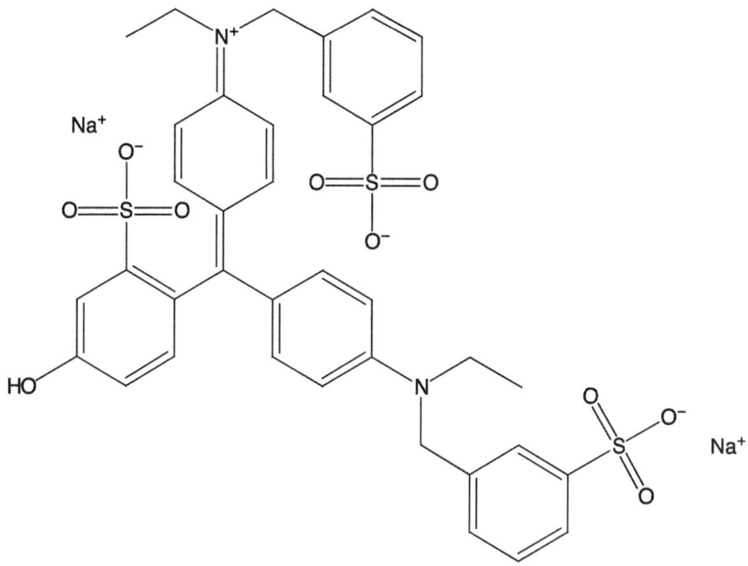

Other names: Fast green FCF, Food green 3, Green no 3, Japan 3
INCI: Cl40253
CAS no: 2353-45-9
Molecular formula: $C_{37}H_{36}N_2O_{10}S_3 \cdot 2Na$
Molecular weight: 810.86
Rank of popularity: 272/502
Intended function: Colourant
Carcinogenic potential: Category 2 (safe to use)

FD & C Red N4

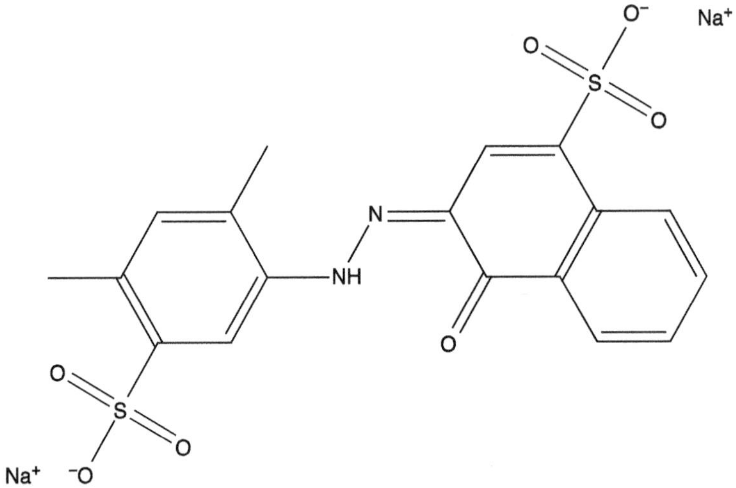

Other names: Food red 1, Ponceau SX, Red no 504
INCI: Cl14700
CAS no: 4548-53-2
Molecular formula: $C_{16}H_{16}N_2O_7S_2 \cdot 2Na$
Molecular weight: 458.41
Rank of popularity: 273/502
Intended function: Colourant

FD & C Red N3

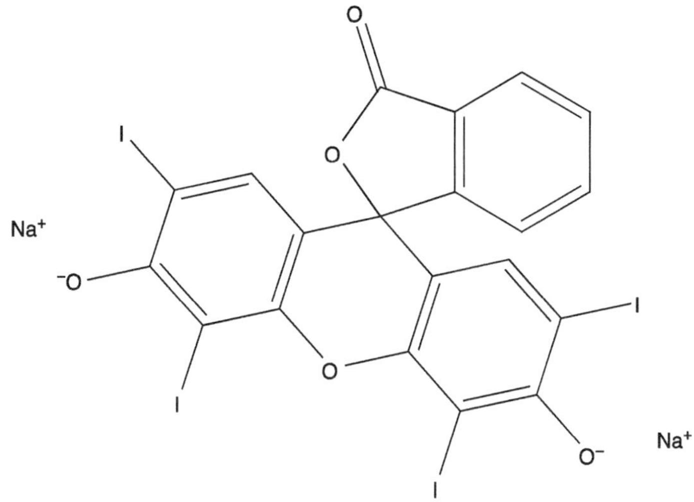

Other names: Acid red 51, Erthyrosine, Food red 14, Japan red 3, Red no 3, Yellow no 201, and 202(1), and 202(2)
INCI: Cl45430
CAS no: 16423-68-0
Molecular formula: $C_{20}H_8I_4O_5 \cdot 2Na$
Molecular weight: 881.87
Rank of popularity: 396/502
Intended function: Colourant

FD & C Yellow N5

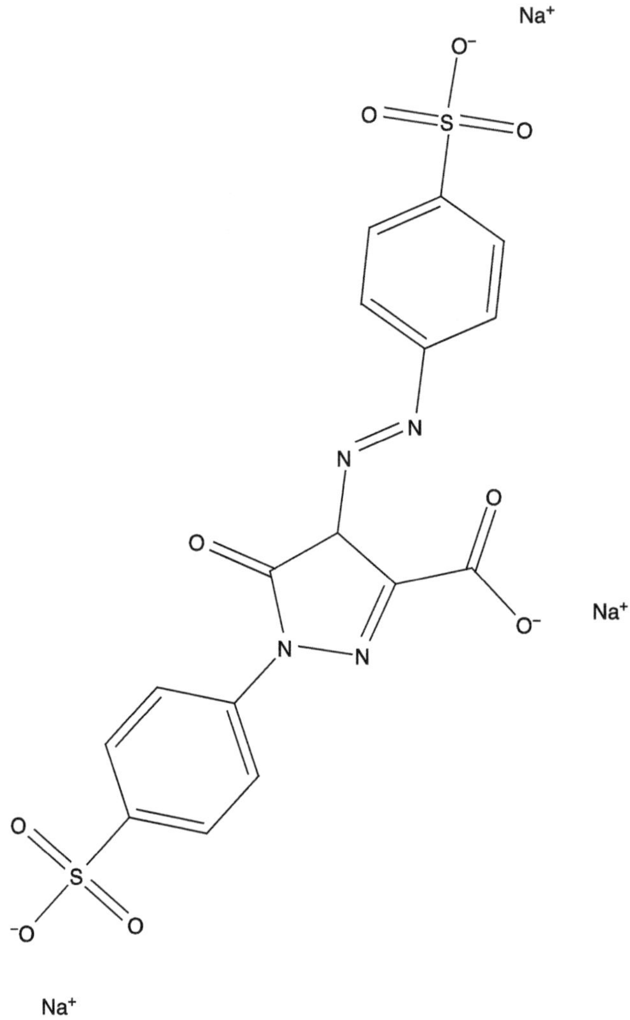

Other names: Food yellow 4, Hydrazine yellow, Tartraphenine, Tartrazin
INCI: Cl19140
CAS no: 1934-21-0/ 12225-21-7
Molecular formula: $C_{16}H_{12}N_4O_9S_2 \cdot 3Na$
Molecular weight: 537.38
Rank of popularity: 67/502
Intended function: Colourant

FD & C Yellow N6

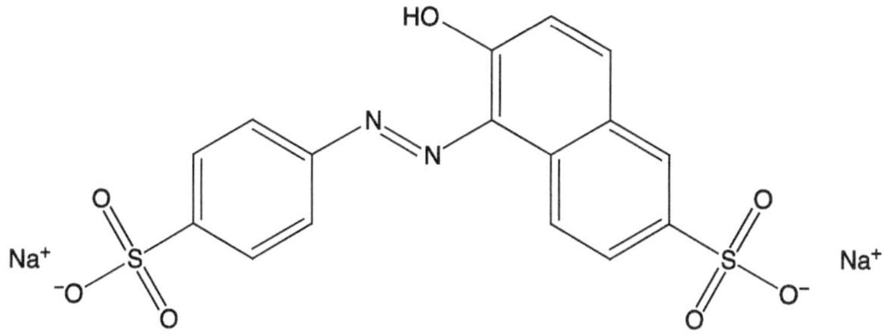

Other names: Sunset yellow
INCI: Cl 15985
CAS no: 2783-94-0
Molecular formula: $C_{16}H_{12}N_2O_7S_2 \cdot 2Na$
Molecular weight: 454.38
Rank of popularity: 274/502
Intended function: Colourant
Allergenic potential: Maximum dose not stated

Ferulic Acid

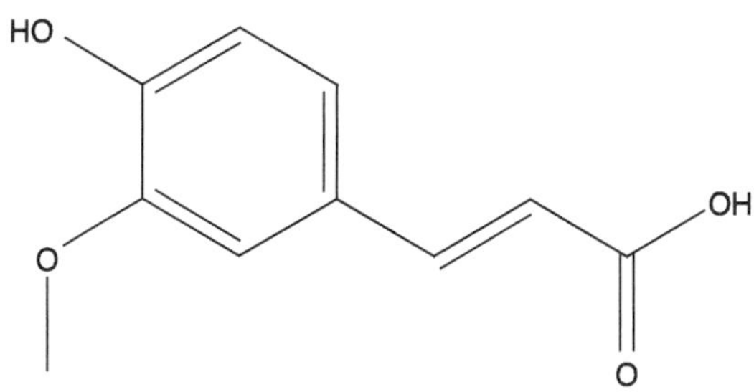

Other names: Coniferic acid
INCI: Ferulic Acid
CAS no: 1135-24-6
Molecular formula: $C_{10}H_{10}O_4$
Molecular weight: 194.18
Rank of popularity: 397/502
Intended function: Preservative
Log P: 0.96

Fragrance

Other names: Fragrance I, Fragrance II
INCI: Fragrance
Rank of popularity: 6/502
Intended function: Fragrance
Allergenic potential: Weak sensitizer (max dose = 58.3 μg/cm^2/hr)

Geraniol

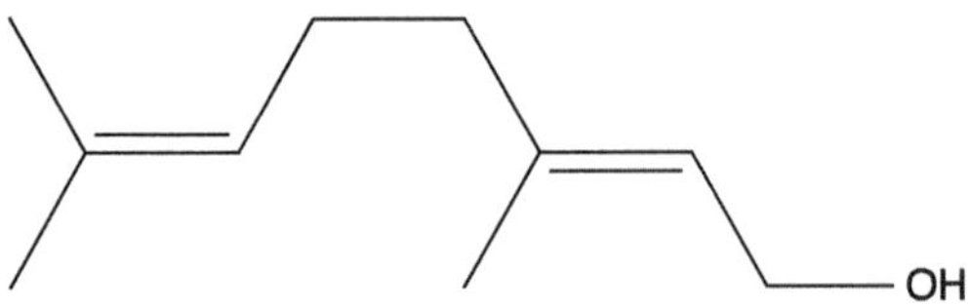

Other names: 3,7-dimethyl-2,6-octadien-1-ol
INCI: Geraniol
CAS no: 106-24-1
Molecular formula: $C_{10}H_{18}O$
Molecular weight: 154.25
Rank of popularity: 398/502
Intended function: Fragrance
Log P: 2.94
Allergenic potential: Very weak sensitizer (max dose = 233 μg/cm^2/hr)

Gluconolactone

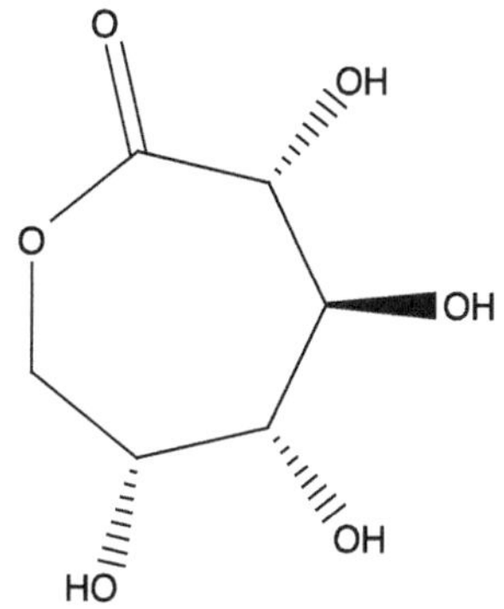

Other names: D-gluconic acid Delta-lactone
INCI: Gluconolactone
CAS no: 90-80-2
Molecular formula: $C_6H_{10}O_6$
Molecular weight: 178.14
Rank of popularity: 75/502
Intended function: Chelating agent, Skin conditioning
Log P: –3.47
Carcinogenic potential: Category 3 (use with precaution)

Glucose

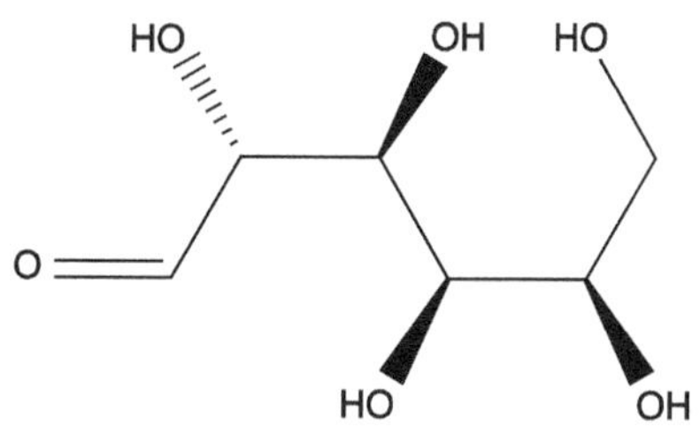

Other names: Dextrose, Destrosum/glucosum
INCI: Glucose
CAS no: 50-99-7(D-form)/ 58367-01-4(dl-alpha)
Molecular formula: $C_6H_{12}O_6$
Molecular weight: 180.16
Rank of popularity: 275/502
Intended function: Flavouring agent, Humectant, Skin conditioning
Log P: –3.29
Carcinogenic potential: Category 3 (use with precaution)

Glucosylrutin

Other names: 4-G-alpha-D-glucopyranosylrutin
INCI: Glucosylrutin
CAS no: 130603-71-3
Molecular formula: $C_{33}H_{40}O_{21}$
Molecular weight: 772.66
Rank of popularity: 276/502
Intended function: Antioxidant
Log P: –1.76

Glutamic Acid

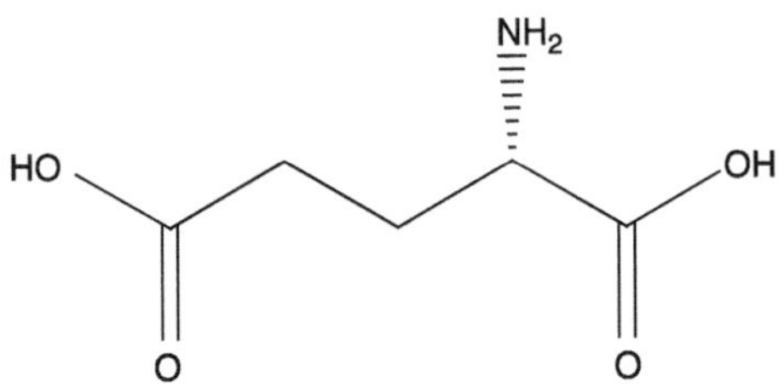

Other names: 2-aminoglutaric acid, 1-aminopentanedioic acid
INCI: Glutamic Acid
CAS no: 56-86-0(L-form)/ 617-65-2(dl-alpha)
Molecular formula: $C_5H_9NO_4$
Molecular weight: 147.13
Rank of popularity: 399/502
Intended function: Hair conditioning, Skin conditioning
Log P: –0.97

Glycadone

INCI: Glycadone
Rank of popularity: 400/502

Glycereth-26

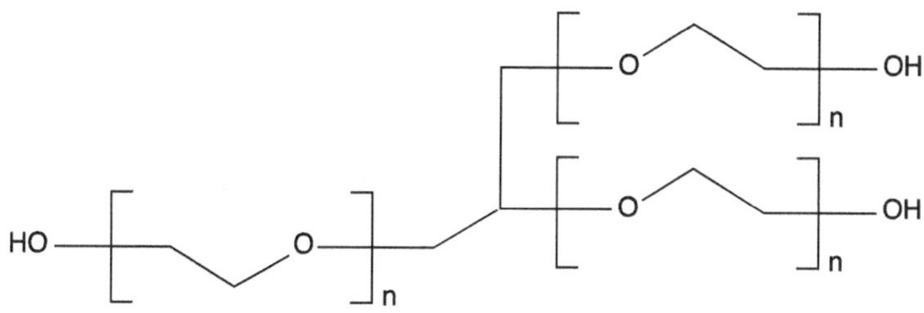

Other names: PEG-26 glyceryl ether, Polyethylene glycol (26) glyceryl ether, Polyoxyethylene (26) glyceryl ether
INCI: Glycereth-26
CAS no: 31694-55-0
Molecular formula: $(C_2H_4O)_n$ $(C_2H_4O)_n$ $(C_2H_4O)_n$ $C_3H_6O_3$ where n=6 or 7
Molecular weight: Approx. 1000
Rank of popularity: 401/502
Intended function: Humectant, Solvent, Viscosity decreasing agent

Glycerin

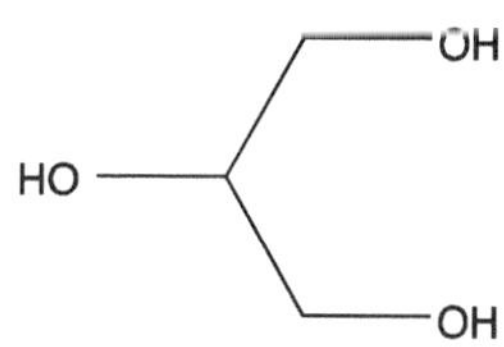

Other names: Glycerine, Glycerol, Glycerolum, Glycyl alcohol, 1,2,3-propanetriol, 1,2,3-trihydroxypropane
INCI: Glycerin
CAS no: 56-81-5
Molecular formula: $C_3H_8O_3$
Molecular weight: 92.09
Rank of popularity: 3/502
Intended function: Denaturant, Fragrance, Hair conditioning, Humectant, Oral care agent, Skin protectant, Viscosity decreasing agent
Log P: –1.85
Carcinogenic potential: Category 2 (safe to use)

Glyceryl Dilaurate

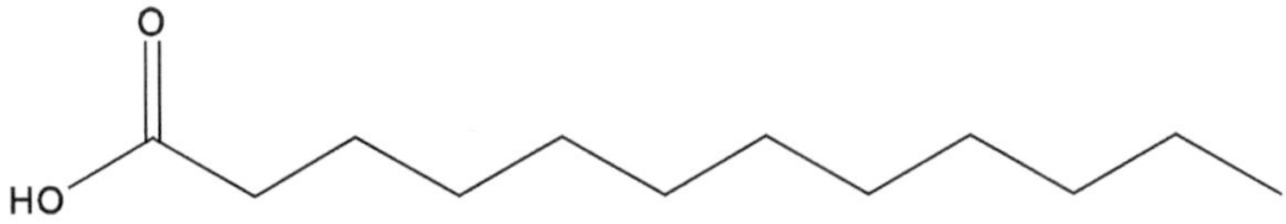

Dodecanoic acid

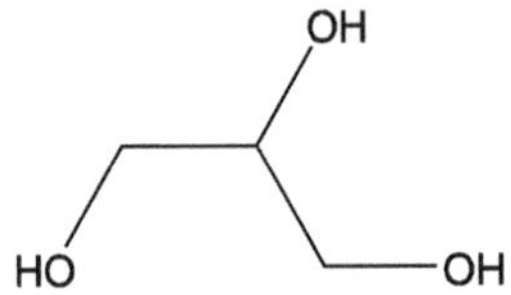

1,2,3-propanetriol

Other names: Dodecanoic acid, diester with 1,2,3-propanetriol , Dilaurin, Dilauroyl glyceride
INCI: Glyceryl Dilaurate
CAS no: 27638-00-2
Molecular formula: $C_{27}H_{52}O_5$
Molecular weight: 456.69
Rank of popularity: 277/502
Intended function: Emollient
Note: Only individual components of the structure are shown.

Glyceryl Distearate

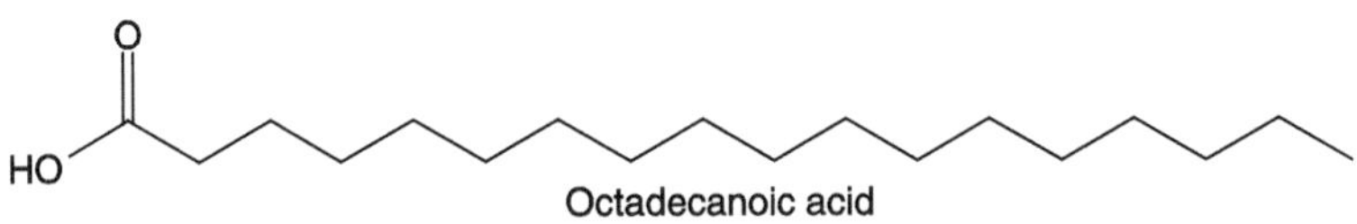

Octadecanoic acid

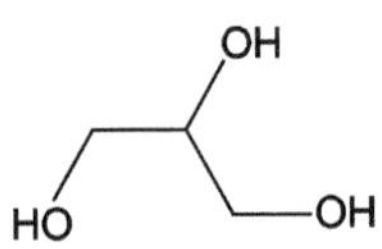

1,2,3-propanetriol

Other names: Octadecanoic acid, diester with 1,2,3-propanetriol, Distearin, Distearoylglycerol, Stearic acid diglyceride
INCI: Glyceryl Distearate
CAS no: 1323-83-7
Molecular formula: $C_{39}H_{76}O_5$
Molecular weight: 625.01
Rank of popularity: 402/502
Intended function: Emollient
Carcinogenic potential: Category 2 (safe to use)
Note: Only individual components of the structure are shown.

Glyceryl Isostearate

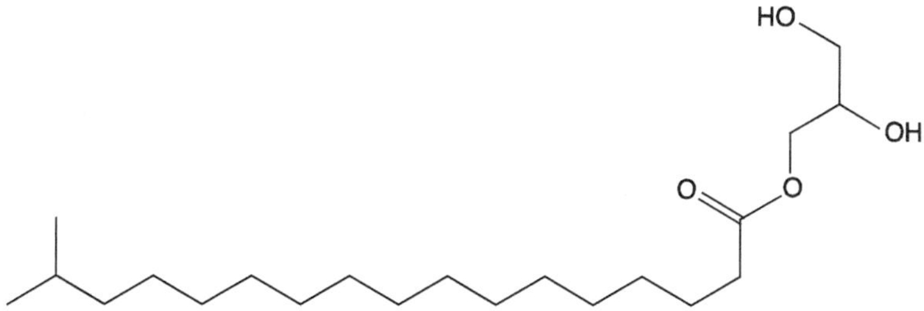

Other names: Glycerol isostearate, Glyceryl monoisostearate, Isostearic acid monoglyceride
INCI: Glyceryl Isostearate
CAS no: 61332-02-3/ 66085-00-5
Molecular formula: $C_{21}H_{42}O_4$
Molecular weight: 358.21
Rank of popularity: 403/502
Intended function: Emollient, Emulsifying agent
Log P: 6.71
Allergenic potential: Very weak sensitizer (max dose = 259 µg/cm²/hr)

Glyceryl Laurate

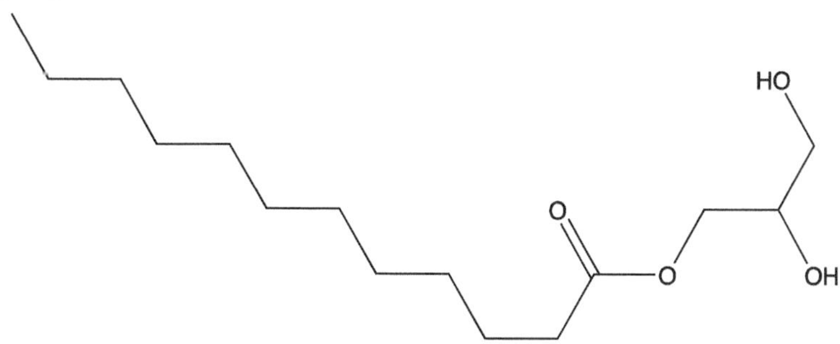

Other names: Glycerin 1-monolaurate, Glycerol 1-laurate, Lauric acid 1-monoglyceride, 1-monododecanoylglycerol, 1-monolaurin
INCI: Glyceryl Laurate
CAS no: 142-18-7/ 27215-38-9/ 37318-95-9
Molecular formula: $C_{15}H_{30}O_4$
Molecular weight: 274.40
Rank of popularity: 164/502
Intended function: Emollient, Emulsifying agent
Log P: 4.03

Glyceryl Oleate

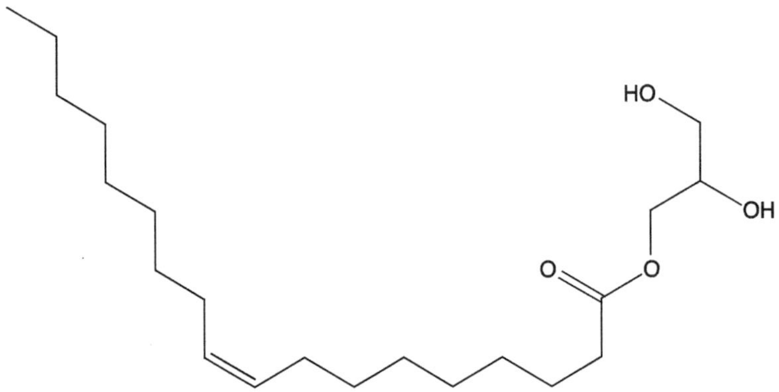

Other names: Glycerine monooleate, Glycerin oleate, Glyceryl monooleate, Glyceryl oleate
INCI: Glyceryl Oleate
CAS no: 111-03-5/ 25496-72-4/ 37220-82-9/ 68424-61-3/ 161403-66-3
Molecular formula: $C_{21}H_{40}O_4$
Molecular weight: 356.54
Rank of popularity: 202/502
Intended function: Emollient, Emulsifying agent, Fragrance
Log P: 6.68

Glyceryl Stearate

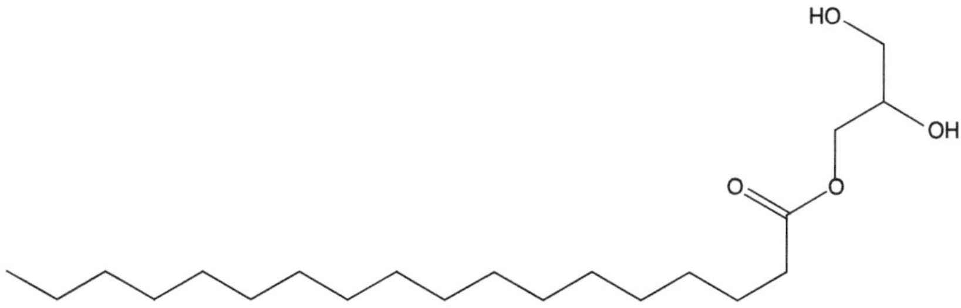

Other names: Glycerin 1-stearate, Glyceroli monostearas, Glyceryl monostearate, Glycerol 1-stearate, Monostearin, Stearic acid 1-monoglyceride
INCI: Glyceryl Stearate
CAS no: 123-94-4/ 11099-07-3/ 31566-31-1/ 85666-92-8
Molecular formula: $C_{21}H_{42}O_4$
Molecular weight: 358.56
Rank of popularity: 10/502
Intended function: Emollient, Emulsifying agent, Fragrance
Log P: 7.09
Carcinogenic potential: Category 2 (safe to use)

Glyceryl Stearate Citrate

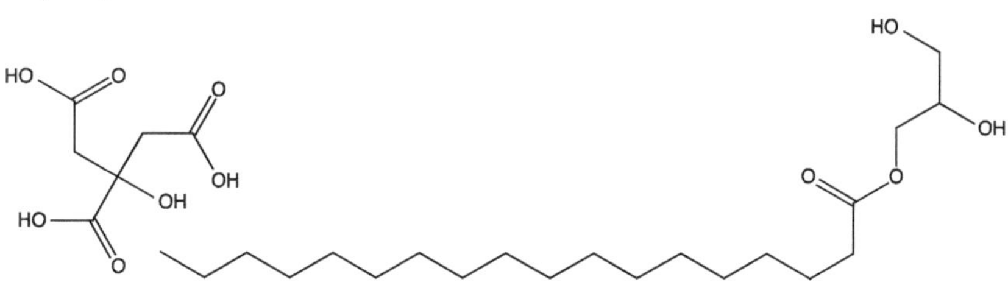

INCI: Glyceryl Stearate Citrate
CAS no: 39175-72-9/ 55840-13-6
Molecular formula: $C_{27}H_{48}O_{10}$
Molecular weight: 532.66
Rank of popularity: 204/502
Intended function: Emollient, Emulsifying agent

Glycine

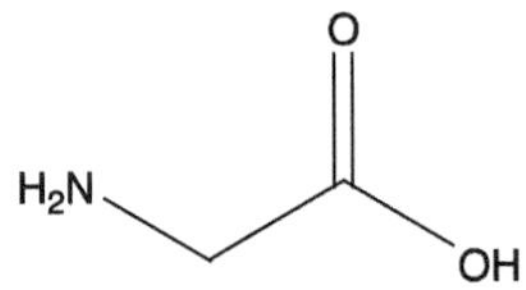

Other names: Aminoacetic acid, Aminoethanoic acid, Glycinum, Glycocoll
INCI: Glycine
CAS no: 56-40-6
Molecular formula: $C_2H_5NO_2$
Molecular weight: 75.07
Rank of popularity: 203/502
Intended function: Buffering agent, Hair conditioning, Skin conditioning
Log P: –0.93

Glycol DE Acetate

Other names: 2-(2-Ethoxyethoxy) ethyl acetate, Ethyldiglycol acetate
INCI: Ethyldiglycol acetate
CAS no: 112-15-2
Molecular formula: C8H16O4
Molecular weight: 176.21
Rank of popularity: 404/502
Intended function: Solvent
Log P: 0.401

Glycol Distearate

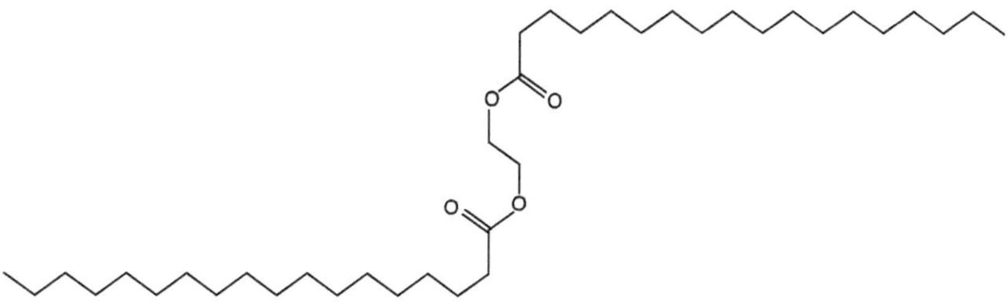

Other names: Ethylene dioctadecanoate, Ethylene glycol distearate
INCI: Glycol Distearate
CAS no: 627-83-8/ 91031-31-1
Molecular formula: $C_{38}H_{74}O_4$
Molecular weight: 594.99
Rank of popularity: 278/502
Intended function: Occlusive agent, Opacifying agent, Viscosity increasing agent
Log P: 16.53

Glycol Montanate

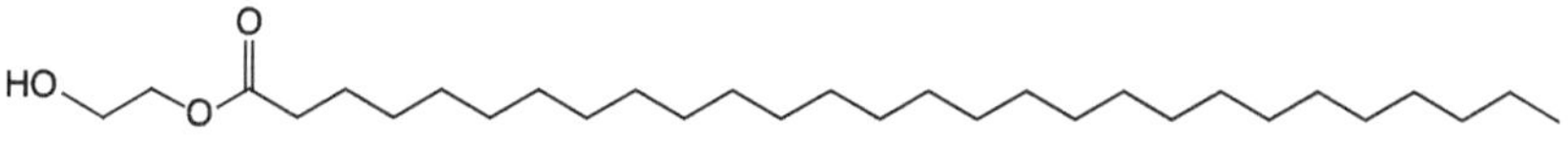

Other names: Ross carnauba wax replacement
INCI: Glycol Montanate
CAS no: 26787-65-5/ 73138-45-1
Molecular formula: $C_{30}H_{59}O_3$
Molecular weight: 468.80
Rank of popularity: 279/502
Intended function: Emollient, Emulsion stabilizer, Opacifying agent
Log P: 12.72

Glycol stearate

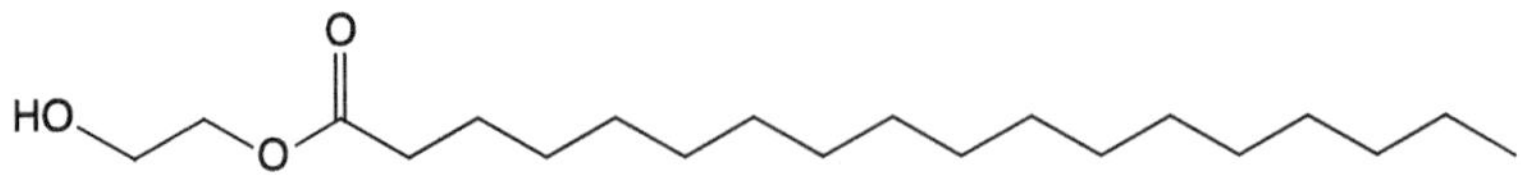

Other names: Ethylene glycol monostearate, Glycol monostearate, 2-hydroxyethyl octadecanoate
INCI: Glycol stearate
CAS no: 111-60-4
Molecular formula: $C_{20}H_{40}O_3$
Molecular weight: 328.53
Rank of popularity: 205/502
Intended function: Emollient, Emulsifying agent, Emulsion stabilizer, Opacifying agent
Log P: 7.63

Glycolic Acid

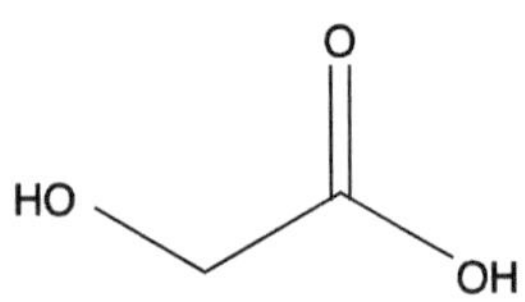

Other names: Hydroxyacetic acid, Hydroxyethanoic acid
INCI: Glycolic Acid
CAS no: 79-14-1
Molecular formula: $C_2H_4O_3$
Molecular weight: 76.05
Rank of popularity: 68/502
Intended function: Exfoliant, ph adjuster
Log P: –1.20
Carcinogenic potential: Category 1 (use within limit on body = 10.0 % w/w)
Allergenic potential: Weak sensitizer (max dose = 3.65 μg/cm^2/hr)

Glycyrrhetinic Acid

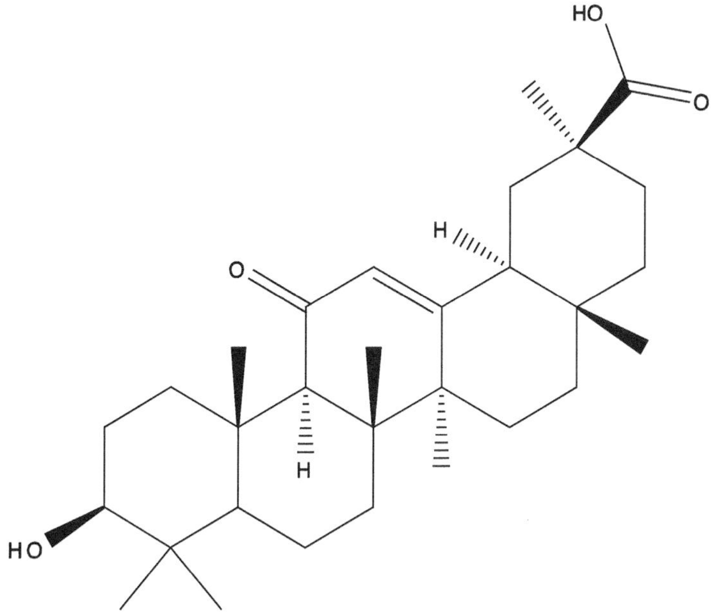

Other names: Enoxolone, Uralenic acid
INCI: Glycyrrhetinic Acid
CAS no: 471-53-4
Molecular formula: $C_{30}H_{46}O_4$
Molecular weight: 470.68
Rank of popularity: 405/502
Intended function: Skin conditioning
Log P: 5.50
Allergenic potential: Weak sensitizer (max dose = 0.729 μg/cm^2/hr)

Guar Gum

Other names: Cyamopsis tetragonoloba (guar) gum
INCI: Cyamopsis tetragonoloba (guar) gum
CAS no: 9000-30-0
Rank of popularity: 207/502
Intended function: Binder, Emulsion stabilizer, Fragrance, Viscosity increasing agent
Carcinogenic potential: Category 2 (safe to use)

Hectorite

Other names: Accofloc HCX; Astratone 40; Bentone CT
INCI: Hectorite
CAS no: 12173-47-6/ 68084-71-9
Molecular formula: $((Mg_{2.67}Li_{0.33})\ Si_4Na_{0.33}[F_{0.5\text{-}1}(OH)_{0-0.5}]_2O_{10})$
Molecular weight: 383.25
Rank of popularity: 406/502
Intended function: Absorbent, Bulking agent, Opacifying agent, Suspending agent, Viscosity increasing agent

Hexyl Cinnamal

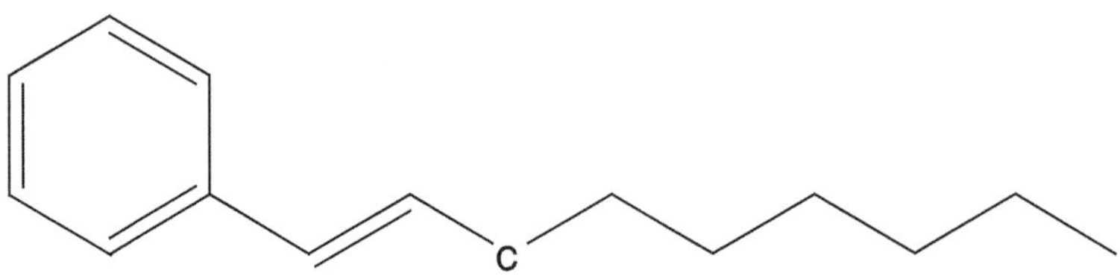

Other names: Alpha-hexylcinnamaldehyde, Hexyl cinnamic aldehyde
INCI: Hexyl Cinnamal
CAS no: 101-86-0
Molecular formula: $C_{15}H_{20}O$
Molecular weight: 216.32
Rank of popularity: 408/502
Intended function: Fragrance
Log P: 4.87
Allergenic potential: Weak sensitizer (max dose = 72.9 μg/cm^2/hr)

Hexyl Laurate

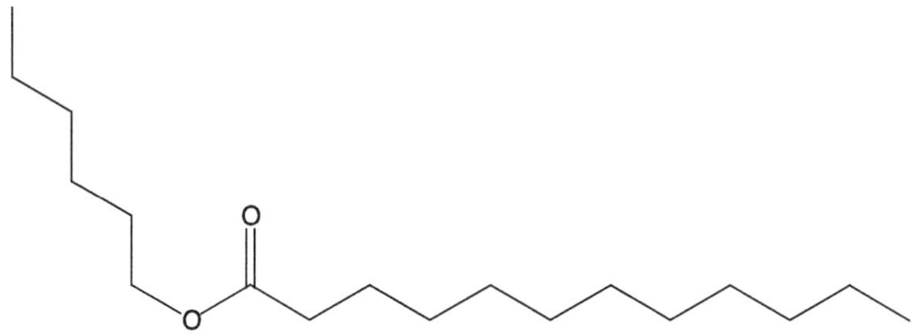

Other names: Dodecanoic acid hexyl ester
INCI: Hexyl Laurate
CAS no: 34316-64-8
Molecular formula: $C_{18}H_{36}O_2$
Molecular weight: 284.48
Rank of popularity: 407/502
Intended function: Emollient, Solvent, Viscosity decreasing agent
Log P: 7.92

Hexylene Glycol

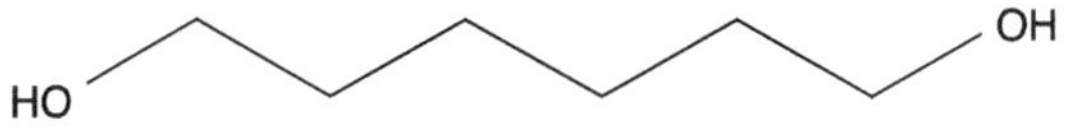

Other names: 2,4-dihydroxy-2-methylpentane, 2-methyl-2,4-pentanediol
INCI: Hexylene Glycol
CAS no: 107-41-5
Molecular formula: $C_6H_{14}O_2$
Molecular weight: 118.17
Rank of popularity: 119/502
Intended function: Fragrance, Solvent, Viscosity decreasing agent
Log P: 0.03
Allergenic potential: Weak sensitizer (max dose = 0.948 μg/cm^2/hr)

Homosalate

Other names: Homomenthyl salicylate, Metahomomenthyl salicylate
INCI: Homosalate
CAS no: 118-56-9
Molecular formula: $C_{16}H_{22}O_3$
Molecular weight: 262.34
Rank of popularity: 120/502
Intended function: Fragrance, UV absorber, UV filter
Log P: 5.95
Carcinogenic potential: Category 3 (use with precaution)
Allergenic potential: Weak sensitizer (max dose = 36.5 μg/cm^2/hr)

Hydrogenated Coco-glycerides

INCI: Hydrogenated Coco-glycerides
CAS no: 91744-42-2
Rank of popularity: 280/502
Intended function: Emollient

Hydrogenated Lanolin

INCI: Hydrogenated Lanolin
CAS no: 8031-44-5
Rank of popularity: 409/502
Intended function: Fragrance, Hair conditioning, Occlusive agent
Allergenic potential: Maximum dose not stated

Hydrogenated Lecithin

Other names: Hydrogenated egg yolk phospholipids
INCI: Hydrogenated Lecithin
CAS no: 92128-87-5
Rank of popularity: 165/502
Intended function: Emulsifying agent, Skin conditioning

Hydrogenated Polydecene

Other names: Hydrogenated 1-decene homopolymer
INCI: Hydrogenated Polydecene
CAS no: 68037-01-4
Rank of popularity: 410/502
Intended function: Emollient

Hydrogenated Polyisobutene

INCI: Hydrogenated Polyisobutene
CAS no: 68937-10-0
Rank of popularity: 140/502
Intended function: Emollient, Viscosity increasing agent
Allergenic potential: Weak sensitizer (max dose = 29.2 $\mu g/cm^2/hr$)

Hydrolysed Collagen

Other names: Collagen hydrolysate, Hydrolysed animal protein
INCI: Hydrolysed Collagen
CAS no: 73049-73-7/ 92113-31-0
Rank of popularity: 208/502
Intended function: Hair conditioning, Nail conditioning, Skin conditioning

Hydrolysed Elastin

Other names: Hydrolysed animal elastin
INCI: Hydrolysed Elastin
CAS no: 73049-73-7/ 100085-10-7
Rank of popularity: 165/502
Intended function: Hair conditioning, Skin conditioning

Hydrolysed Silk

Other names: Silk hydrolysate
INCI: Hydrolysed Silk
CAS no: 73049-73-7/ 96690-41-4
Rank of popularity: 281/502
Intended function: Hair conditioning, Skin conditioning

Hydroxyethyl acrylate/ sodium acryloyldimethyl taurate copolymer

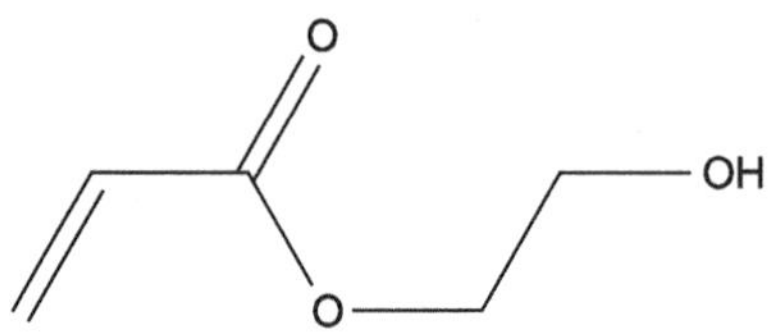

INCI: Hydroxyethyl acrylate/ sodium acryloyldimethyl taurate copolymer
CAS no: 111286-86-3
Rank of popularity: 411/502
Intended function: Emulsion stabilizer, Opacifying agent, Suspending agent, Viscosity increasing agent
Note: The structure does not represent the polymer. Only individual components are shown.

Hydroxyethylcellulose

Other names: Cellulose hydroxyethylate, Hyetellose, H.E. cellulose
INCI: Hydroxyethylcellulose
CAS no: 9004-62-0
Rank of popularity: 50/502
Intended function: Binder, Emulsion stabilizer, Film former, Viscosity increasing agent

Hydroxymethylglycinate

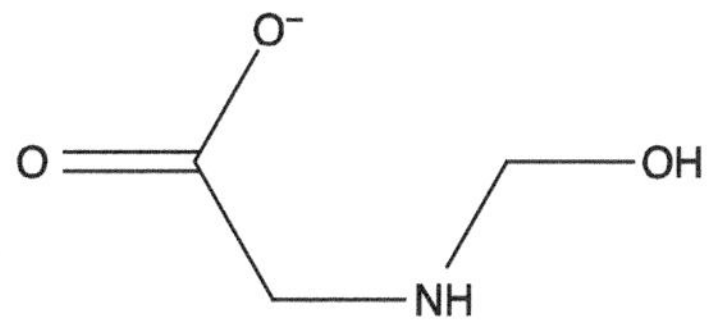

Other names: Sodium Hydroxymethylglycinate
INCI: Sodium Hydroxymethylglycinate
CAS no: 70161-44-3
Molecular formula: $C_3H_7NO_3$. Na
Molecular weight: 128.07
Rank of popularity: 412/502
Intended function: Hair conditioning, Preservative
Log P: 0.78

Hydroxypalmitoyl Sphinganine

INCI: Hydroxypalmitoyl Sphinganine
Molecular formula: $C_{34}H_{69}NO_4$
Molecular weight: 555.91
Rank of popularity: 413/502
Intended function: Hair conditioning, Skin conditioning

Hydroxypropyl Methylcellulose

Other names: Carbohydrate gum, Hypromellose
INCI: Hydroxypropyl Methylcellulose
CAS no: 9004-65-3
Rank of popularity: 121/502
Intended function: Adhesive agent, Binder, Emulsion stabilizer, Film former, Viscosity increasing agent

Imidurea

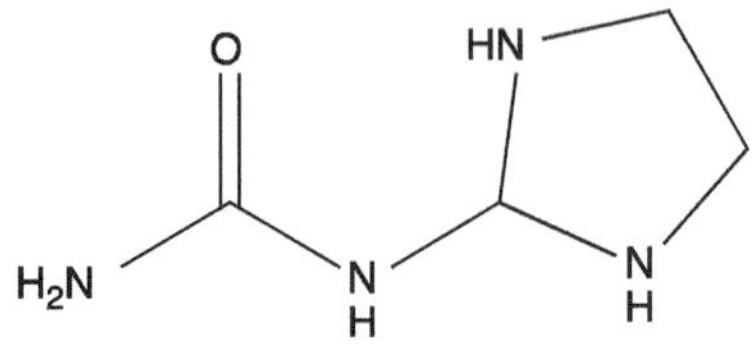

Imidazolidinyl urea

Other names: Imidazolidinyl urea
INCI: Imidazolidinyl urea
CAS no: 39236-46-9
Molecular formula: $C_{11}H_{16}N_8O_8$
Molecular weight: 388.29
Rank of popularity: 58/502
Intended function: Preservative
Log P: –4.93
Allergenic potential: Weak sensitizer (max dose = 14.6 μg/cm²/hr)

Iodopropynyl Butylcarbamate

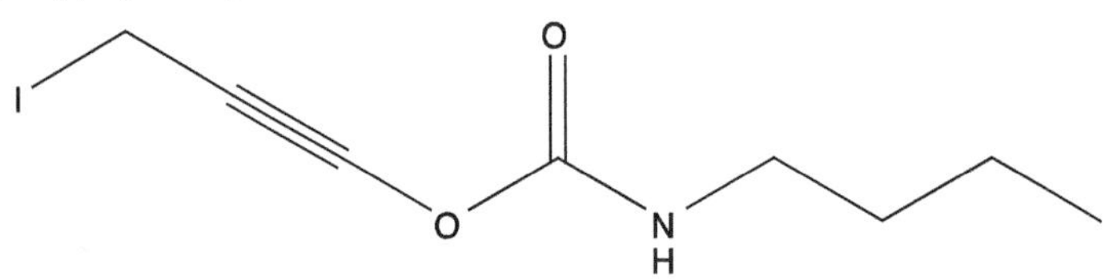

Other names: Butyl-3-iodo-2-propynylcarbamate, IPBC
INCI: Iodopropynyl Butylcarbamate
CAS no: 55406-53-6
Molecular formula: $C_8H_{12}INO_2$
Molecular weight: 281.09
Rank of popularity: 59/502
Intended function: Preservative
Log P: 3.38
Allergenic potential: Weak sensitizer (max dose = 0.72 μg/cm²/hr)

Iron Oxides (CI77492)

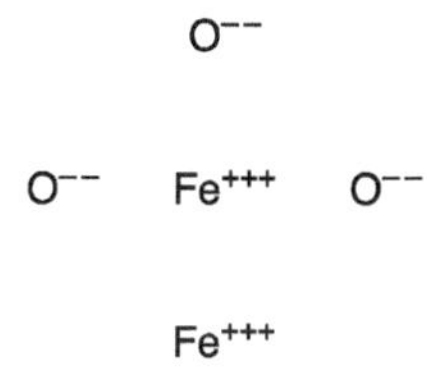

Other names: Black oxide of iron, Brown iron oxide, CI 77489,77491,77492,77499, Iron oxide Rd 10-34-PC-2045, Pigment black 11, Pigment brown 6, and 7, Pigment red 101, and 102, Pigment yellow 42, and 43, Red iron oxide, Synthetic iron oxide, Yellow iron oxide
INCI: Iron Oxides
CAS no: 51274-00-1/1309-37-1/ 1309-38-2/ 1317-61-9/ 1345-25-1/ 1332-37-2/ 12227-89-3/ 20344-49-4/ 52357-70-7/ 64294-91-3
Molecular formula: Fe_2O_3
Molecular weight: 177.71
Rank of popularity: 209/502
Intended function: Colourant
Log P: 0.21
Carcinogenic potential: Category 2 (safe to use)
Allergenic potential: Weak sensitizer (max dose = 5.83 μg/cm²/hr)

Isobutane

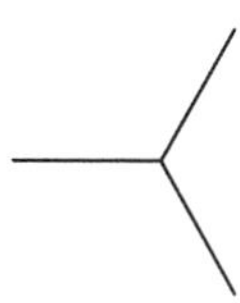

Other names: 1,1-dimethylethane, 2-methylpropane, Trimethylmethane
INCI: Isobutane
CAS no: 75-28-5
Molecular formula: C_4H_{10}
Molecular weight: 58.12
Rank of popularity: 284/502
Intended function: Propellant
Log P: 2.59

Isobutylparaben

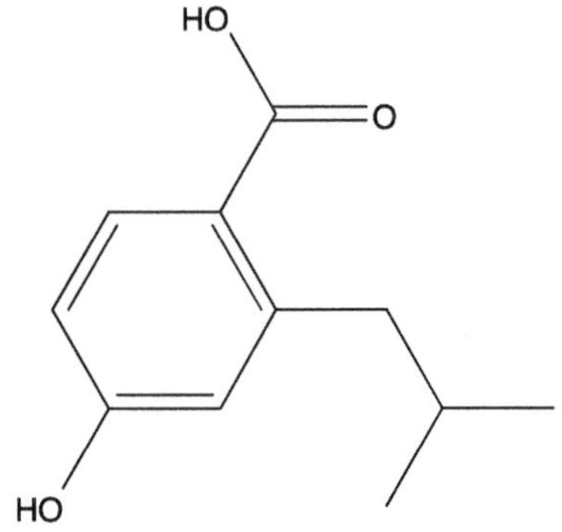

Other names: Isobutyl parahydroxybenzoate
INCI: Isobutylparaben
CAS no: 4247-02-3
Molecular formula: $C_{11}H_{14}O_3$
Molecular weight: 194.23
Rank of popularity: 35/502
Intended function: Preservative
Log P: 3.26
Allergenic potential: Maximum dose not stated

Isoceteth-20

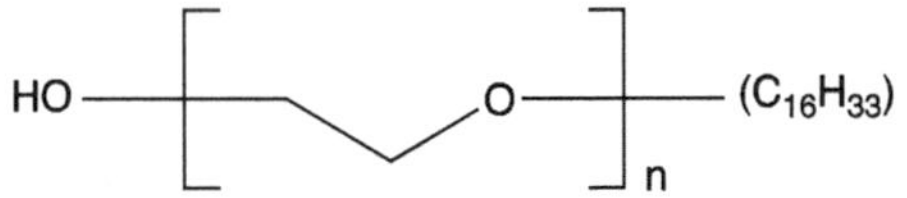

Other names: PEG-20 isocetyl ether, Polyethylene glycol 1000 isocetyl ether, Polyoxyethylene (20) isocetyl ether
INCI: Isoceteth-20
CAS no: 69364-63-2
Molecular formula: $(C_2H_4O)_n \cdot C_{16}H_{34}O$
Rank of popularity: 282/502
Intended function: Emulsifying agent, Solubilizing agent

Isocetyl Stearate

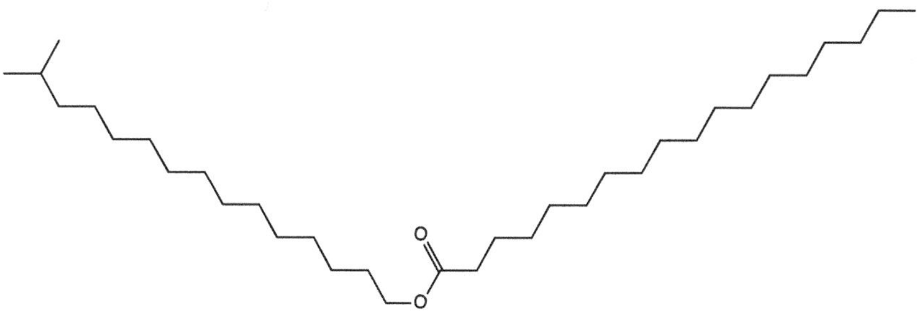

Other names: Isohexadecyl stearate, Octadecanoic acid isocetyl ester
INCI: Isocetyl Stearate
CAS no: 25339-09-7
Molecular formula: $C_{34}H_{68}O_2$
Molecular weight: 508.90
Rank of popularity: 141/502
Intended function: Emollient

Isodecyl Neopentanoate

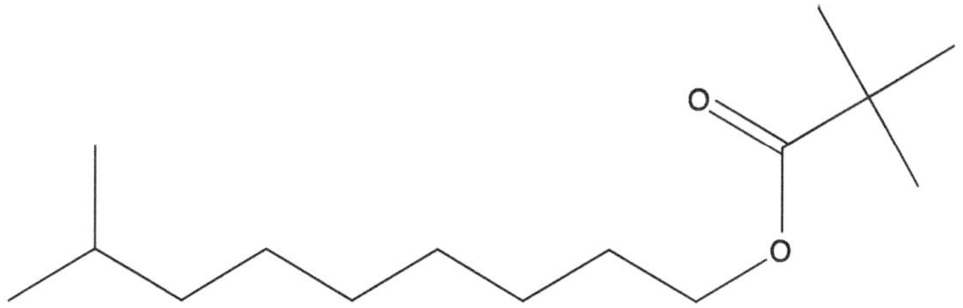

Other names: Isodecyl trimethylacetate
INCI: Isodecyl Neopentanoate
CAS no: 60209-82-7
Molecular formula: $C_{15}H_{30}O_2$
Molecular weight: 242.39
Rank of popularity: 166/502
Intended function: Emollient

Isododecane

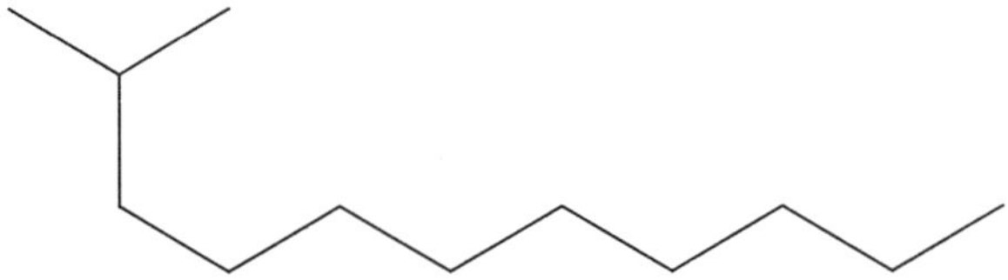

Other names: 1,1-dineopentylethylene
INCI: Isododecane
CAS no: 141-70-8/ 13475-82-6/ 31807-55-3/ 93685-81-5
Molecular formula: $C_{12}H_{26}$
Molecular weight: 170.33
Rank of popularity: 167/502
Intended function: Emollient, Fragrance, Solvent, Viscosity decreasing agent

Isohexadecane

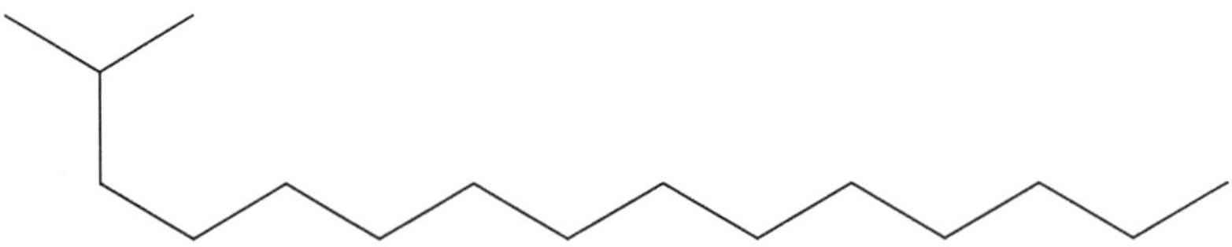

Other names: 2,2,4,4,6,6,8 heptamethylnonane
INCI: Isohexadecane
CAS no: 4390-04-9/ 60908-77-2/ 93685-80-4
Molecular formula: $C_{16}H_{34}$
Molecular weight: 226.44
Rank of popularity: 70/502
Intended function: Emollient, Solvent
Log P: 7.94

Isononyl Isononanoate

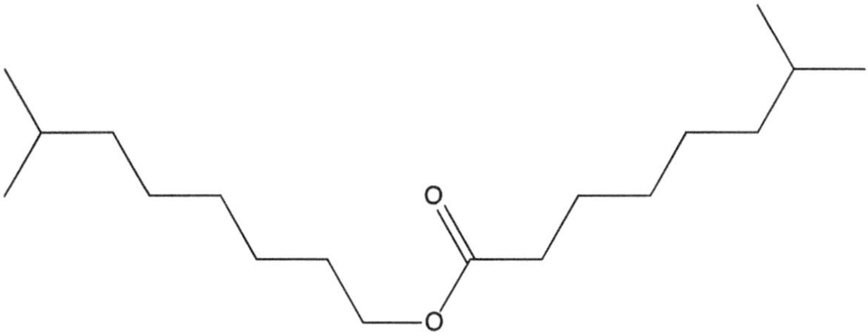

INCI: Isononyl Isononanoate
CAS no: 42131-25-9/59219-71-5
Molecular formula: $C_{18}H_{36}O_2$
Molecular weight: 286.46
Rank of popularity: 76/502
Intended function: Emollient
Allergenic potential: Very weak sensitizer (max dose = 146 μg/cm^2/hr)

Isopropyl Alcohol

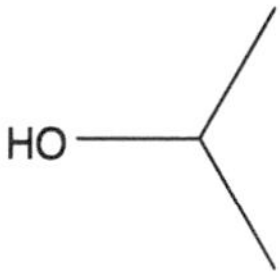

Other names: 2-hydroxypropane, isopropanol, 1-methylethanol, 2-propanol
INCI: Isopropyl Alcohol
CAS no: 67-63-0
Molecular formula: $C_3H_8O_3$
Molecular weight: 60.10
Rank of popularity: 283/502
Intended function: Antifoaming agent, Fragrance, Solvent, Viscosity decreasing agent
Log P: 0.17
Allergenic potential: Weak sensitizer (max dose = 72.9 μg/cm^2/hr)

Isopropyl Isostearate

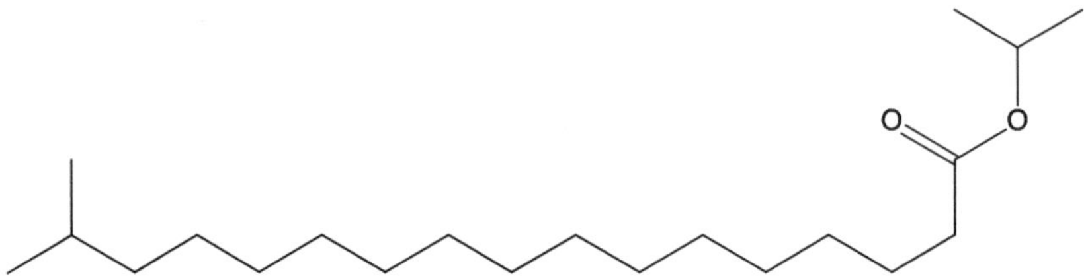

INCI: Isopropyl Isostearate
CAS no: 31478-84-9/ 68171-33-5
Molecular formula: $C_{21}H_{42}O_2$
Molecular weight: 326.56
Rank of popularity: 414/502
Intended function: Binder, Emollient
Log P: 9.14

Isopropyl Lanolate

Other names: Lanolin fatty acid isopropyl ester
INCI: Isopropyl lanolate
CAS no: 63393-93-1
Rank of popularity: 415/502
Intended function: Antistatic agent, Binder, Emollient, Emulsifying agent
Allergenic potential: Very weak sensitizer (max dose = 146 μg/cm^2/hr)

Isopropyl Myristate

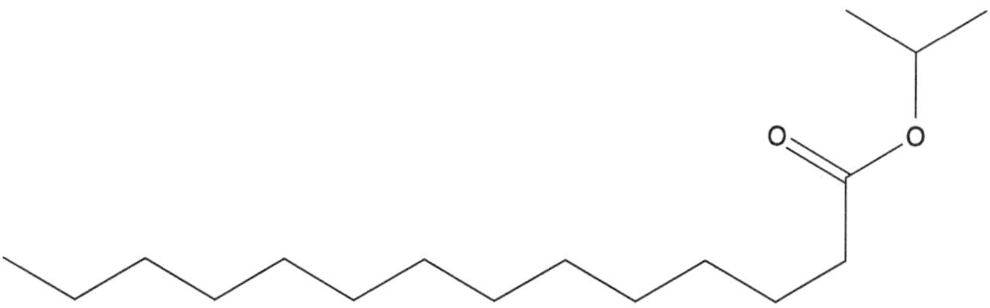

Other names: IPM, Isopropylis myristas, Isopropyl tetradeconoate, 1-methylethyl tetradecanoate
INCI: Isopropyl Myristate
CAS no: 110-27-0
Molecular formula: $C_{17}H_{34}O_2$
Molecular weight: 270.45
Rank of popularity: 77/502
Intended function: Binder, Emollient, Fragrance
Log P: 7.25
Allergenic potential: Weak sensitizer (max dose = 72.9 $\mu g/cm^2/hr$)

Isopropyl Palmitate

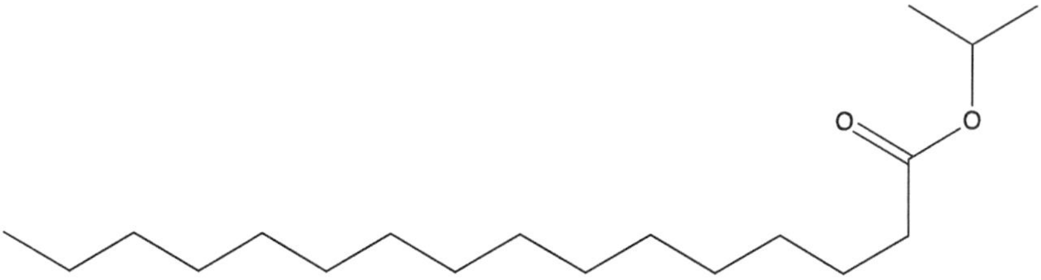

Other names: IPP, Isopropyl-n-hexadecanoate, Isopropylpalmitat
INCI: Isopropyl Palmitate
CAS no: 142-91-6
Molecular formula: $C_{19}H_{38}O_2$
Molecular weight: 298.50
Rank of popularity: 41/502
Intended function: Binder, Emollient
Log P: 8.27

Isopropyl Stearate

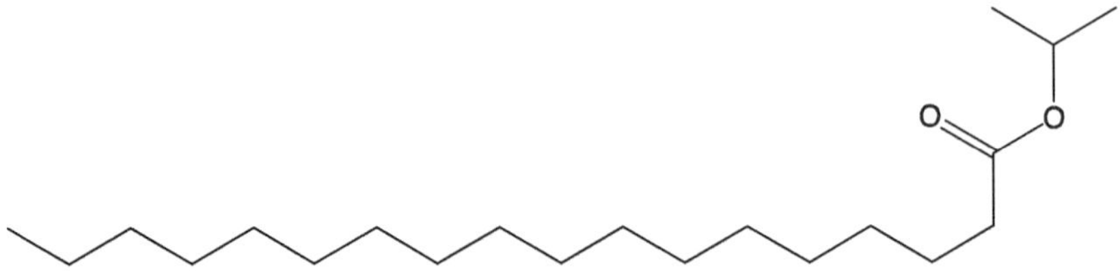

Other names: Isopropyl octadecanoate, 1-methylethyl octadecanoate
INCI: Isopropyl Stearate
CAS no: 112-10-7
Molecular formula: $C_{21}H_{42}O_2$
Molecular weight: 326.56
Rank of popularity: 210/502
Intended function: Binder, Emollient
Log P: 9.29
Allergenic potential: Weak sensitizer (max dose = 7.29 μg/cm²/hr)

Isopropylparaben

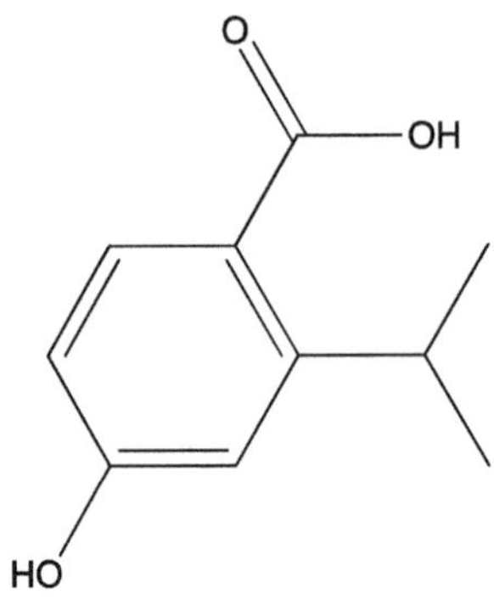

Other names: Isopropyl p-hydroxybenzoate, 1-methylethyl-4-hydroxybenzoate
INCI: Isopropylparaben
CAS no: 4191-73-5
Molecular formula: $C_{10}H_{12}O_3$
Molecular weight: 180.20
Rank of popularity: 168/502
Intended function: Preservative
Log P: 2.75
Carcinogenic potential: Category 1 (use within limit on body = 21.8 %w/w; face >100 %w/w; hands >100 %w/w)
Allergenic potential: Weak sensitizer (max dose = 7.29 μg/cm²/hr)

Isoquercitrin

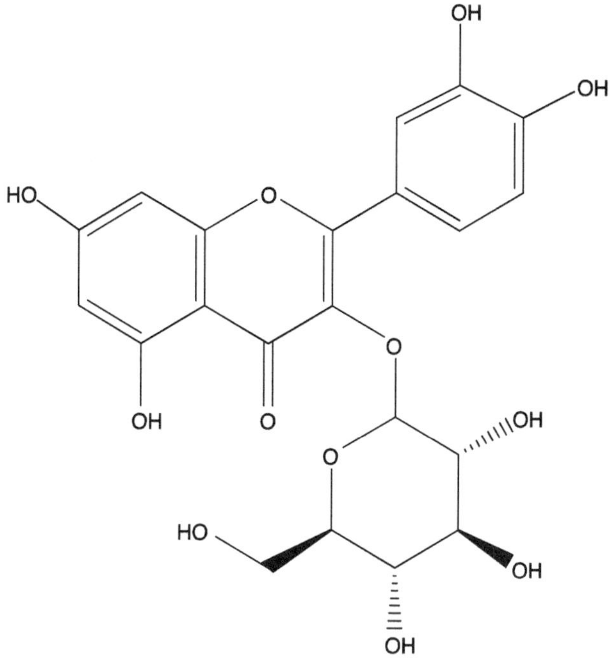

INCI: Isoquercitrin
CAS no: 21637-25-2
Molecular formula: $C_{21}H_{20}O_{12}$
Molecular weight: 464.38
Rank of popularity: 285/502
Intended function: Antioxidant
Log P: 0.05

Isostearic Acid

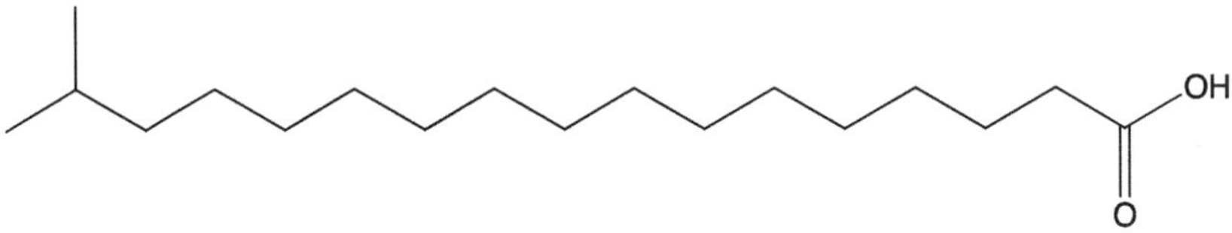

Other names: Isooctadecanoic acid, 16-methylheptadecanoic acid
INCI: Isostearic Acid
CAS no: 2724-58-5/ 30399-84-9
Molecular formula: $C_{18}H_{36}O_2$
Molecular weight: 284.48
Rank of popularity: 286/502
Intended function: Binder, Cleansing agent
Log P: 7.67

Kaolin

Other names: Bolus alba, China clay, Cl77004, Kaolinum, Kaolite, Pigment white 19
INCI: Kaolin
CAS no: 1332-58-7
Rank of popularity: 287/502
Intended function: Abrasive, Absorbent, Anticaking agent, Bulking agent, Opacifying agent, Skin protectant, Slip modifier

Kojic acid

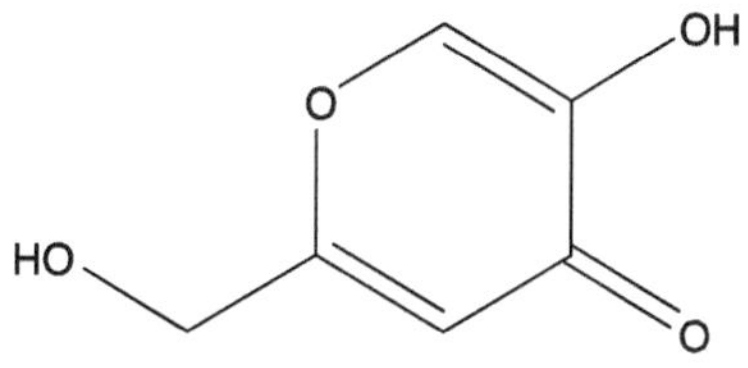

INCI: Kojic acid
CAS no: 501-30-4
Molecular formula: $C_6H_6O_4$
Molecular weight: 142.11
Rank of popularity: 211/502
Intended function: Antioxidant
Log P: −0.66
Carcinogenic potential: Category 3 (use with precaution)
Allergenic potential: Weak sensitizer (max dose = 0.729 μg/cm²/hr)

Lactic acid

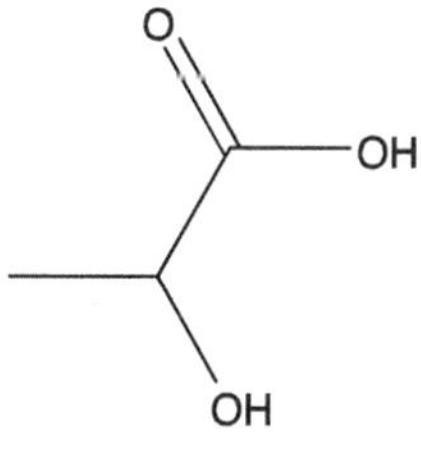

Other names: Acidum lacticum, 2-hydroxypropanoic acid
INCI: Lactic acid
CAS no: 50-21-5/ 79-33-4
Molecular formula: $C_3H_6O_3$
Molecular weight: 90.08
Rank of popularity: 78/502
Intended function: Exfoliant, pH adjuster, Fragrance, Humectant, Skin conditioning
Log P: −0.85
Carcinogenic potential: Category 3 (use with precaution)
Allergenic potential: Weak sensitizer (max dose = 14.6 μg/cm²/hr)

Lactobionic acid

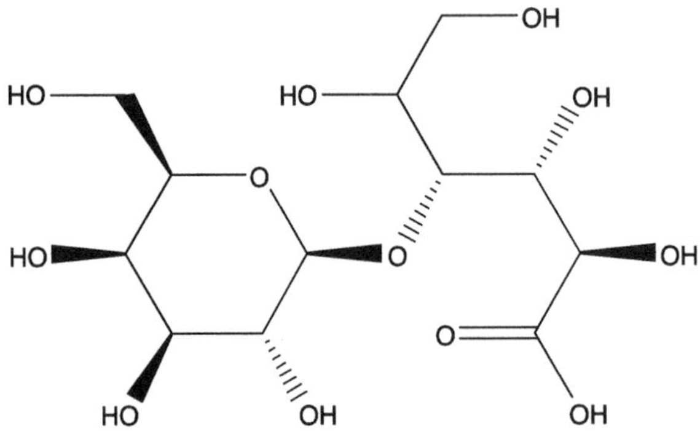

Other names: D-lactobionic acid
INCI: Lactobionic acid
CAS no: 96-82-2
Molecular formula: $C_{12}H_{22}O_{12}$
Molecular weight: 358.30
Rank of popularity: 212/502
Intended function: pH adjuster
Log P: –3.85

Lactoyl ethanolamine

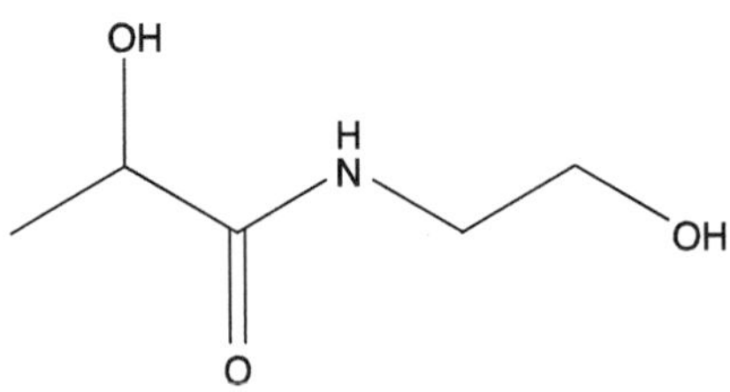

Other names: Lactic acid monoethanolamide
INCI: Lactamide MEA
CAS no: 5422-34-3
Molecular formula: $C_5H_{11}NO_3$
Molecular weight: 133.15
Rank of popularity: 288/502
Intended function: Foam booster, Hair conditioning, Humectant, Viscosity increasing agent
Log P: –1.27

Lanolin

Other names: Adeps lanae, Anhydrous lanolin, Hard lanolin, Wool fat, Wool wax
INCI: Lanolin
CAS no: 8006-54-0 (anhydrous)
Rank of popularity: 169/502
Intended function: Emollient, Emulsifying agent, Emulsion stabilizer, Hair conditioning, Skin protectant
Allergenic potential: Very weak sensitizer (max dose = 219 $\mu g/cm^2/hr$)

Lanolin alcohol

Other names: Alcoholes adipis lanae, Wool wax alcohol
INCI: Lanolin alcohol
CAS no: 8027-33-6
Rank of popularity: 112/502
Intended function: Binder, Emulsion stabilizer, Hair conditioning, Viscosity increasing agent
Allergenic potential: Very weak sensitizer (max dose = 219 $\mu g/cm^2/hr$)

Laureth-17

Rank of popularity: 289/502
Intended function: Cleansing agent, Solubilizing agent

Laureth-23

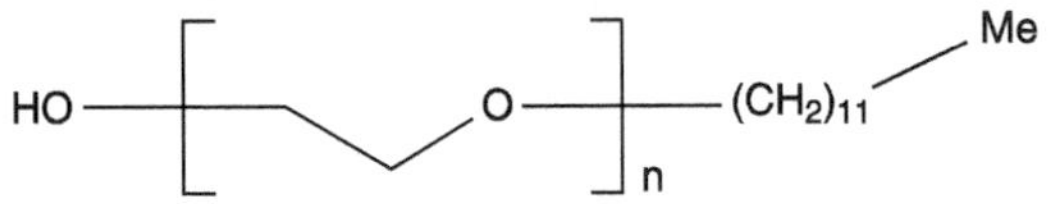

Other names: PEG-23 lauryl ether, Polyethylene glycol (23) lauryl ether
INCI: Laureth-23
CAS no: 9002-92-0
Molecular formula: $(C_2 H_4 O)_n C_{12} H_{26} O$
Rank of popularity: 416/502
Intended function: Cleansing agent, Solubilizing agent
Log P: 4.81
Allergenic potential: Weak sensitizer (max dose = 21.9 μg/cm^2/hr)

Laureth-3

Other names: Lauryl triglycol ether, PEG-3 lauryl ether, Polyethylene glycol (3) lauryl ether
INCI: Laureth-3
CAS no: 3055-94-5
Molecular formula: $C_{18}H_{38}O_4$
Molecular weight: 318.49
Rank of popularity: 417/502
Intended function: Emulsifying agent
Log P: 4.44

Laureth-7

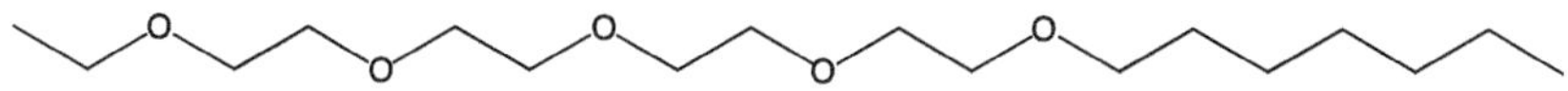

Other names: Hyptaethylene glycol dodecyl ether, PEG-7 lauryl ether, Polyethyleneglycol(7)laurylether,3,6,9,12,15,18,21-Heptaoxatritriacontan-1-ol
INCI: Laureth-7
CAS no: 3055-97-8
Molecular formula: $C_{26}H_{54}O_8$
Molecular weight: 494.70
Rank of popularity: 60/502
Intended function: Emulsifying agent
Log P: 3.50

Lauryl lactate

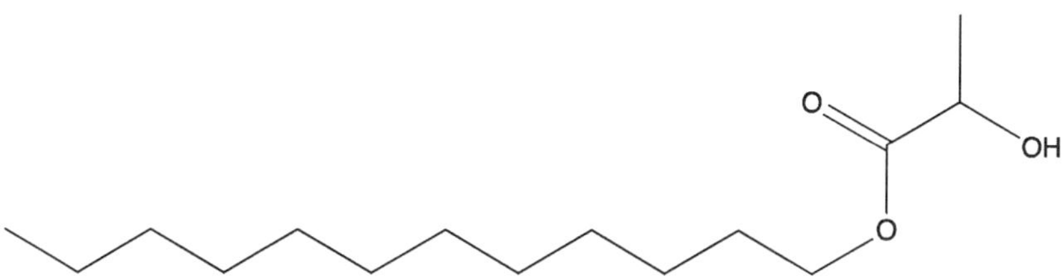

Other names: Dodecyl 2-hydroxypropanoate, Dodecyl lactate
INCI: Lauryl lactate
CAS no: 6283-92-7
Molecular formula: $C_{15}H_{30}O_3$
Molecular weight: 258.40
Rank of popularity: 418/502
Intended function: Emollient, Fragrance
Log P: 5.06

Lauryl PEG/PPG-18/18 methicone
INCI: Lauryl PEG/PPG-18/18 methicone
Molecular formula: alkoxylated derivative of Lauryl Methicone containing an average of 18 moles of ethylene oxide and 18 moles of propylene oxide
Rank of popularity: 419/502
Intended function: Skin conditioning

Lauryl Pyrrolidone

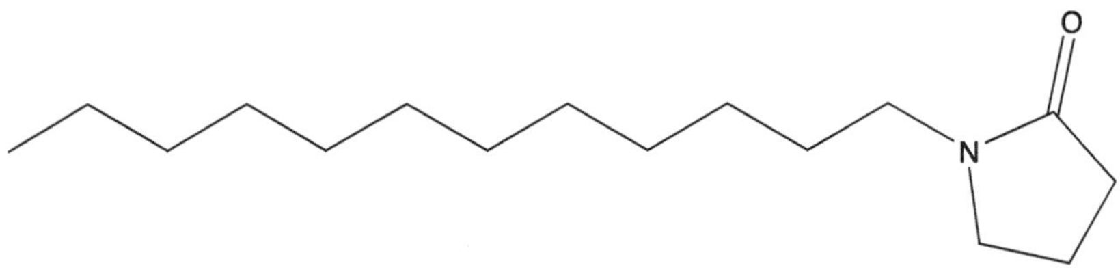

Other names: 1-dodecyl-2-pyrrolidone
INCI: Lauryl Pyrrolidone
CAS no: 2687-96-9
Molecular formula: $C_{16}H_{31}NO$
Molecular weight: 253.42
Rank of popularity: 420/502
Intended function: Cleansing agent, Hair conditioning
Log P: 4.97

Lecithin

Other names: Egg yolk lecithin, Soybean lecithin
INCI: Lecithin
CAS no: 8002-43-5/ 8030-76-0/ 93685-90-6
Rank of popularity: 53/502
Intended function: Emulsifying agent, Skin conditioning

Limonene

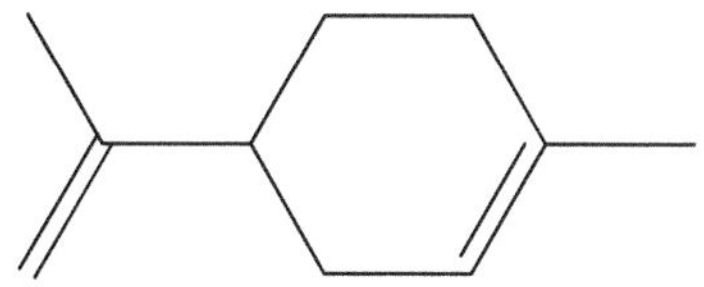

Other names: D-limonene, L-limonene
INCI: Limonene
CAS no: 138-86-3(dl-alpha)/ 5989-27-5(d-alpha)
Molecular formula: $C_{10}H_{15}$
Molecular weight: 136.23
Rank of popularity: 170/502
Intended function: Fragrance, Solvent
Log P: 4.55
Allergenic potential: Weak sensitizer (max dose = 14.6 μg/cm^2/hr)

Linalool

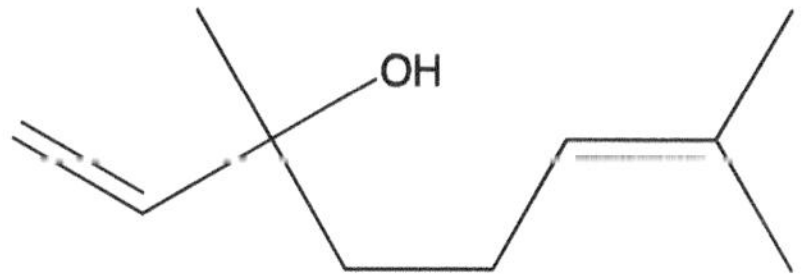

Other names: Linalyl alcohol
INCI: Linalool
CAS no: 78-70-6
Molecular formula: $C_{10}H_{18}O$
Molecular weight: 154.25
Rank of popularity: 142/502
Intended function: Fragrance
Log P: 2.80
Allergenic potential: Weak sensitizer (max dose = 72.9 μg/cm^2/hr)

Locust Bean Gum

Other names: Algaroba, Carob flour, Ceratonia
INCI: Ceratonia siliqua gum
CAS no: 9000-40-2
Rank of popularity: 421/502
Intended function: Adhesive, Binder, Emulsion stabilizer, Fragrance, Viscosity increasing agent

Lyral

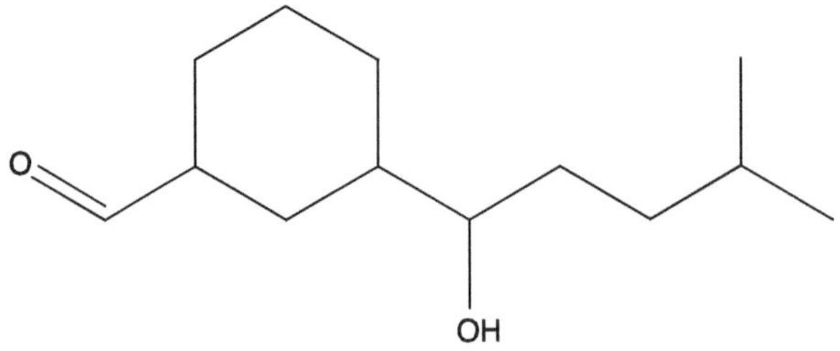

INCI: Hydroxyisohexyl 3-cyclohexane carboxaldehyde
CAS no: 31906-04-4
Molecular formula: $C_{13}H_{22}O_2$
Molecular weight: 210.31
Rank of popularity: 422/502
Intended function: Fragrance
Log P: 2.42
Allergenic potential: Weak sensitizer (max dose = 36.5 μg/cm^2/hr)

Madecassoside

INCI: Madecassoside
CAS no: 34540-22-2
Molecular formula: $C_{48}H_{78}O_{20}$
Molecular weight: 975.12
Rank of popularity: 423/502
Intended function: Antioxidant, Skin conditioning, Skin protectant
Log P: −1.34

Magnesium Aluminium Silicate

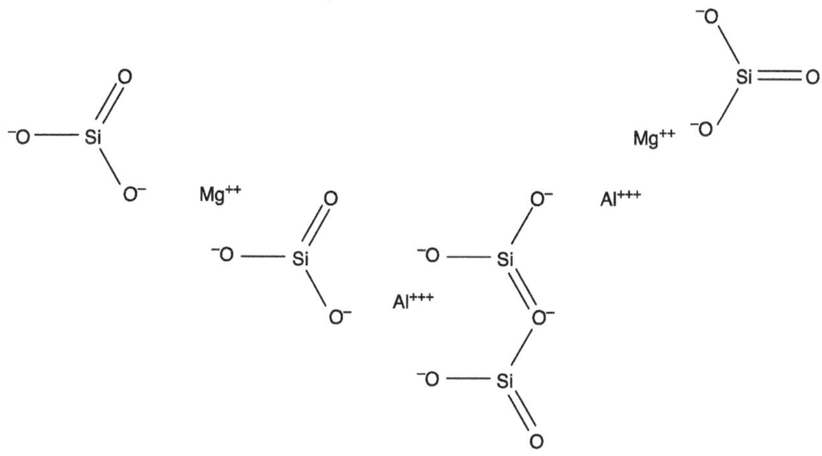

Other names: Aluminium magnesium silicon dioxide
INCI: Magnesium Aluminium Silicate
CAS no: 12199-37-0/ 12511-31-8
Rank of popularity: 40/502
Intended function: Absorbent, Anticaking agent, Opacifying agent, Slip modifier, Viscosity increasing agent

Magnesium Ascorbyl Phosphate

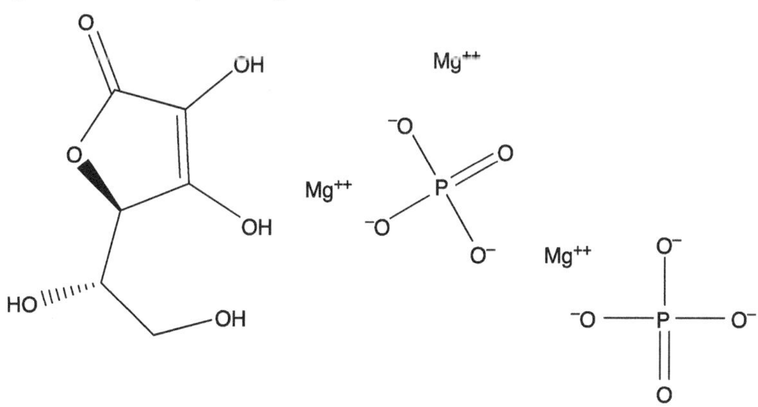

Other names: Magnesium L-ascorbyl-2-phosphate
INCI: Magnesium Ascorbyl Phosphate
CAS no: 113170-55-1/ 114040-31-2
Molecular formula: $C_6H_8O_9P$. 3/2Mg
Molecular weight: 272.30
Rank of popularity: 290/502
Intended function: Antioxidant

Magnesium Silicate Hydroxide

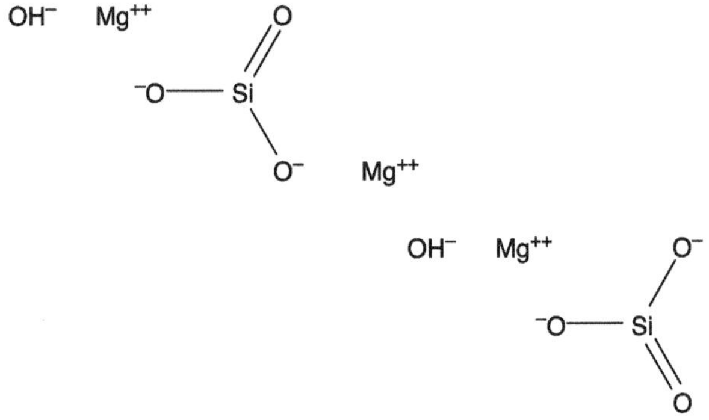

Other names: Cosmetic talc, French chalk
INCI: Talc
CAS no: 14807-96-6
Molecular formula: $H_2\ O_3$ Si. 3/4 Mg
Molecular weight: 96.32
Rank of popularity: 291/502
Intended function: Abrasive agent, Absorbent, Anticaking agent, Bulking agent, Opacifying agent, Skin protectant, Slip modifier
Carcinogenic potential: Category 2 (safe to use)

Magnesium Stearate

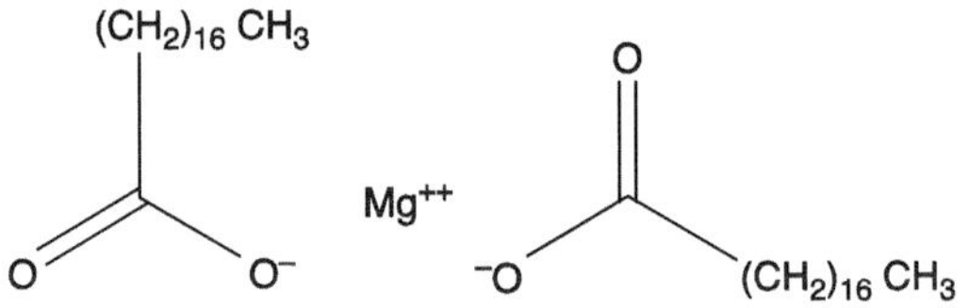

Other names: Magnesii stearas, Magnesium octadecanoate
INCI: Magnesium Stearate
CAS no: 557-04-0
Molecular formula: $C_{18}H_{36}O_2$. 1/2Mg
Molecular weight: 296.61
Rank of popularity: 213/502
Intended function: Anticaking agent, Bulking agent, Colourant, Skin conditioning, Viscosity increasing agent

Magnesium Sulphate

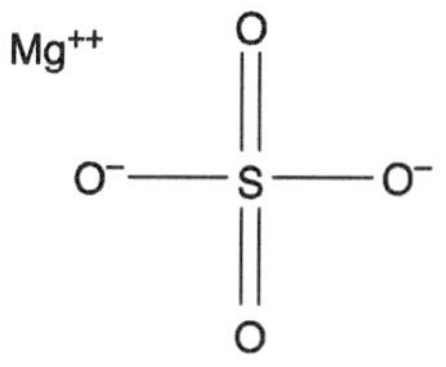

Other names: Anhydrous magnesium sulfate, Epsom salt, Magnesii sulfas
INCI: Magnesium sulfate
CAS no: 7487-88-9
Molecular formula: $H_2O_4S \cdot Mg$
Molecular weight: 122.39
Rank of popularity: 102/502
Intended function: Bulking agent

Mandelic Acid

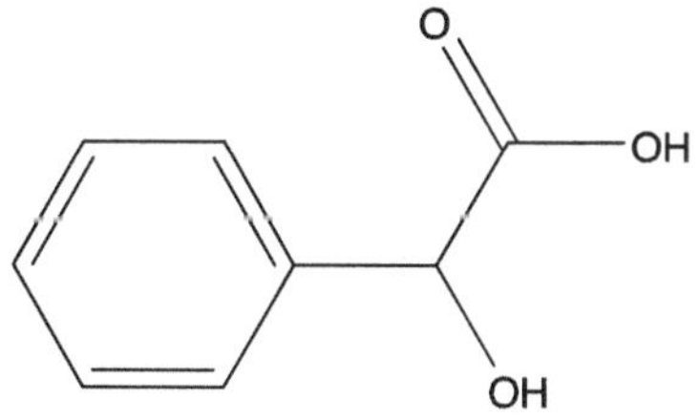

Other names: Almond acid, Amygdalic acid, Alpha-hydroxybenzeneacetic acid, 2-phenylglycolic acid
INCI: Mandelic Acid
CAS no: 90-64-2
Molecular formula: $C_8H_8O_3$
Molecular weight: 152.15
Rank of popularity: 424/502
Intended function: Cosmetic biocide
Log P: 0.55

Manganese Gluconate

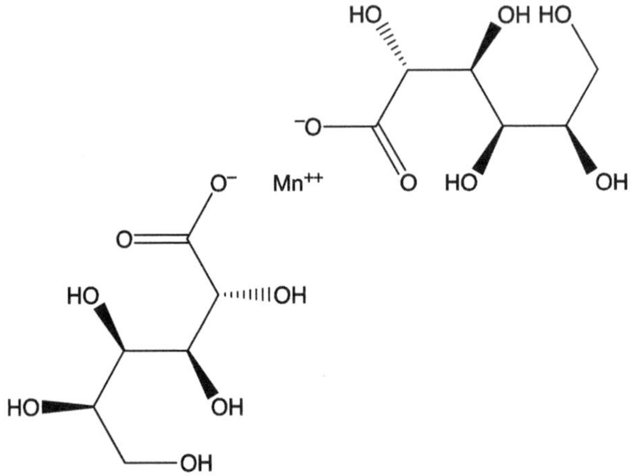

INCI: Manganese Gluconate
CAS no: 6485-39-8
Molecular formula: $C_{12}H_{24}O_{14}{\cdot}Mn$
Molecular weight: 447.24
Rank of popularity: 425/502
Intended function: Skin conditioning

Mannitol

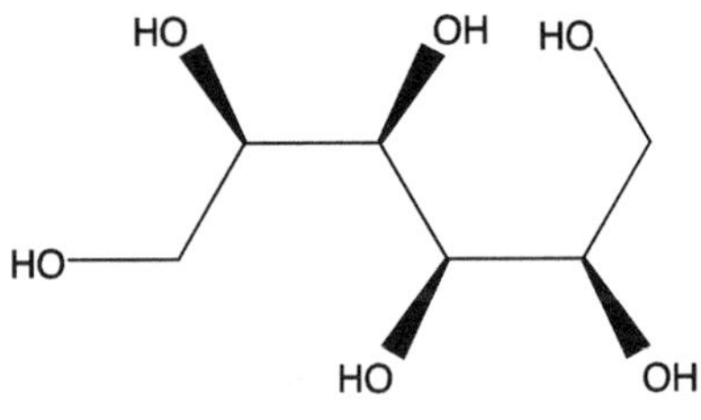

Other names: Manna sugar, D-mannitol, Mannitolum
INCI: Mannitol
CAS no: 69-65-8/ 87-78-5
Molecular formula: $C_6H_{14}O_6$
Molecular weight: 182.17
Rank of popularity: 292/502
Intended function: Binder, Flavouring agent, Humectant
Log P: –3.26

Menthyl Anthranilate

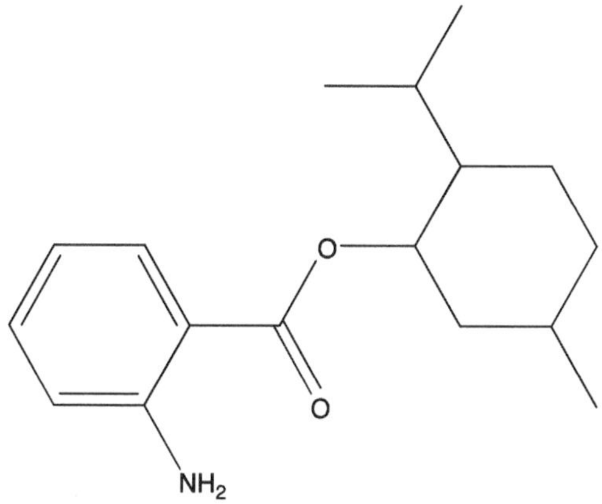

INCI: Menthyl Anthranilate
CAS no: 134-09-8
Molecular formula: $C_{17}H_{25}NO_2$
Molecular weight: 275.39
Rank of popularity: 426/502
Intended function: UV absorber
Log P: 6.09
Carcinogenic potential: Category 3 (use with precaution)
Allergenic potential: Weak sensitizer (max dose = 7.29 μg/cm²/hr)

Methyl Acetyl Ricinoleate

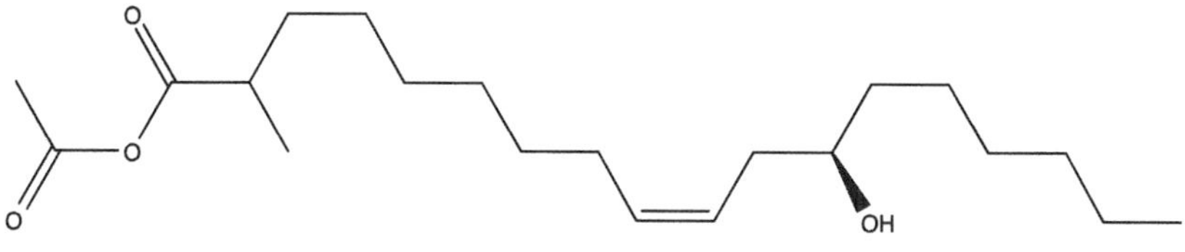

INCI: Methyl Acetyl Ricinoleate
CAS no: 140-03-4
Molecular formula: $C_{21}H_{38}O_4$
Molecular weight: 354.52
Rank of popularity: 214/502
Intended function: Emollient
Log P: 6.91

Methyl Dihydroxybenzoate

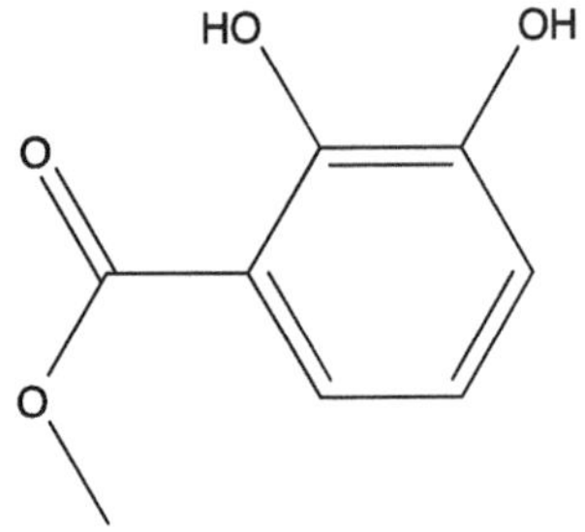

Other names: Methyl gentisate
INCI: Methyl Dihydroxybenzoate
CAS no: 2150-46-1
Molecular formula: $C_8H_8O_4$
Molecular weight: 168.15
Rank of popularity: 427/502
Intended function: Chelating agent
Log P: 1.78

Methyl Ether

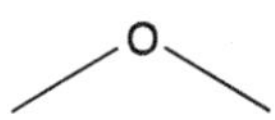

Other names: Dimethyl oxide, Methoxymethane, Oxybismethane
INCI: Dimethyl ether
CAS no: 115-10-6
Molecular formula: C_2H_6O
Molecular weight: 46.07
Rank of popularity: 428/502
Intended function: Propellant, Solvent, Viscosity decreasing agent
Log P: 0.02

Methyl Gluceth-20

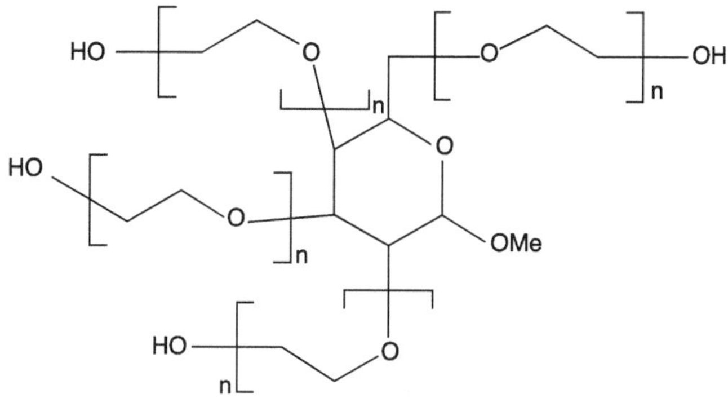

INCI: Methyl Gluceth-20
CAS no: 68239-42-9
Molecular formula: $(C_2H_4O)_n(C_2H_4O)_n(C_2H_4O)_nC_7H_{14}O_6$
Rank of popularity: 215/502
Intended function: Humectant

Methyl Glucose Sesquistearate

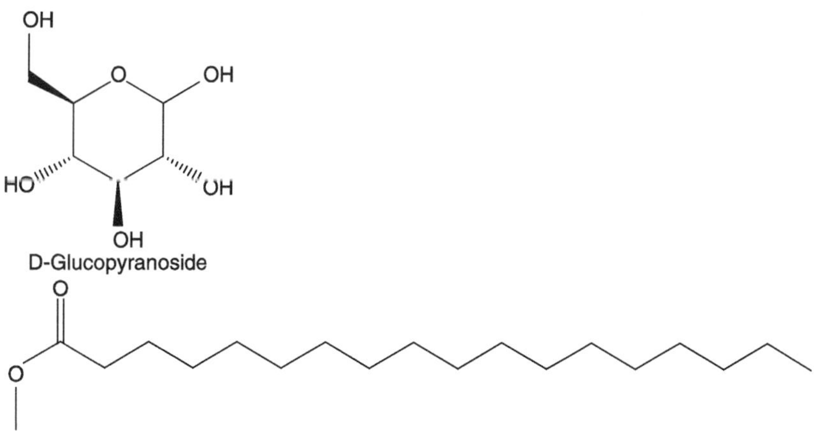

Other names: D-Glucopyranoside, methyl, octadecanoate (2:3)
INCI: Methyl Glucose Sesquistearate
CAS no: 68936-95-8
Molecular formula: C18H36O2 · 2/3 C7H14O6
Molecular weight: 413.93
Rank of popularity: 429/502
Intended function: Emollient
Note: Only individual components of the structure are shown.

Methyl Methacrylate Crosspolymer

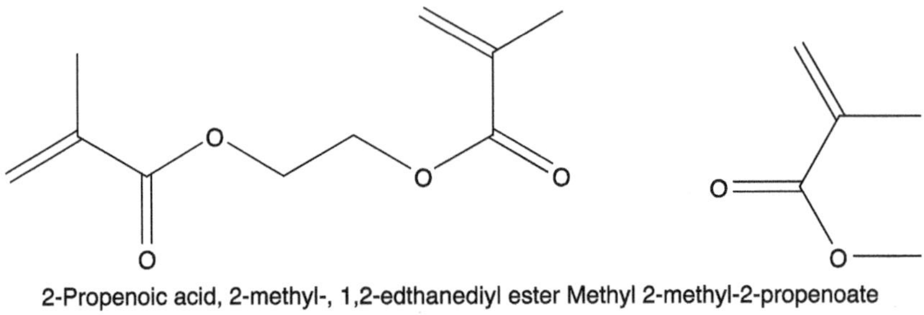

Other names: 2-Propenoic acid, 2-methyl-, 1,2-ethanediyl ester, polymer with methyl 2-methyl-2-propenoate
INCI: Methyl Methacrylate Crosspolymer
CAS no: 25777-71-3
Rank of popularity: 214/502
Intended function: Film former, Viscosity increasing agent
Allergenic potential: Weak sensitizer (max dose = 10.9 μg/cm^2/hr)

Methyl Stearate

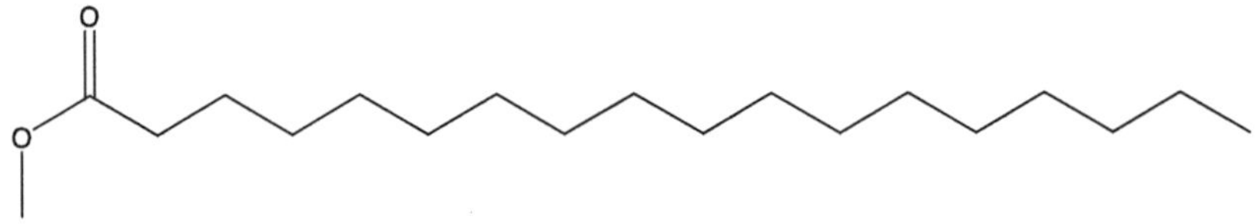

Other names: Methyl octadecanoate
INCI: Methyl Stearate
CAS no: 112-61-8
Molecular formula: $C_{19}H_{38}O_2$
Molecular weight: 298.50
Rank of popularity: 430/502
Intended function: Emollient, Fragrance
Log P: 8.43
Note: The structure does not represent the polymer. Only individual components are shown.

Methylchloroisothiazolinone

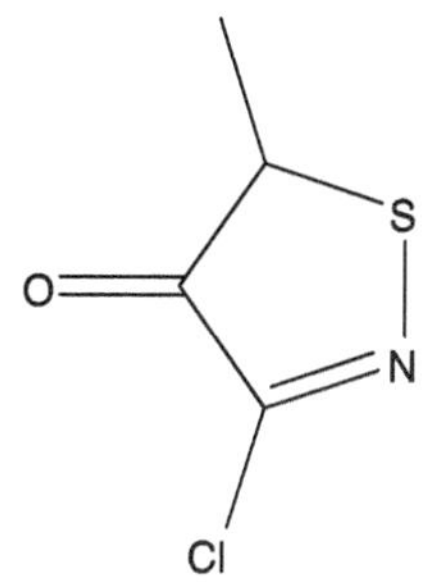

INCI: Methylchloroisothiazolinone
CAS no: 26172-55-4
Molecular formula: C_4H_4ClNOS
Molecular weight: 149.60
Rank of popularity: 103/502
Intended function: Preservative
Log P: 0.49
Allergenic potential: Moderate sensitizer (max dose = 0.0729 μg/cm²/hr)

Methyldibromo glutaronitrile

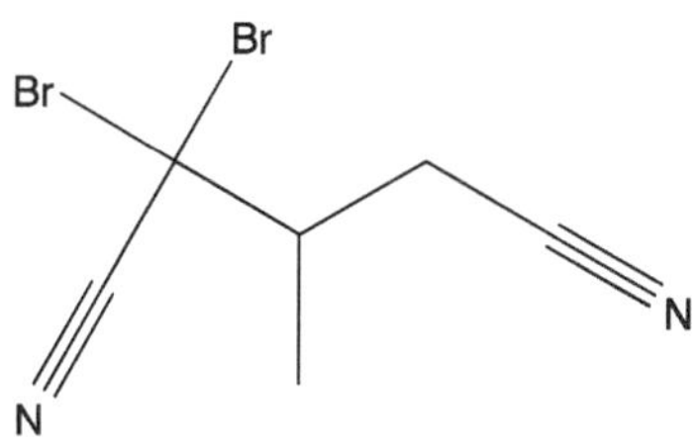

Other names: 1,2-dibromo-2,4-dicyanobutane
INCI: Methyldibromo glutaronitrile
CAS no: 35691-65-7
Molecular formula: $C_6H_6Br_2N_2$
Molecular weight: 265.93
Rank of popularity: 143/502
Intended function: Preservative
Log P: 1.52
Allergenic potential: Moderate sensitizer (max dose = 0.101 μg/cm²/hr)

Methylene Blue

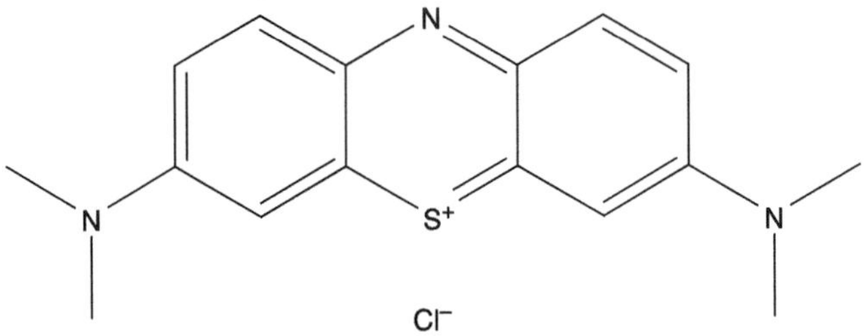

Other names: Cl52015 methylene blue, Solvent blue 8, basic blue 9, Tetramethylthionine chloride
INCI: Basic blue 9
CAS no: 61-73-4
Molecular formula: $C_{16}H_{18}N_3S$. Cl
Molecular weight: 319.85
Rank of popularity: 431/502
Intended function: Hair colourant
Carcinogenic potential: Category 3 (use with precaution)
Allergenic potential: Maximum dose not stated

Methylisothiazolinone

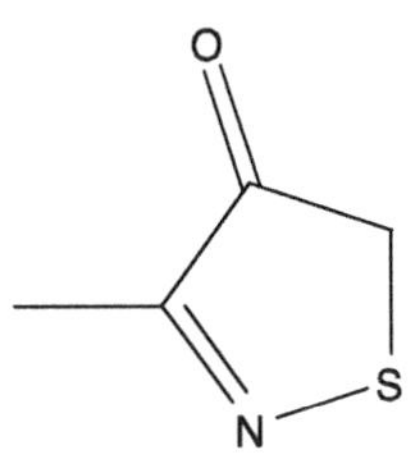

INCI: Methylisothiazolinone
CAS no: 2682-20-4
Molecular formula: C_4H_5NOS
Molecular weight: 115.15
Rank of popularity: 104/502
Intended function: Preservative
Log P: 0.12
Allergenic potential: moderate sensitizer (max dose = 0.00729 $\mu g/cm^2/hr$)

Methylparaben

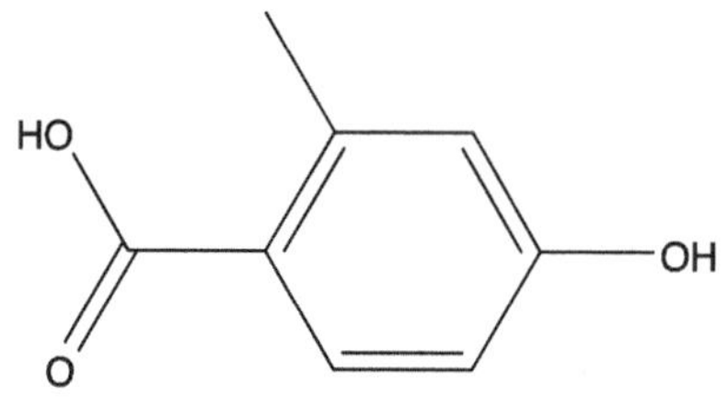

Other names: Methyl-4-hydroxybenzoate, Methyl parahydroxybenzoate, p-carbomethoxyphenol
INCI: Methylparaben
CAS no: 99-76-3
Molecular formula: $C_8H_8O_3$
Molecular weight: 152.15
Rank of popularity: 2/502
Intended function: Fragrance, Preservative
Log P: 1.88
Carcinogenic potential: Category 3 (use with precaution)
Allergenic potential: Weak sensitizer (max dose = 21.9 $\mu g/cm^2/hr$)

Mica

Other names: Cl77019, Golden mica, Muscovite mica, Pigment white 20, Sericite GMS-C, and GMS-2C, and MK-A, and MK-B
INCI: Mica
CAS no: 12001-26-2
Rank of popularity: 216/502
Intended function: Colourant, Opacifying agent

Microcrystalline Wax

Other names: Cera microcristallina, Hydrocarbon waxes microcyst, Petroleum wax microcrystalline
INCI: Microcrystalline Wax
CAS no: 63231-60-7/ 64742-42-3
Rank of popularity: 171/502
Intended function: Binder, Bulking agent, Emulsion stabilizer, Viscosity increasing agent
Allergenic potential: Maximum dose not stated

Myreth-3 Myristate

Other names: PEG-3 myristyl ether myristate, Polyethylene glycol (3) myristyl ether myristate
INCI: Myreth-3 Myristate
CAS no: 59686-68-9
Molecular formula: $C_{34}H_{68}O_5$
Molecular weight: 556
Rank of popularity: 432/502
Intended function: Emollient

Myristic Acid

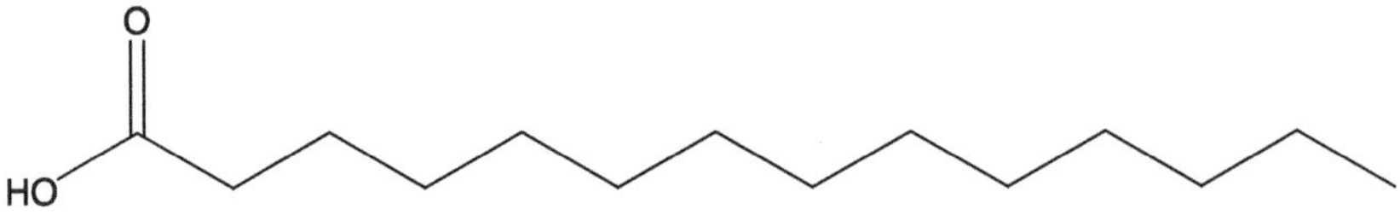

Other names: Tetradecanoic acid
INCI: Myristic Acid
CAS no: 544-63-8
Molecular formula: $C_{14}H_{28}O2$
Molecular weight: 228.37
Rank of popularity: 89/502
Intended function: Cleansing agent, Fragrance, Opacifying agent
Log P: 5.79
Carcinogenic potential: Category 1 (use within limit on body=26.0 %w/w; face >100 %w/w; hands >100 %w/w)

Myristyl Alcohol

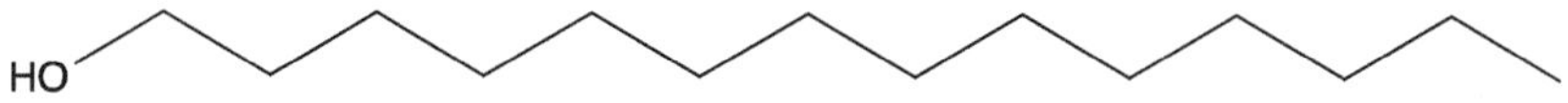

Other names: 1-hydroxytetradecane, Tetradecanol, Tetradecyl alcohol
INCI: Myristyl Alcohol
CAS no: 112-72-1
Molecular formula: $C_{14}H_{30}O$
Molecular weight: 214.39
Rank of popularity: 293/502
Intended function: Emollient, Emulsion stabilizer, Foam booster, Fragrance, Viscosity increasing agent
Log P: 5.93

Myristyl Lactate

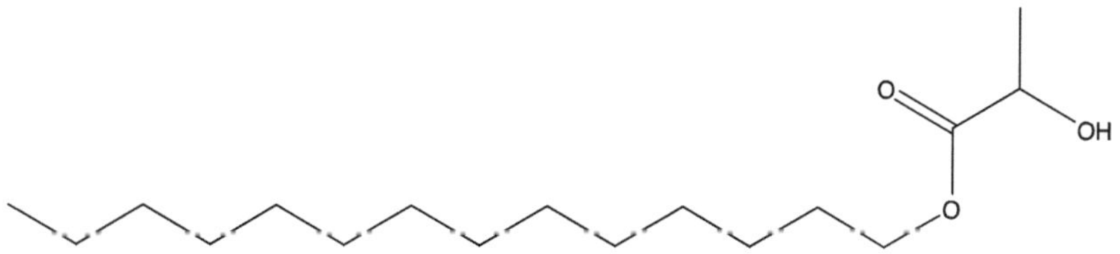

Other names: Tetradecyl lactate
INCI: Myristyl Lactate
CAS no: 1323-03-1
Molecular formula: $C_{17}H_{34}O_3$
Molecular weight: 286.45
Rank of popularity: 172/502
Intended function: Emollient
Log P: 6.08

Myristyl Myristate

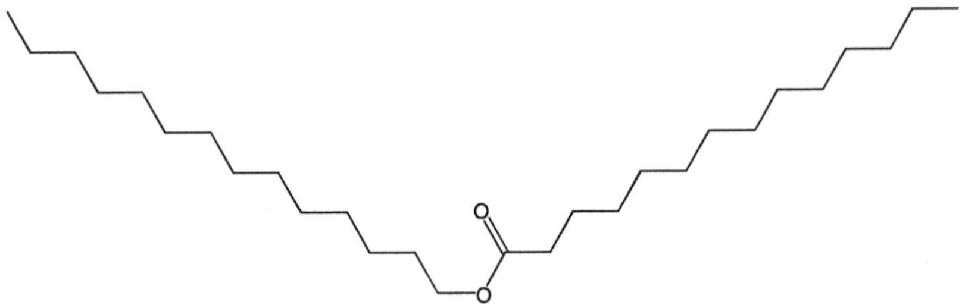

Other names: Tetradecyl tetradecanoate
INCI: Myristyl Myristate
CAS no: 3234-85-3
Molecular formula: $C_{28}H_{56}O_2$
Molecular weight: 424.74
Rank of popularity: 113/502
Intended function: Occlusive agent
Log P: 13.01
Allergenic potential: Weak sensitizer (max dose = 58.3 μg/cm²/hr)

N-acetyl Ethanolamine

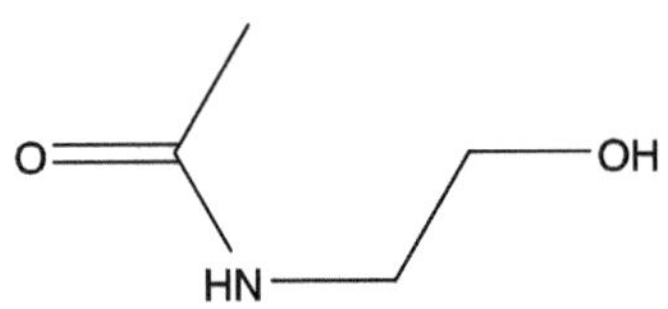

Other names: N-acetyl-2-aminoethanol, Acetylcolamine
INCI: Acetamide MEA
CAS no: 142-26-7
Molecular formula: $C_4H_9NO_2$
Molecular weight: 103.12
Rank of popularity: 294/502
Intended function: Foam booster, Hair conditioning, Humectant, Viscosity increasing agent
Log P: −1.3

Niacinamide (Vit B3)

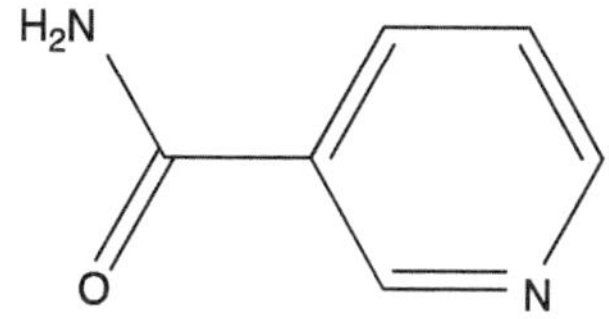

Other names: Nicotinamide vitamin B3
INCI: Niacinamide
CAS no: 98-92-0
Molecular formula: $C_6H_6N_2O$
Molecular weight: 122.12
Rank of popularity: 106/502
Intended function: Hair conditioning, Skin conditioning
Log P: –0.37

Nitrilotriacetic Acid

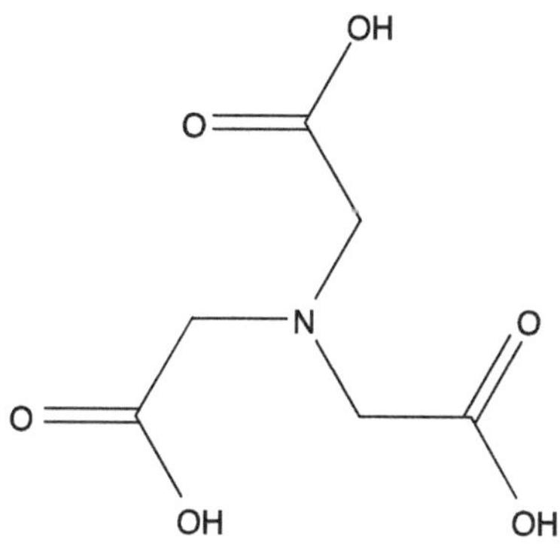

Other names: N,N-Bis(carboxymethyl)glycine, NTA, Tris(carboxymethyl) amine
INCI: Nitrilotriacetic Acid
CAS no: 139-13-9
Molecular formula: $N(CH_2COOH)_3$
Molecular weight: 191.14
Rank of popularity: 433/502
Intended function: Chelating agent
Log P: 0.03
Carcinogenic potential: Category 2 (safe to use)

Nylon-12

Other names: Dodecalactam polymer, Laurolactum polymer, Polydodecanamide, Polyauramide
INCI: Nylon-12
CAS no: 25038-74-8
Molecular formula: $(C_{12}H_{23}NO)_n$
Rank of popularity: 144/502
Intended function: Bulking agent, Opacifying agent

Octadecene/ MA Copolymer

INCI: Octadecene/ MA Copolymer
CAS no: 25266-02-8
Molecular formula: $(C_{18}H_{36} .C_4H_2O_3)_n$
Rank of popularity: 173/502
Intended function: Emulsion stabilizer, Film former, Viscosity increasing agent

Octisalate

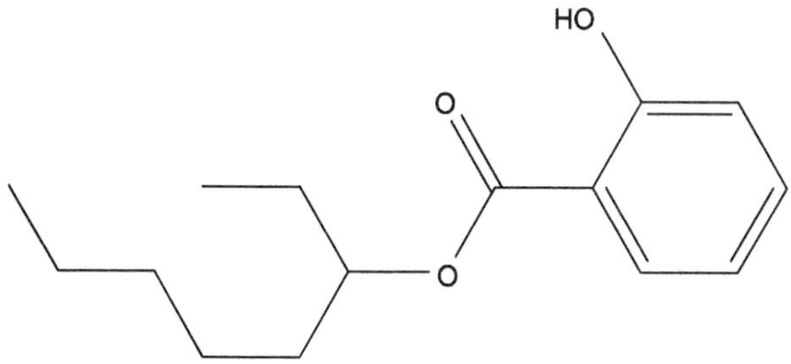

Other names: Ethylhexyl salicylate, Octyl salicylate
INCI: Ethylhexyl salicylate
CAS no: 118-60-5
Molecular formula: $C_{15}H_{22}O_3$
Molecular weight: 250.33
Rank of popularity: 55/502
Intended function: Fragrance, UV absorber, UV filter
Log P: 5.93
Allergenic potential: Weak sensitizer (max dose = 36.5 μg/cm^2/hr)

Octocrylene

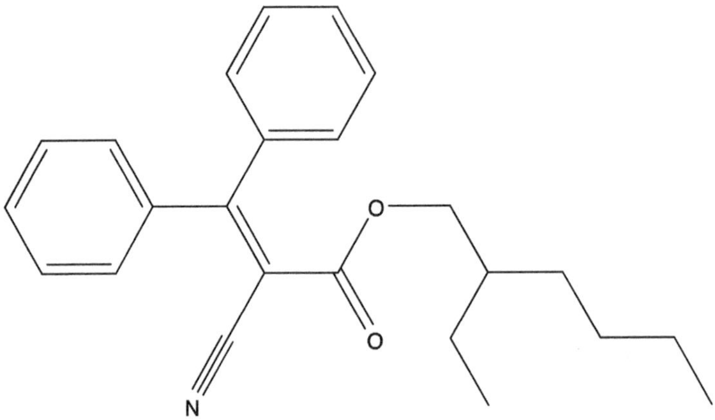

Other names: UV absorber-3
INCI: Octocrylene
CAS no: 6197-30-4
Molecular formula: $C_{24}H_{27}NO_2$
Molecular weight: 361.48
Rank of popularity: 37/502
Intended function: UV absorber, UV filter
Log P: 6.89
Carcinogenic potential: Category 2 (safe to use)
Allergenic potential: Weak sensitizer (max dose = 72.9 μg/cm²/hr)

Octoxynol-11

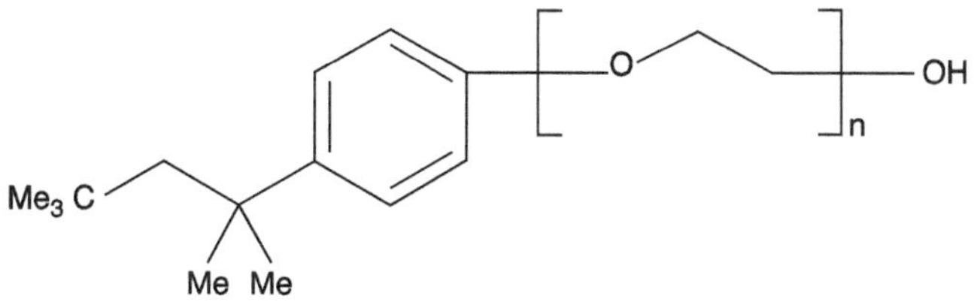

Other names: Octoxinol, PEG-11 octyl phenyl ether, Polyethylene glycol (11) octyl ether
INCI: Octoxynol-11
CAS no: 9002-93-1/ 9004-87-9/ 9036-19-5/ 108437-62-3
Molecular formula: $C_{36}H_{66}O_{12}$
Molecular weight: 690.90
Rank of popularity: 434/502
Intended function: Emulsifying agent

Octyl Dimethyl PABA

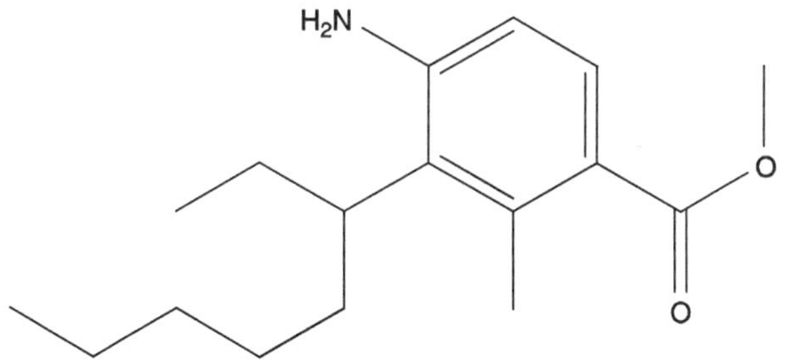

Other names: Octyl Dimethyl PABA, Ethylhexyl dimethyl para amino benzoic acid
INCI: Ethylhexyl dimethyl PABA
CAS no: 21245-02-3/ 58817-05-3
Molecular formula: $C_{17}H_{27}NO_2$
Molecular weight: 277.40
Rank of popularity: 295/502
Intended function: UV absorber, UV filter
Log P: 5.41
Carcinogenic potential: Category 2 (safe to use)
Allergenic potential: Weak sensitizer (max dose = 36.5 μg/cm²/hr)

Octyl Hydroxystearate

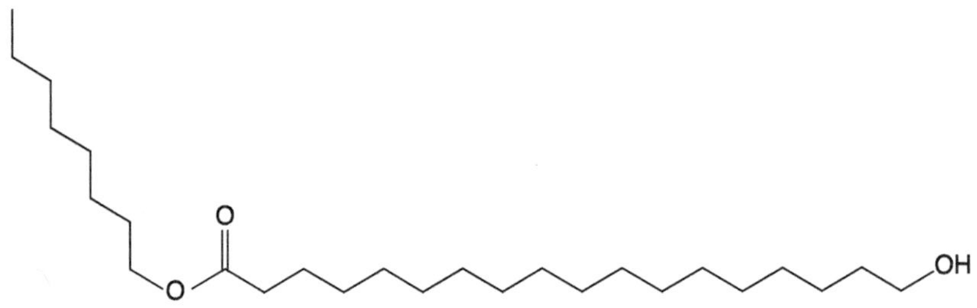

Other names: Ethylhexyl hydroxystearate
INCI: Ethylhexyl hydroxystearate
CAS no: 29383-26-4/ 29710-25-6
Molecular formula: $C_{26}H_{52}O_3$
Molecular weight: 412.68
Rank of popularity: 218/502
Intended function: Emollient

Octyl Methoxycinnamate

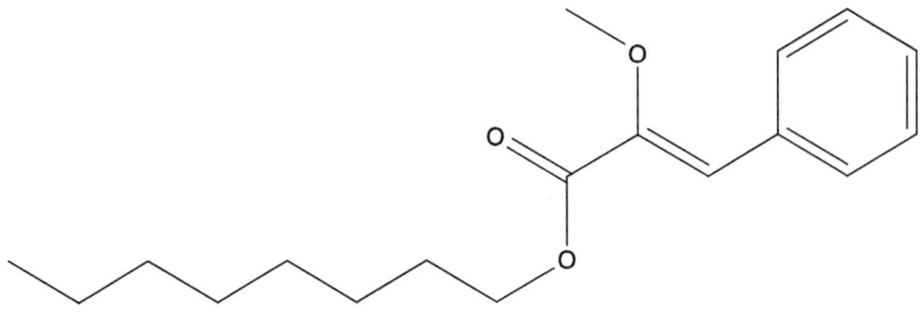

Other names: Octinoxate, Octyl methoxycinnamate, Ethylhexyl methoxycinnamate
INCI: Ethylhexyl methoxycinnamate
CAS no: 5466-77-3
Molecular formula: $C_{18}H_{26}O_3$
Molecular weight: 176.17
Rank of popularity: 15/502
Intended function: UV absorber, UV filter
Log P: 1.32
Allergenic potential: Weak sensitizer (max dose = 14.6 μg/cm²/hr)

Octyldodecanol

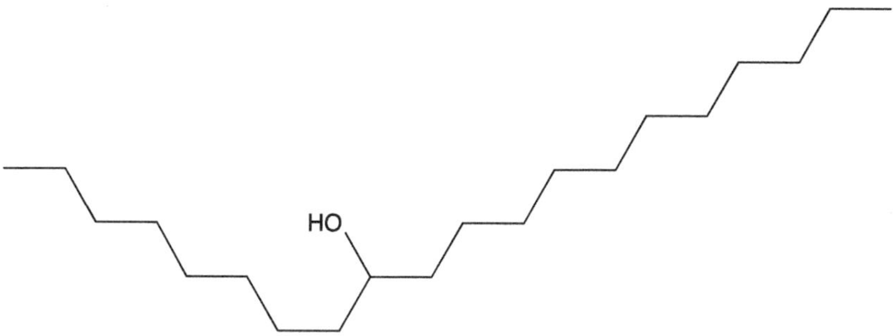

Other names: 2-octyldodecanol, Octyl dodecanolum
INCI: Octyldodecanol
CAS no: 5333-42-6
Molecular formula: $C_{20}H_{42}O$
Molecular weight: 298.55
Rank of popularity: 145/502
Intended function: Emollient, Emulsion stabilizer, Fragrance
Log P: 8.83
Allergenic potential: Very weak sensitizer (max dose = 219 μg/cm^2/hr)

Octyldodecyl Myristate

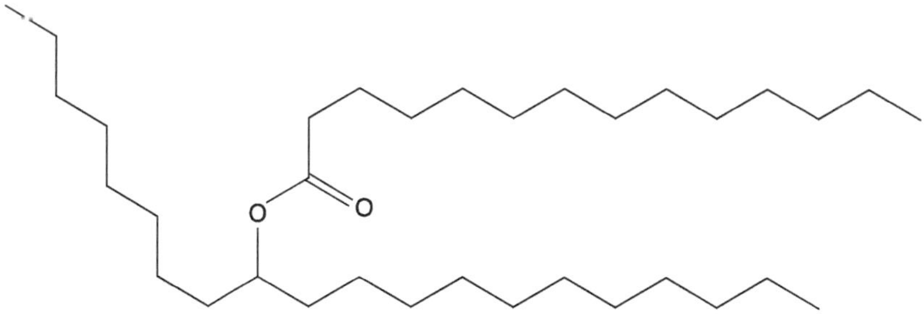

Other names: 2-octyldodecyl myristate, Tetradecanoic acid octyldodecyl ester
INCI: Octyldodecyl Myristate
CAS no: 22766-83-2/ 83826-43-1
Molecular formula: $C_{34}H_{68}O_2$
Molecular weight: 508.90
Rank of popularity: 435/502
Intended function: Occlusive agent
Log P: 15.91

Octyldodecyl Neopentanoate

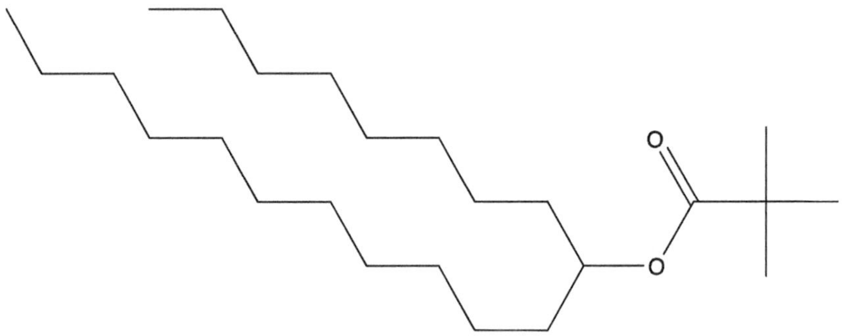

INCI: Octyldodecyl Neopentanoate
CAS no: 158567-66-9
Molecular formula: $C_{25}H_{50}O_2$
Molecular weight: 382.66
Rank of popularity: 122/502
Intended function: Emollient
Log P: 11.07

O-Cymen-5-ol

Other names: 4-Isopropyl-3-methylphenol
INCI: O-Cymen-5-ol
CAS no: 3228-02-2
Molecular formula: $(CH_3)_2CHC_6H_3(CH_3)OH$
Molecular weight: 150.22
Rank of popularity: 219/502
Intended function: Cosmetic biocide, Fragrance, Preservative
Log P: 3.28

Oleth-3

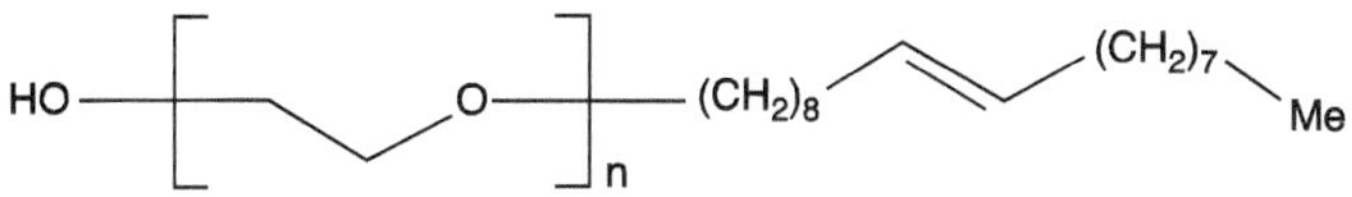

Other names: PEG-3 oleyl ether, Polyethylene glycol (3) oleyl ether, Triethylene glycol oleyl ether
INCI: Oleth-3
CAS no: 5274-66-8/ 9004-98-2(generic)/ 96459-08-4
Molecular formula: $C_{24}H_{48}O_4$
Molecular weight: 400.64
Rank of popularity: 436/502
Intended function: Emulsifying agent, Fragrance
Log P: 7.09

Oxybenzone

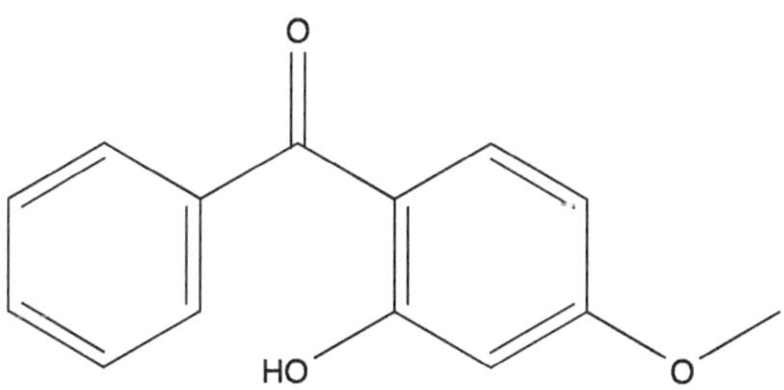

Other names: Benzophenone-3
INCI: Benzophenone-3
CAS no: 131-57-7
Molecular formula: $C_{14}H_{12}O_3$
Molecular weight: 228.24
Rank of popularity: 32/502
Intended function: UV absorber, UV filter
Log P: 4.00
Carcinogenic potential: Category 3 (use with precaution)
Allergenic potential: Weak sensitizer (max dose = 21.9 µg/cm^2/hr)

Oxynex ST

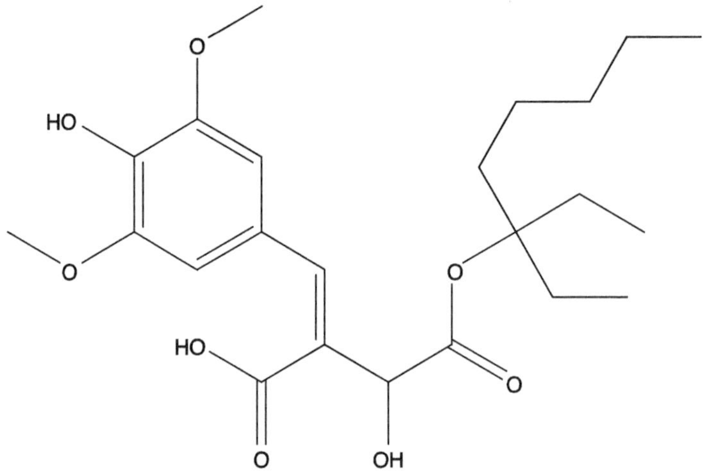

Other names: Diethylhexyl syringylidenemaloate
INCI: Diethylhexyl syringylidenemaloate
CAS no: 444811-29-4
Molecular formula: $C_{28}H_{44}O_7$
Molecular weight: 492.64
Rank of popularity: 437/502
Intended function: Skin protectant
Log P: 8.78

Ozokerite

Other names: Earth wax, Fossil wax, Mineral wax, Ozocerite
INCI: Ozokerite
CAS no: 12198-93-5
Rank of popularity: 296/502
Intended function: Binder, Emulsion stabilizer, Viscosity increasing agent

Palmitic Acid

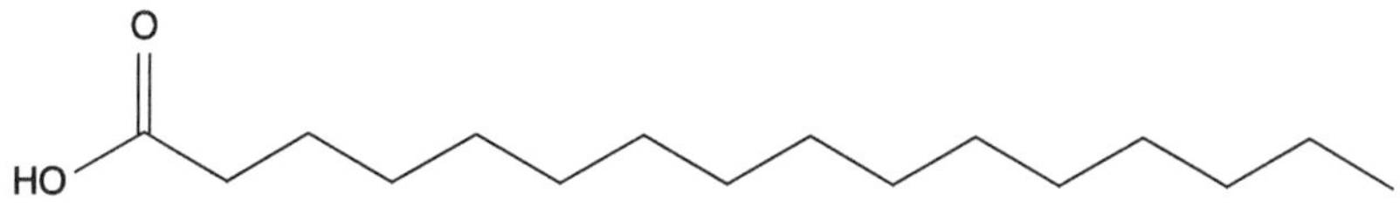

Other names: Cetylic acid, n-hexadecanoic acid
INCI: Palmitic Acid
CAS no: 57-10-3
Molecular formula: $C_{16}H_{32}O_2$
Molecular weight: 256.42
Rank of popularity: 83/502
Intended function: Cleansing agent, Emulsifying agent, Fragrance, Opacifying agent
Log P: 6.81
Allergenic potential: Maximum dose not stated

Panthenol (Vit B5)

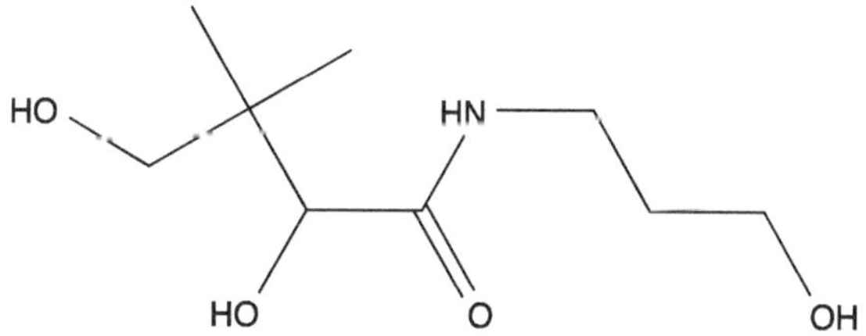

Other names: Dexpanthenol, Pantothenol, Pantothenyl alcohol, Provitamin B5
INCI: Panthenol
CAS no: 81-13-0 (D-form) / 16485-10-2
Molecular formula: $C_9H_{19}NO_4$
Molecular weight: 205.25
Rank of popularity: 18/502
Intended function: Hair conditioning, Skin conditioning
Log P: –0.99
Allergenic potential: Weak sensitizer (max dose = 3.65 $\mu g/cm^2/hr$)

Panthenyl Triacetate

INCI: Panthenyl Triacetate
CAS no: 94089-18-6/ 98133-47-2
Molecular formula: $C_{15}H_{25}NO_7$
Molecular weight: 331.36
Rank of popularity: 438/502
Intended function: Hair conditioning
Log P: 0.84

Paraffin

Other names: High melting point paraffin, Low melting point paraffin, Paraffin wax, Petroleum wax
INCI: Paraffin
CAS no: 8002-74-2
Rank of popularity: 174/502
Intended function: Fragrance, Occlusive agent, Viscosity increasing agent
Carcinogenic potential: Category 2 (safe to use)

PCA (pyrrolidonecarboxylic acid)

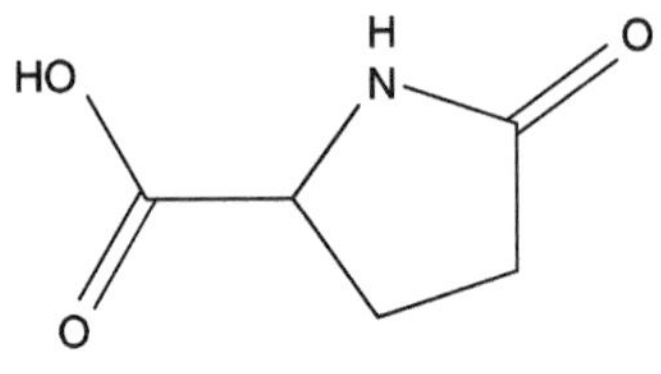

Other names: Glutimic acid, Glutiminic acid, Pidolic acid, L-pyroglutamic acid
INCI: PCA
CAS no: 98-79-3/149-87-1(dl-alpha)
Molecular formula: $C_5H_7NO_3$
Molecular weight: 129.11
Rank of popularity: 439/502
Intended function: Humectant
Log P: –1.35
Allergenic potential: Maximum dose not stated

PEG 5 Glyceryl Stearate

Other names: Polyethylene glycol (5) glyceryl monostearate
INCI: PEG-5 Glyceryl Stearate
Molecular formula: $C_{31}H_{62}O_9$
Molecular weight: 578.81
Rank of popularity: 440/502
Intended function: Emulsifying agent

PEG/PPG-18/18 Dimethicone

INCI: PEG/PPG-18/18 Dimethicone
Rank of popularity: 441/502
Intended function: Emulsifying agent

PEG/PPG-20/6 dimethicone

INCI: PEG/PPG-20/6 dimethicone
Rank of popularity: 442/502
Intended function: Emulsifying agent

PEG-100

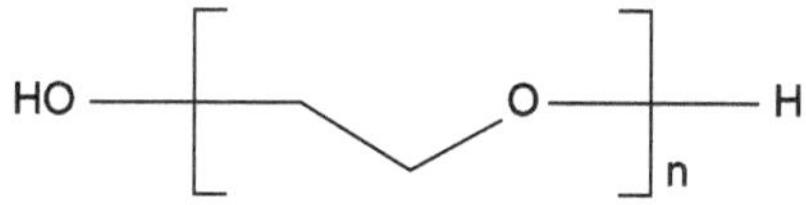

Other names: Macrogol, Polyethylene (1000)
INCI: PEG-100
CAS no: 25322-68-3
Molecular formula: $(C_2H_4O)_n\ H_2O$
Rank of popularity: 443/502
Intended function: Binder, Humectant, Solvent

PEG-100 Stearate

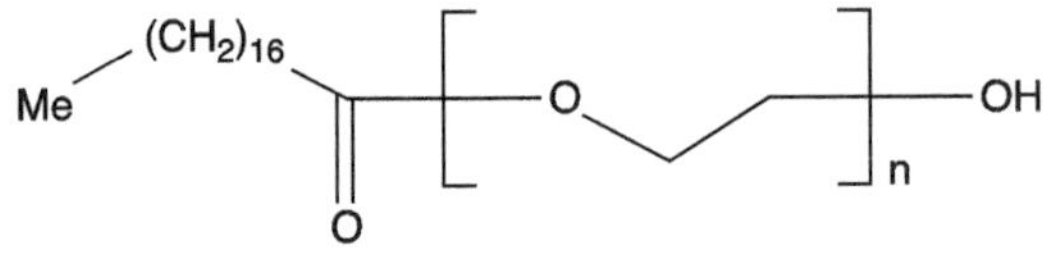

Other names: Polyethylene glycol (100) monostearate
INCI: PEG-100 Stearate
CAS no: 9004-99-3
Molecular formula: $(C_2H_4O)_n\ C_{18}H_{36}O_2$
Rank of popularity: 19/502
Intended function: Cleansing agent

PEG-12

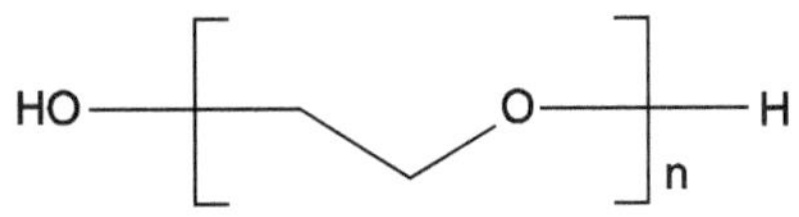

Other names: Dodecaethylene glycol, Polyethylene glycol 600
INCI: PEG-12
CAS no: 6790-09-6/ 25322-68-3
Molecular formula: $C_{24}H_{50}O_{13}$
Molecular weight: 546.64
Rank of popularity: 220/502
Intended function: Humectant, Solvent

PEG-15 Stearyl Ether

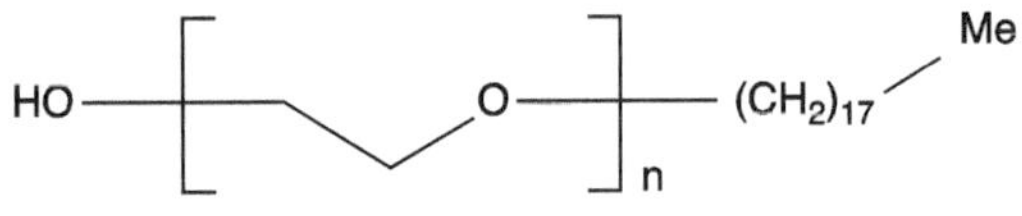

Other names: PEG-15 stearyl ether, Polyethylene glycol (15) stearyl ether
INCI: Steareth-15
CAS no: 9005-00-9 (generic)
Molecular formula: $(C_2H_4O)_n\ C_{18}H_{38}O$
Rank of popularity: 444/502
Intended function: Cleansing agent, Emulsifying agent

PEG-150 Distearate

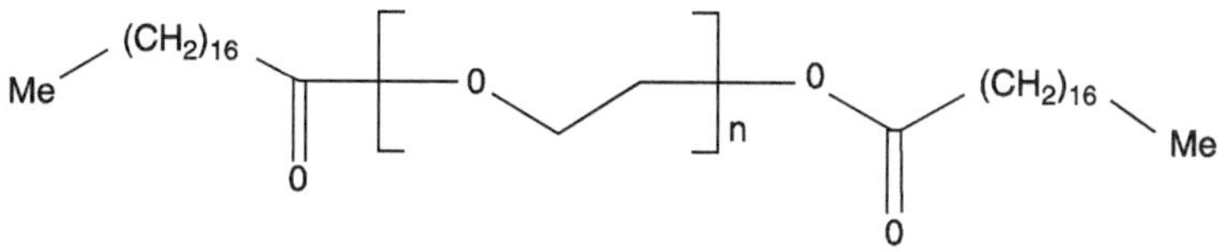

Other names: Polyethylene glycol 6000 distearate
INCI: PEG-150 Distearate
CAS no: 9005-08-7
Molecular formula: $(C_2H_4O)_n\ C_{36}H_{70}O_3$
Rank of popularity: 445/502
Intended function: Cleansing agent, Solubilizing agent

PEG-20

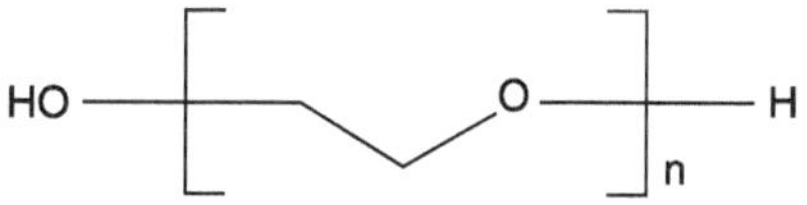

Other names: Macrogol, Polyethylene glycol 1000
INCI: PEG 20
CAS no: 25322-68-3(generic)
Molecular formula: $(C_2H_4O)_n\ H_2O$
Rank of popularity: 297/502
Intended function: Humectant, Solvent

PEG-20 Esters

Rank of popularity: 298/502

PEG-20 Methyl Glucose Sesquistearate

Other names: PEG-20 methyl glucoside sesquistearate, Polyethylene glycol 1000 methyl glucose sesquistearate
INCI: PEG-20 Methyl Glucose Sesquistearate
Rank of popularity: 446/502
Intended function: Emollient, Emulsifying agent

PEG-20 Stearate

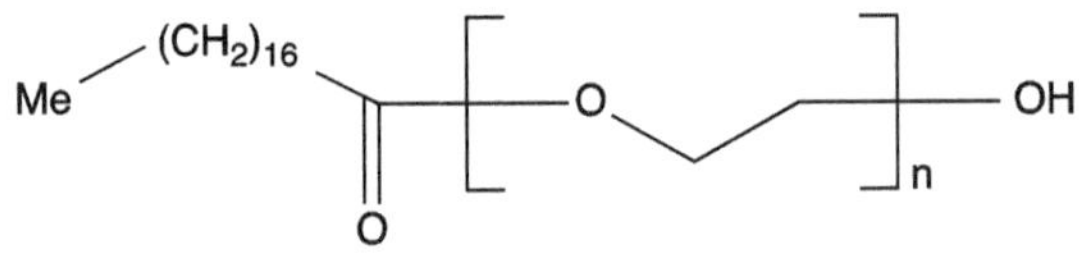

Other names: Polyethylene glycol 1000 monostearate
INCI: PEG-20 Stearate
CAS no: 9004-99-3
Molecular formula: $(C_2H_4O)_n\ C_{18}H_{36}O_2$
Rank of popularity: 175/502
Intended function: Cleansing agent, Emulsifying agent, Solubilizing agent

PEG-22/Dodecyl Glycol Copolymer

INCI: PEG-22/Dodecyl Glycol Copolymer
CAS no: 78336-31-9
Rank of popularity: 299/502
Intended function: Emulsion stabilizer, Emollient
Allergenic potential: Weak sensitizer (max dose = 14.6 μg/cm^2/hr)

PEG-30 Dipolyhydroxystearate

Other names: Polyethylene glycol (30) dipolyhydroxystearate
INCI: PEG-30 Dipolyhydroxystearate
Rank of popularity: 300/502
Intended function: Emulsifying agent

PEG-32

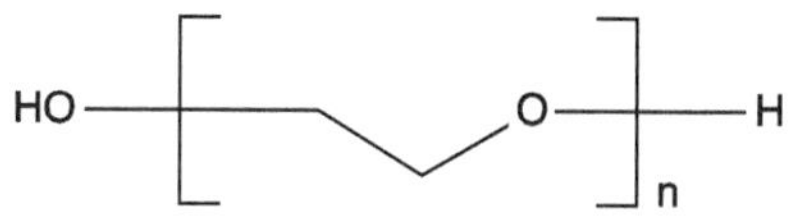

Other names: Macrogol, Polyethylene glycol 1540
INCI: PEG-32
CAS no: 25322-68-3
Molecular formula: $(C_2H_4O)_n\ H_2O$
Rank of popularity: 447/502
Intended function: Binder, Humectant, Solvent

PEG-4

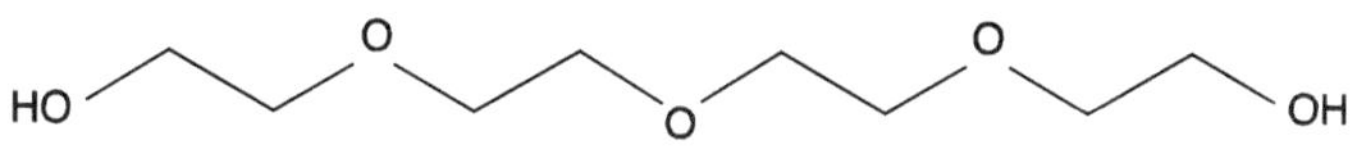

Other names: Polyethylene glycol 200, Tetraethylene glycol
INCI: PEG-4
CAS no: 112-60-7/ 25322-68-3
Molecular formula: $C_8H_{18}O_5$
Molecular weight: 194.23
Rank of popularity: 221/502
Intended function: Humectant, Solvent
Log P: –1.88
Allergenic potential: Maximum dose not stated

PEG-4 Dilaurate

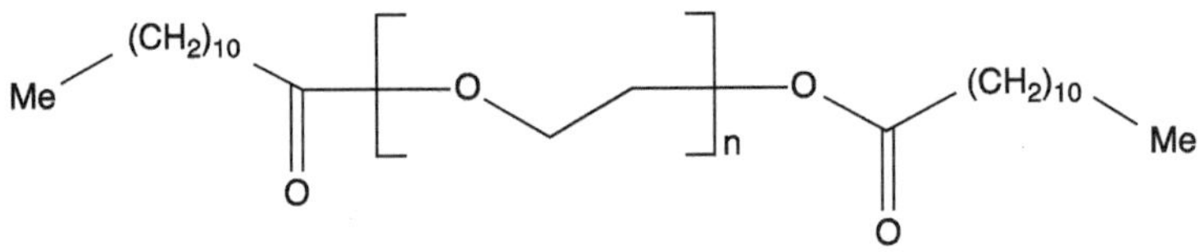

Other names: Polyethylene glycol 200 dilaurate
INCI: PEG-4 Dilaurate
CAS no: 9005-02-1
Molecular formula: $C_{32}H_{62}O_7$
Molecular weight: 558.83
Rank of popularity: 448/502
Intended function: Cleansing agent, Emulsifying agent
Allergenic potential: Maximum dose not state

PEG-4 Laurate

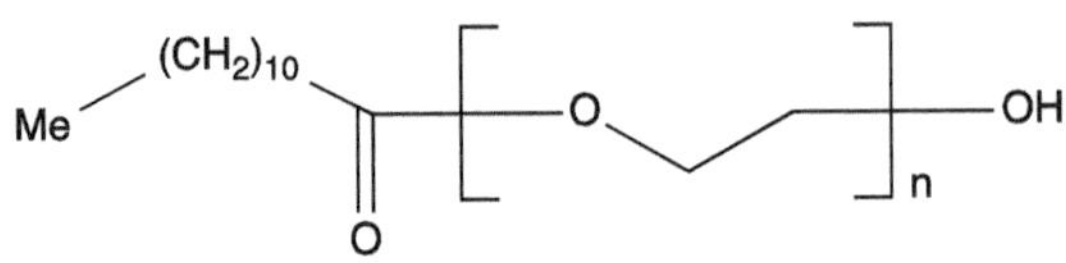

Other names: Polyethylene glycol 200 monolaurate, Tetraethylene glycol laurate
INCI: PEG-4 Laurate
CAS no: 9004-81-3
Molecular formula: $C_{20}H_{40}O_6$
Molecular weight: 376.52
Rank of popularity: 301/502
Intended function: Cleansing agent, Emulsifying agent

PEG-40 Stearate

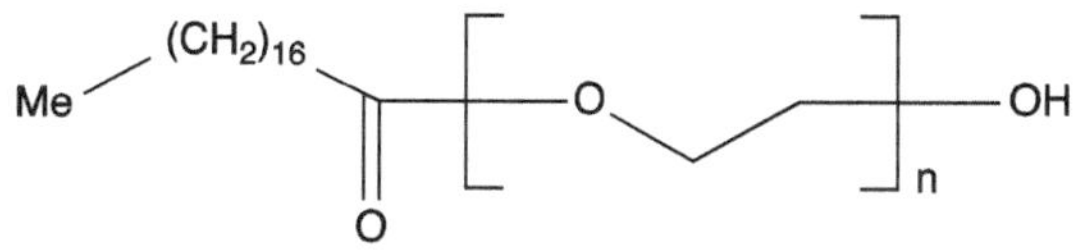

Other names: Macrogol stearate 2000, Polyethylene glycol 2000 monostearate polyoxyl 40 stearate, Stearethate 40
INCI: PEG-40 Stearate
CAS no: 9004-99-3
Molecular formula: $(C_2H_4O)_n$ $C_{18}H_{36}O_2$
Rank of popularity: 105/502
Intended function: Cleansing agent, Solubilizing agent

PEG-6

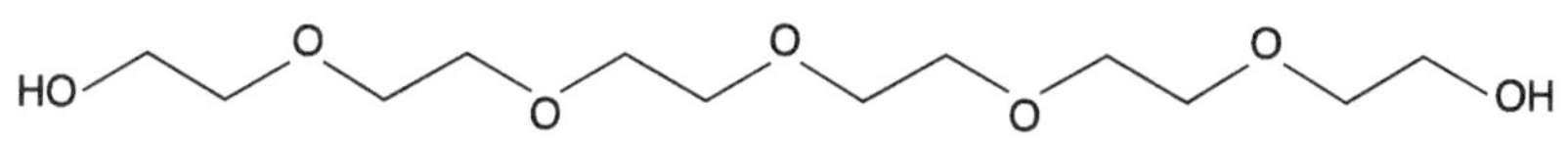

Other names: Hexaethylene glycol, Polyethylene glycol 300
INCI: PEG-6
CAS no. 2615-15-8/25332-68-3(generic)
Molecular formula: $C_{12}H_{26}O_7$
Molecular weight: 282.33
Rank of popularity: 449/502
Intended function: Humectant, Solvent
Log P: –2.35
Allergenic potential: Maximum dose not stated

PEG-6 Stearate

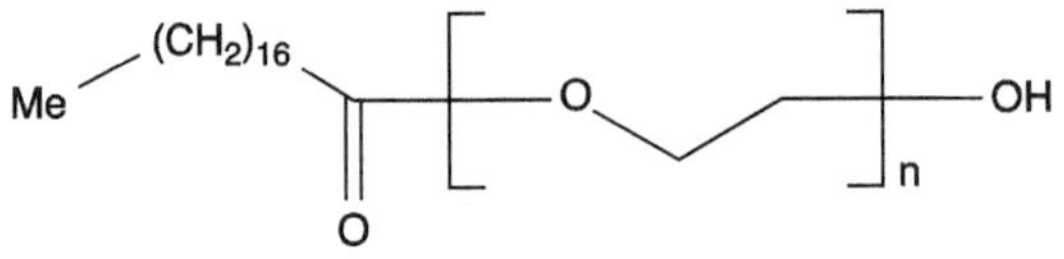

Other names: Polyethylene glycol 300 monostearate
INCI: PEG-6 Stearate
CAS no: 9004-99-3/ 10108-28-8
Molecular formula: $C_{30}H_{60}O_8$
Molecular weight: 548.79
Rank of popularity: 450/502
Intended function: Cleansing agent, Emulsifying agent
Log P: 6.62

PEG-7 Glyceryl Cocoate

Other names: Macrogoli 7 glyceroli cococas, Polyethylene glycol (7) glyceryl monococoate
INCI: PEG-7 Glyceryl Cocoate
CAS no: 66105-29-1/ 68201-46-7
Rank of popularity: 146/502
Intended function: Emollient, Emulsifying agent

PEG-8

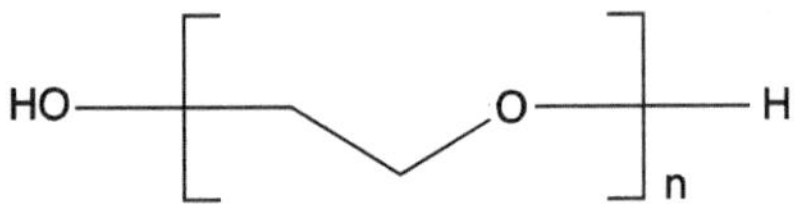

Other names: Octaethylene glycol, Polyethylene glycol 400
INCI: PEG-8
CAS no: 5117-19-1 / 25322-68-3
Molecular formula: $C_{16}H_{34}O_9$
Molecular weight: 370.44
Rank of popularity: 125/502
Intended function: Humectant, Solvent
Log P: −2.82
Allergenic potential: Weak sensitizer (max dose = 21.9 $\mu g/cm^2/hr$)

PEG-8 Distearate

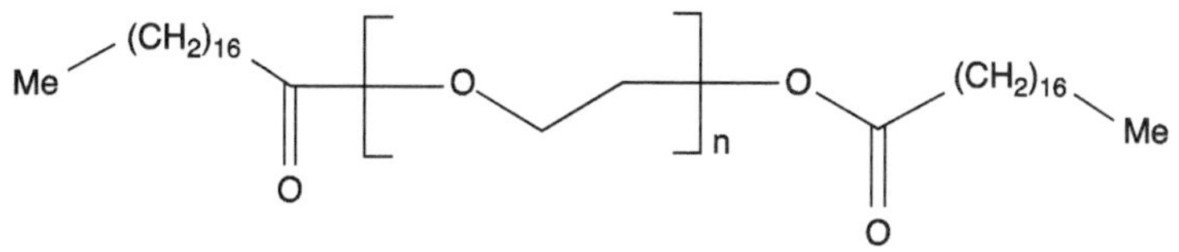

Other names: Polyethylene glycol 400 distearate
INCI: PEG-8 Distearate
CAS no: 9005-08-7
Molecular formula: $C_{52}H_{102}O_{11}$
Molecular weight: 903.35
Rank of popularity: 451/502
Intended function: Cleansing agent, Emulsifying agent

Pentaerythrityl Tetraisostearate

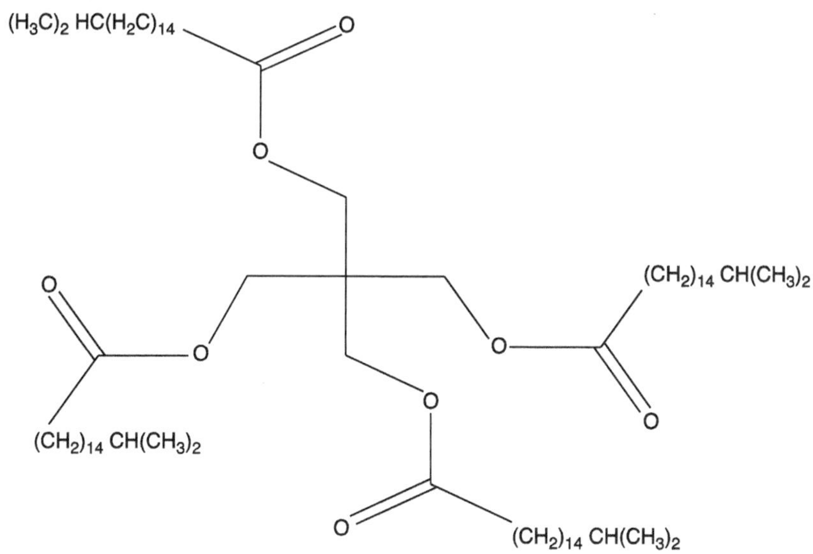

Other names: Pentaerythritol tetraisooctanoate, Pentaerythritol tetraisostearate
INCI: Pentaerythrityl Tetraisostearate
CAS no: 62125-22-8
Molecular formula: $C_{77}H_{148}O_8$
Molecular weight: 1201.99
Rank of popularity: 452/502
Intended function: Binder, Occlusive agent, Viscosity increasing agent

Pentasodium Ethylenediamine Tetramethylene Phosphonate

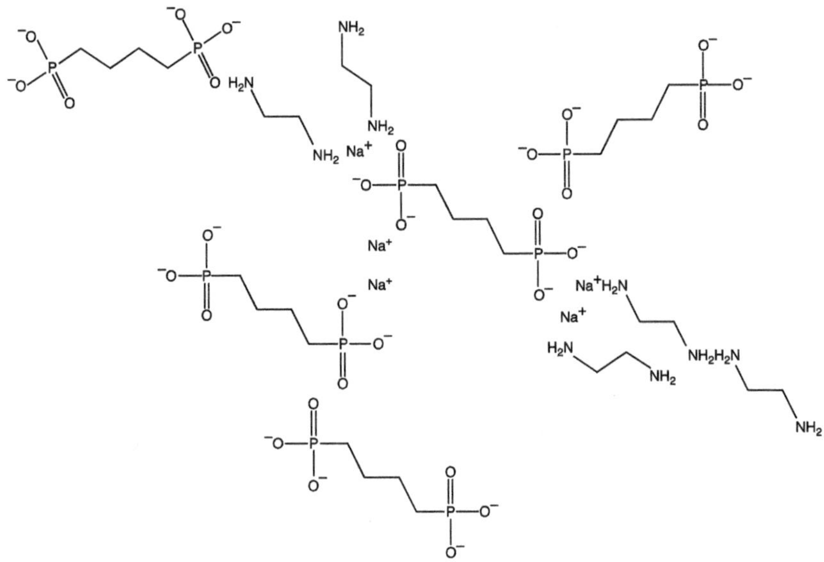

INCI: Pentasodium Ethylenediamine Tetramethylene Phosphonate
CAS no: 7651-99-2
Molecular formula: $C_6H_{15}N_2O_{12}P_4Na_5$
Molecular weight: 551.06
Rank of popularity: 302/502
Intended function: Chelating agent

Pentylene Glycol

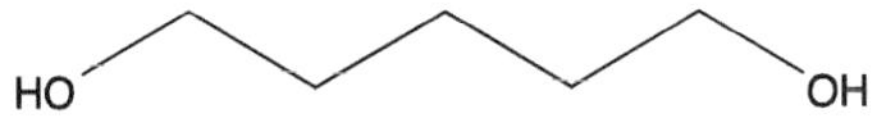

Other names: 1,2-dihydroxypentane, 1,2-pentanediol
INCI: Pentylene Glycol
CAS no: 5343-92-0
Molecular formula: $C_5H_{12}O_2$
Molecular weight: 104.15
Rank of popularity: 177/502
Intended function: Skin conditioning, Solvent
Log P: 0.01

Phenol

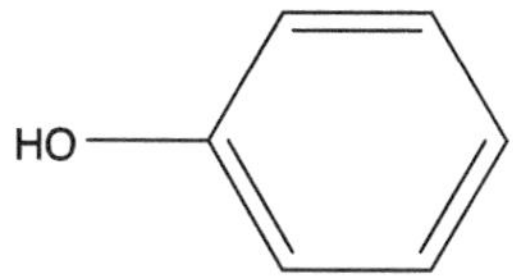

Other names: Benzenol, Hydroxybenzene, Oxybenzene, Phenolum, Phenyl alcohol
INCI: Phenol
CAS no: 108-95-2
Molecular formula: C_6H_6O
Molecular weight: 94.11
Rank of popularity: 458/502
Intended function: Cosmetic biocide, Denaturant, Deodorant, Exfoliant, Fragrance, Preservative
Log P: 1.54
Carcinogenic potential: Category 3 (use with precaution)

Phenoxyethanol

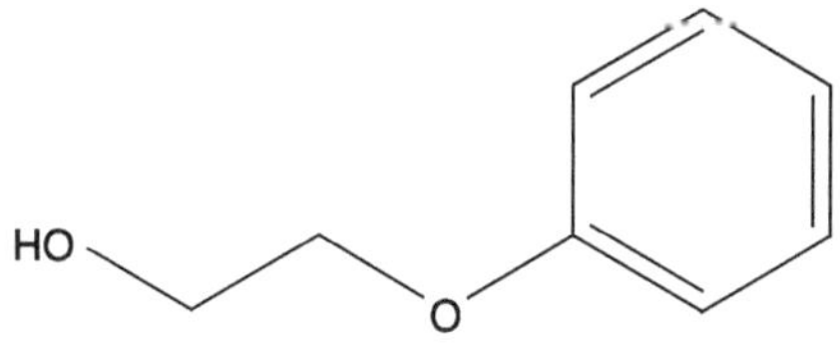

Other names: 2-phenoxyethanol, Phenoxyethanolum, Phenoxytol
INCI: Phenoxyethanol
CAS no: 122-99-6
Molecular formula: $C_8H_{10}O_2$
Molecular weight: 138.16
Rank of popularity: 7/502
Intended function: Fragrance, Preservative
Log P: 1.25
Allergenic potential: Weak sensitizer (max dose = 7.29 µg/cm^2/hr)

Phenylbenzimidozole sulfonic acid

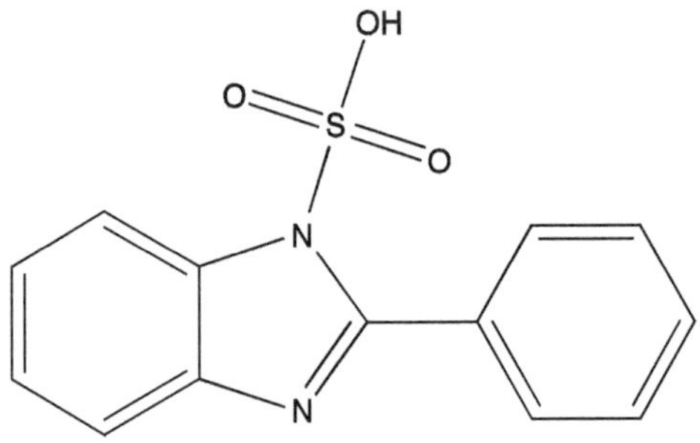

Other names: Ensulizole, 2-phenyl-5-sulfobenzimidazole
INCI: Phenylbenzimidozole sulfonic acid
CAS no: 27503-81-7
Molecular formula: $C_{13}H_{10}N_2O_3S$
Molecular weight: 274.30
Rank of popularity: 176/502
Intended function: UV absorber, UV filter
Log P: –0.23
Carcinogenic potential: Category 3 (use with precaution)
Allergenic potential: Weak sensitizer (max dose = 36.5 μg/cm²/hr)

Pink Australian Clay

Rank of popularity: 453/502
Intended function: Bulking agent

Piroctone Olamine

Other names: 1-Hydroxy-4-methyl-6-(2,4,4-trimethylpentyl)-2(1*H*)-pyridone ethanolammonium salt
INCI: Piroctone Olamine
CAS no: 68890-66-4
Molecular formula: $C_{14}H_{23}NO_2$. C_2H_7NO
Molecular weight: 298.42
Rank of popularity: 454/502
Intended function: Cosmetic biocide, Preservative

Poloxamer 182

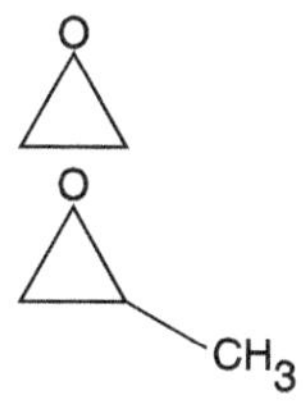

Other names: Poloxalene, Poloxamer
INCI: Poloxamer 182
CAS no: 9003-11-6
Molecular formula: $HO(C_2H_4O)_a(C_3H_6O)_b(C_2H_4O)_aH$
Rank of popularity: 455/502
Intended function: Cleansing agent, Solubilizing agent
Note: The structure does not represent the polymer. Only individual components are shown.

Poloxamer 188

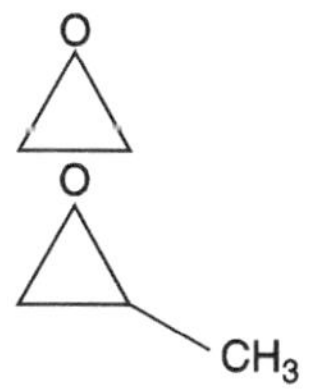

Other names: Poloxalene, Poloxamer, Poloxalkol
INCI: Poloxamer 188
CAS no: 9003-11-6
Molecular formula: $HO\ (C_2H_4O)_a(C_3H_6O)_b(C_2H_4O)_aH$
Molecular weight: average 8400
Rank of popularity: 303/502
Intended function: Cleansing agent
Note: The structure does not represent the polymer. Only individual components are shown.

Polyacrylamide

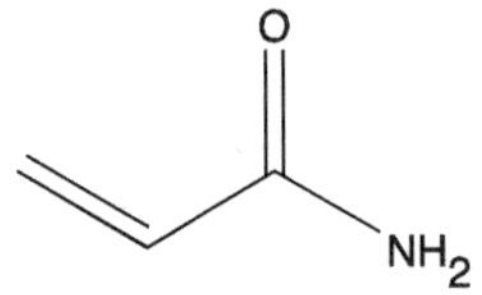

Other names: Arcylamide homopolymer, 2-Propenamide, homopolymer
INCI: Polyacrylamide
CAS no: 9003-05-8
Molecular formula: $(C_3H_5NO)_x$
Rank of popularity: 42/502
Intended function: Antistatic agent, Binder, Film former, Hair fixative
Note: The structure does not represent the polymer. Only individual components are shown.

Polyacrylate-3

INCI: Polyacrylate-3
Rank of popularity: 456/502
Intended function: Viscosity decreasing agent

Polyacrylic Acid

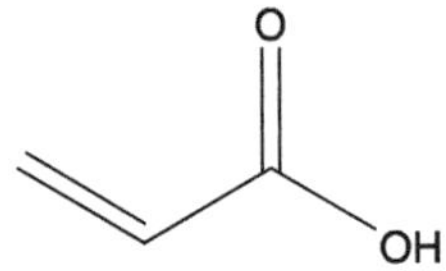

2-Propenoic acid

Other names: Arcylic acid homopolymer, Acrylic acid resin, Carbopol 907, Carboxypolymethane, 2-Propenoic acid, homopolymer
INCI: Polyacrylic Acid
CAS no: 9003-01-4
Molecular formula: $(C_3H_4O_2)_x$
Rank of popularity: 457/502
Intended function: Binder, Emulsion stabilizer, Film former, Viscosity increasing agent
Note: The structure does not represent the polymer. Only individual components are shown.

Polyaminopropyl Biguanide

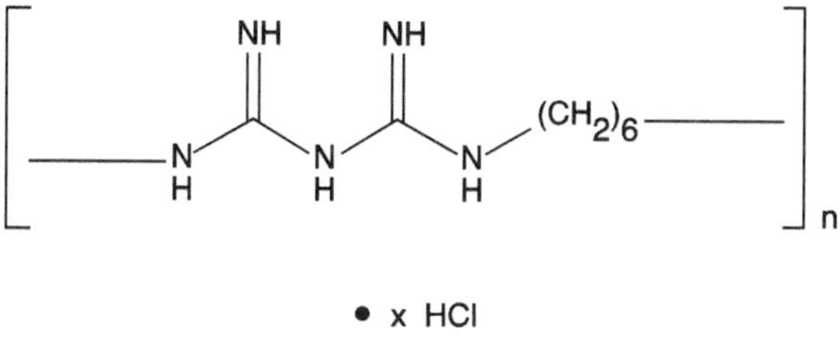

Other names: Polihexanide
INCI: Polyaminopropyl Biguanide
CAS no: 32289-58-0/ 133029-32-0
Molecular formula: $(C_8H_{17}N_5)_n \cdot xClH$
Rank of popularity: 304/502
Intended function: Preservative

Polybutene

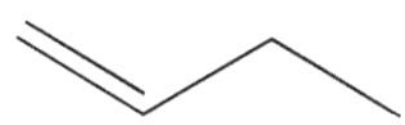

Other names: 1-butene homopolymer
INCI: Polybutene
CAS no: 9003-28-5/ 9003-29-6
Molecular formula: $(C_4H_8)_x$
Rank of popularity: 459/502
Intended function: Binder, Epilating agent, Viscosity increasing agent
Note: The structure does not represent the polymer. Only individual components are shown.

Polyethylene

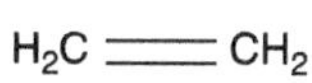

Other names: Ethene homopolymer, Polyethylene powder, Synthetic wax
INCI: Polyethylene
CAS no: 9002-88-4
Rank of popularity: 124/502
Intended function: Abrasive agent, Adhesive agent, Binder, Bulking agent, Emulsion stabilizer, Film former, Oral care agent, Viscosity increasing agent
Note: The structure does not represent the polymer. Only individual components are shown.

Polyglyceryl-2 Dipolyhydroxystearate

INCI: Polyglyceryl-2 Dipolyhydroxystearate
Rank of popularity: 222/502
Intended function: Occlusive agent

Poly-glyceryl-2 Sesquiisostearate

Other names: Diglyceryl sesquiisostearate
INCI: Polyglyceryl-2 Sesquiisostearate
Rank of popularity: 460/502
Intended function: Emollient, Emulsifying agent

Polyglyceryl-3 Diisostearate

Other names: Triglycerin diisostearate, Triglyceryl diisostearate
INCI: Polyglyceryl-3 Diisostearate
CAS no: 63705-03-3/ 66082-42-6
Rank of popularity: 123/502
Intended function: Emollient, Emulsifying agent

Polyglyceryl-3 Distearate

Other names: Triglycerin distearate, Triglyceryl distearate
INCI: Poly-glyceryl-3 Distearate
CAS no: 9009-32-9/ 34423-19-5
Molecular formula: $C_{18} H_{36} O_2 . x (C_3 H_8 O_3)x$
Rank of popularity: 305/502
Intended function: Emollient, Emulsifying agent

Polyglyceryl-3 Methylglucose Distearate

INCI: Polyglyceryl-3 Methylglucose Distearate
Rank of popularity: 223/502
Intended function: Emollient, Emulsifying agent

Polyglyceryl-4 Isostearate

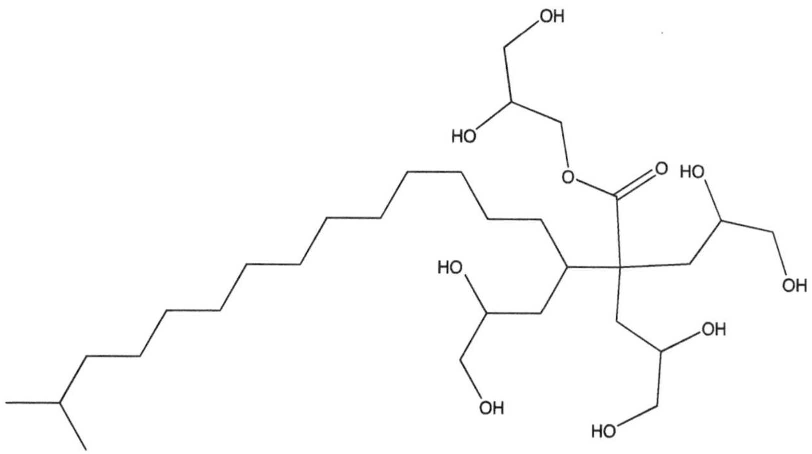

Other names: Tetraglyceryl monoisostearate, Isooctadecanoic acid, monoester with tetraglycerol
INCI: Polyglyceryl-4 Isostearate
CAS no: 63705-03-3/ 91824-88-3
Molecular formula: $C_{18} H_{36} O_2$. 1/2 $(C_3 H_8 O_3)_x$
Rank of popularity: 461/502
Intended function: Emollient, Emulsifying agent

Polyglyceryl methacrylate

CAS no: 96614-21-0
Rank of popularity: 462/502
Intended function: Film former

Polyhydroxystearic Acid

Other names: Polyhydroxyoctadecanoic acid
INCI: Polyhydroxystearic Acid
CAS no: 27924-99-8/ 58128-22-6
Rank of popularity: 178/502
Intended function: Suspending agent

Polymethyl Methacrylate

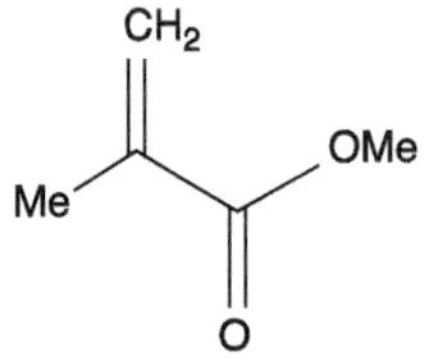

Other names: PMMA, Poly (methacrylic acid methyl ester)
INCI: Polymethyl Methacrylate
CAS no: 9011-14-7
Molecular formula: $(C_5H_8O_2)_x$
Molecular weight: Average of 350 000
Rank of popularity: 84/502
Intended function: Film former
Note: The structure does not represent the polymer. Only individual components are shown.

Polymethylsilsesquioxane

INCI: Polymethylsilsesquioxane
CAS no: 68554-70-1
Rank of popularity: 464/502
Intended function: Opacifying agent

Polyphosphorylchlorine

INCI: Polyphosphorylchlorine
CAS no: 67881-99-6
Rank of popularity: 465/502
Intended function: Film former

Polypropylene Glycol-2

CAS no: 25323-30-2
Rank of popularity: 479/502
Intended function: Humectant
Allergenic potential: Maximum dose not stated

Polyquaternium-10

Other names: Quaterium-42
INCI: Polyquaternium-10
CAS no: 53568-66-4/ 54351-50-7/ 55353-19-0/ 68610-92-4/ 81859-24-7
Rank of popularity: 114/502
Intended function: Antistatic agent, Film former, Hair fixative
Allergenic potential: Maximum dose not stated

Polyquaternium-22

Other names: Acrylic acid-diallyldimethylammonium chloride polymer
INCI: Polyquaternium-22
CAS no: 53694-17-0
Rank of popularity: 466/502
Intended function: Antistatic agent, Film former, Hair fixative

Polyquaternium-39

INCI: Polyquaternium-39
CAS no: 25136-75-8
Rank of popularity: 463/502
Intended function: Antistatic agent, Film former, Hair fixative

Polyquaternium-7

Other names: Quaterium-41
INCI: Polyquaternium-7
CAS no: 26590-05-6
Rank of popularity: 467/502
Intended function: Antistatic agent, Film former, Hair fixative

Polysorbate 20

Other names: Polysorbatum 20, Sorbimarcogol laurate 300, Tween® 20
INCI: Polysorbate 20
CAS no: 9005-64-5
Molecular weight: 354.57
Rank of popularity: 48/502
Intended function: Emulsifying agent, Fragrance, Solubilizing agent
Log P: 6.99
Allergenic potential: Weak sensitizer (max dose = 36.5 μg/cm^2/hr)

Polysorbate 60

Other names: Polysorbatum 60, Sorbimarcogol laurate 300, Tween® 60
INCI: Polysorbate 60
CAS no: 9005-67-8
Molecular weight: 438.73
Rank of popularity: 107/502
Intended function: Emulsifying agent, Fragrance, Solubilizing agent
Log P: 9.78
Allergenic potential: Weak sensitizer (max dose = 36.5 μg/cm^2/hr)

Polysorbate 80

Other names: Polysorbatum 80, Sorbimarcogol laurate 300, Tween® 80
INCI: Polysorbate 80
CAS no: 9005-65-6
Molecular weight: 605.00
Rank of popularity: 147/502
Intended function: Denaturant, Emulsifying agent, Fragrance, Solubilizing agent
Log P: 5.30
Carcinogenic potential: Category 2 (safe to use)
Allergenic potential: Weak sensitizer (max dose = 36.5 μg/cm^2/hr)

Polysorbate Blend

Rank of popularity: 468/502
Intended function: Denaturant, Emulsifying agent, Fragrance, Solubilizing agent
Allergenic potential: Maximum dose not stated

Polyvinyl Alcohol

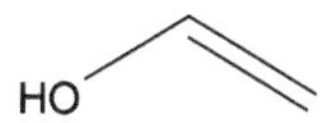

Ethenol

Other names: Ethenol homopolymer
INCI: Polyvinyl Alcohol
CAS no: 9002-89-5/ 25213-24-5
Molecular formula: $[-CH_2CHOH-]_n$
Molecular weight: 89 000-98 000
Rank of popularity: 469/502
Intended function: Binder, Film former, Viscosity increasing agent
Allergenic potential: Wery weak sensitizer (max dose = 94.8 μg/cm²/hr)
Note: The structure does not represent the polymer. Only individual components are shown.

Polyvinylpyrrolidone

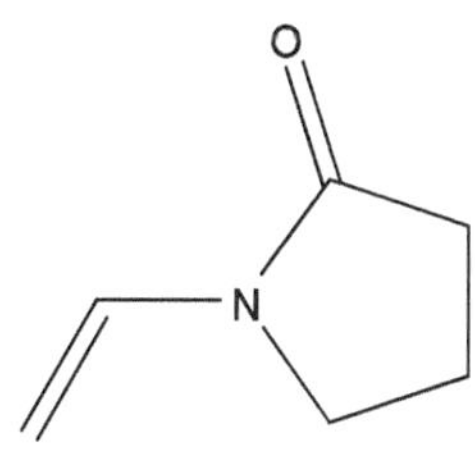

1-Ethenyl-2-pyrrolidinone

Other names: Crospovidone, Polyvinylpyrrolidone, Povidone, Povidonum, 1-Ethenyl-2-pyrrolidinone homopolymer
INCI: PVP
CAS no: 9003-39-8
Molecular formula: $(C_6H_9NO)_x$
Molecular weight: Average of 40 000
Rank of popularity: 470/502
Intended function: Binder, Emulsion stabilizer, Film former, Hair fixative, Suspending agent
Allergenic potential: Weak sensitizer (max dose = 72.9 μg/cm²/hr)
Note: The structure does not represent the polymer. Only individual components are shown.

Potassium Alum

Other names: Alum, Alumen, Aluminium potassium sulfate, Exsiccated alum
INCI: Potassium Alum
CAS no: 7784-24-9
Molecular formula: KAl (SO4)2
Molecular weight: 258.21
Rank of popularity: 471/502
Intended function: Astringent

Potassium Cetyl Phosphate

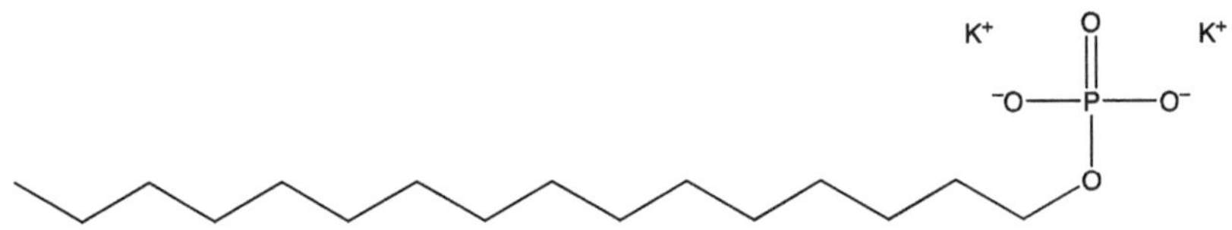

INCI: Potassium Cetyl Phosphate
CAS no: 17026-85-6/ 19035-79-1
Molecular formula: $C_{16}\,H_{35}\,O_4\,P\cdot x\,K$
Rank of popularity: 61/502
Intended function: Emulsifying agent

Potassium Hydroxide

$K^+ \quad OH^-$

Other names: Caustic potash, Kalii hydroxidum
INCI: Potassium Hydroxide
CAS no: 1310-58-3
Molecular formula: HKO
Molecular weight: 56.10
Rank of popularity: 306/502
Intended function: pH adjuster

Potassium Phosphate

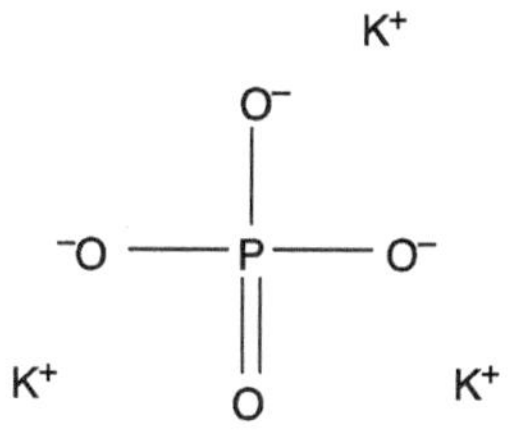

Other names: Monobasic potassium phosphate
INCI: Potassium Phosphate
CAS no: 7778-77-0/ 16068-46-5
Molecular formula: $H_3O_4P.K$
Molecular weight: 137.09
Rank of popularity: 487/502
Intended function: pH adjuster
Carcinogenic potential: Category 2 (safe to use)

Potassium Sorbate

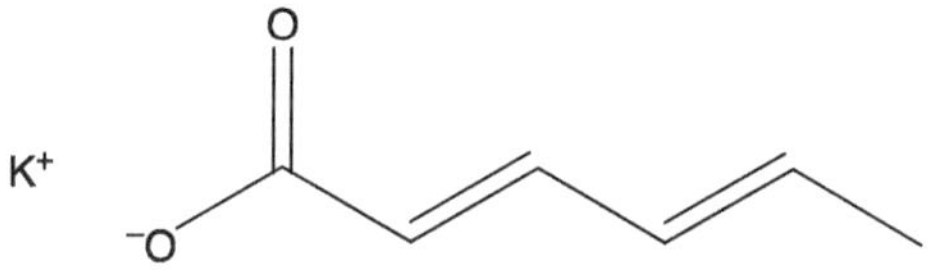

INCI: Potassium Sorbate
CAS no: 590-00-1/ 24634-61-5
Molecular formula: $C_6H_8O_2$. K
Molecular weight: 152.22
Rank of popularity: 90/502
Intended function: Fragrance, Preservative
Carcinogenic potential: Category 3 (use with precaution)
Allergenic potential: Maximum dose not stated

PPG-15 Stearyl Ether

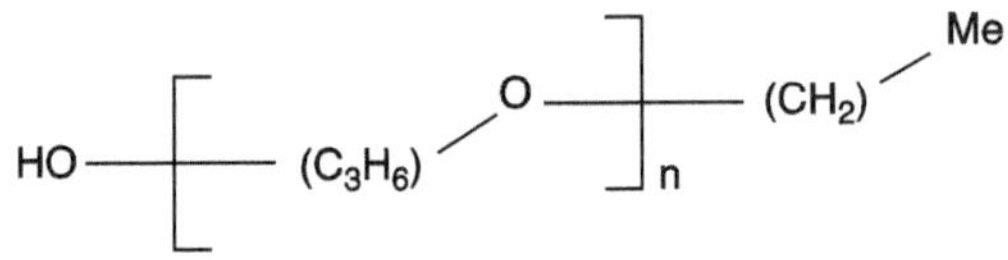

Other names: Polyoxypropylene (15) stearyl ether
INCI: PPG-15 Stearyl Ether
CAS no: 25231-21-4
Molecular formula: $(C_3H_6O)_n\ C_{18}H_{38}O$
Rank of popularity: 472/502
Intended function: Emollient

PPG-15 Stearyl Ether Benzoate

Other names: Polyoxypropylene (15) stearyl ether benzoate
INCI: PPG-15 Stearyl Ether Benzoate
Rank of popularity: 473/502
Intended function: Emollient

PPG-1-PEG9 Lauryl Glycol Ether

INCI: PPG-1-PEG9 Lauryl Glycol Ether
Rank of popularity: 474/502
Intended function: Emulsifying agent

PPG-26 Buteth-26

INCI: PPG-26 Buteth-26
CAS no: 9038-95-3/ 9065-63-8
Rank of popularity: 475/502
Intended function: Emulsifying agent, Fragrance, Hair conditioning, Skin conditioning

Promulgen™ D

Other names: Cetearyl Alcohol (and) Ceteareth 20
INCI: Cetearyl Alcohol (and) Ceteareth 20
CAS no: 69072-97-5
Rank of popularity: 476/502
Intended function: Emulsifying agent

Propyl Gallate

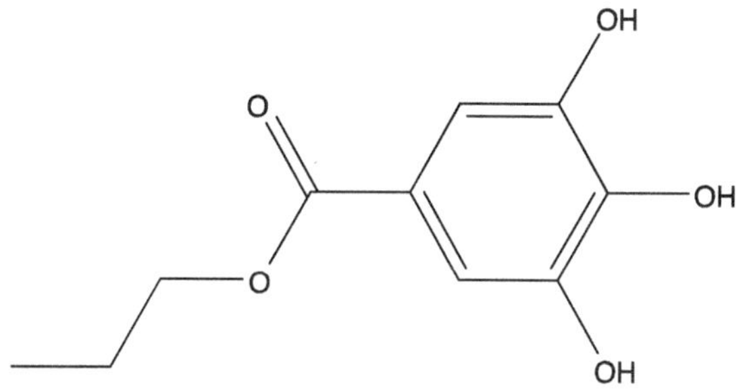

Other names: 3,4,5-Trihydroxybenzoic acid propyl ester, Tenox PG
INCI: Propyl Gallate
CAS no: 121-79-9
Molecular formula: $C_{10}H_{12}O_5$
Molecular weight: 212.20
Rank of popularity: 307/502
Intended function: Antioxidant, Fragrance
Log P: 1.78
Allergenic potential: Moderate sensitizer (max dose = 0.0255 μg/cm^2/hr)

Propylene Carbonate

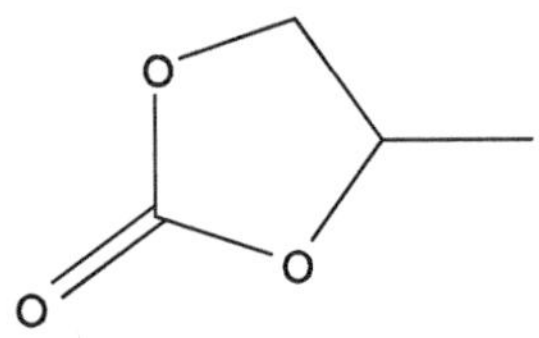

Other names: 1,2-Propanediol cyclic carbonate, 4-Methyl-1,3-dioxolan-2-one
INCI: Propylene Carbonate
Molecular formula: $C_4H_6O_3$
Molecular weight: 102.09
Rank of popularity: 308/502
Intended function: Solvent, Viscosity decreasing agent
Log P: –0.41
Allergenic potential: Weak sensitizer (max dose = 3.94 μg/cm²/hr)

Propylene Glycol

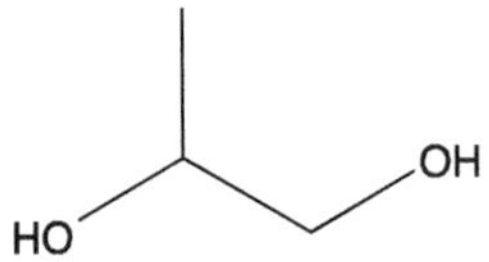

Other names: Methylethyl glycol, 1,2-propanediol
INCI: Propylene Glycol
CAS no: 57-55-6
Molecular formula: $C_3H_8O_2$
Molecular weight: 76.09
Rank of popularity: 9/502
Intended function: Fragrance, Humectant, Skin conditioning, Solvent, Viscosity decreasing
Log P: –1.01
Allergenic potential: Weak sensitizer (max dose = 3.33 μg/cm²/hr)

Propylene Glycol Ceteth-3 Acetate

Other names: Propylene glycol polyethylene glycol (3) cetyl ether acetate
INCI: Propylene Glycol Ceteth-3 Acetate
CAS no: 93385-03-6
Molecular formula: $C_{27}H_{54}O_6$
Molecular weight: 474.71
Rank of popularity: 477/502
Intended function: Emollient
Log P: 7.42

Propylene Glycol Dicaprylate

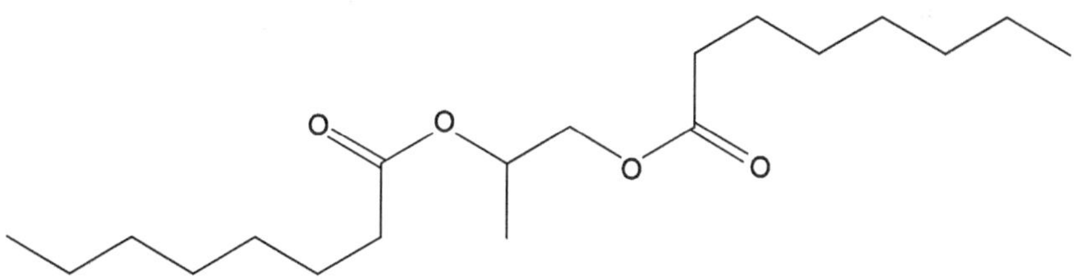

INCI: Propylene Glycol Dicaprylate
CAS no: 7384-98-7
Molecular formula: $C_{19}H_{36}O_4$
Molecular weight: 328.49
Rank of popularity: 309/502
Intended function: Occlusive agent, Viscosity increasing agent
Log P: 6.69
Allergenic potential: Weak sensitizer (max dose = 16.7 μg/cm^2/hr)

Propylene Glycol Laurate

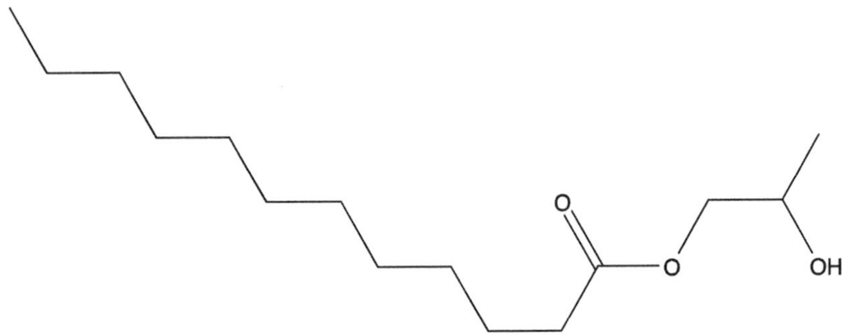

Other names: Lauroglycol, Propylene glycol monododecanoate, Propylene glycol monolaurate
INCI: Propylene Glycol Laurate
CAS no: 142-55-2/ 27194-74-7/ 37321-62-3/ 199282-83-2
Molecular formula: $C_{15}H_{30}O_3$
Molecular weight: 258.40
Rank of popularity: 310/502
Intended function: Emollient, Emulsifying agent
Log P: 4.93

Propylene Glycol Stearate

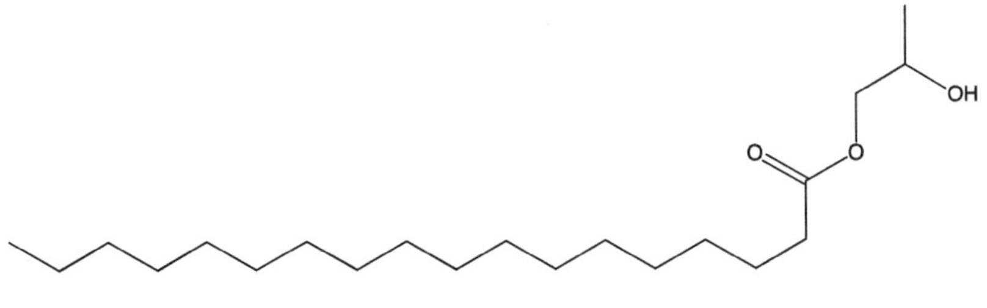

Other names: Propylene glycol monooctadecanoate, Propylene glycol monostearate, Propylenglycoli monostearas
INCI: Propylene Glycol Stearate
CAS no: 142-75-6/ 1323-39-3
Molecular formula: $C_{21}H_{42}O_3$
Molecular weight: 342.56
Rank of popularity: 311/502
Intended function: Emollient, Emulsifying agent, Fragrance
Log P: 7.98

Propylene

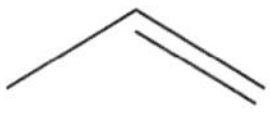

Other names: Propene, Methylethylene
INCI: 1-Propene
CAS no: 115-07-1
Molecular formula: C_3H_6
Molecular weight: 42.0797
Rank of popularity: 478/502
Log P: 1.827

Propylparaben

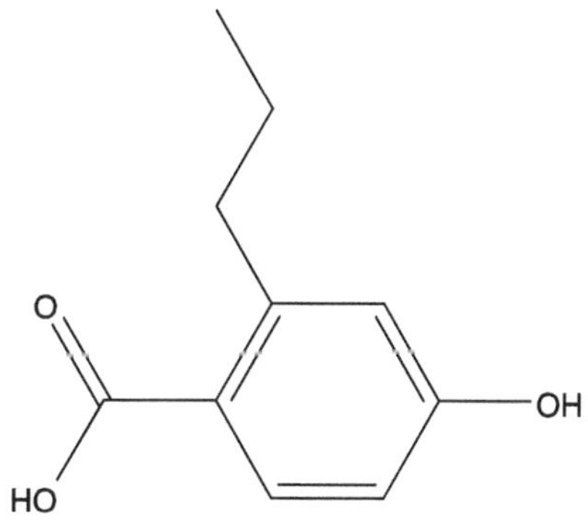

Other names: Propyl p-hydroxybenzoate, Propyl parahydroxybenzoate
INCI: Propylparaben
CAS no: 94-13-3
Molecular formula: $C_{10}H_{12}O_3$
Molecular weight: 180.20
Rank of popularity: 5/502
Intended function: Fragrance, Preservative
Log P: 2.90
Carcinogenic potential: Category 3 (use with precaution)
Allergenic potential: Weak sensitizer (max dose = 21.9 μg/cm^2/hr)

Quaternium-15

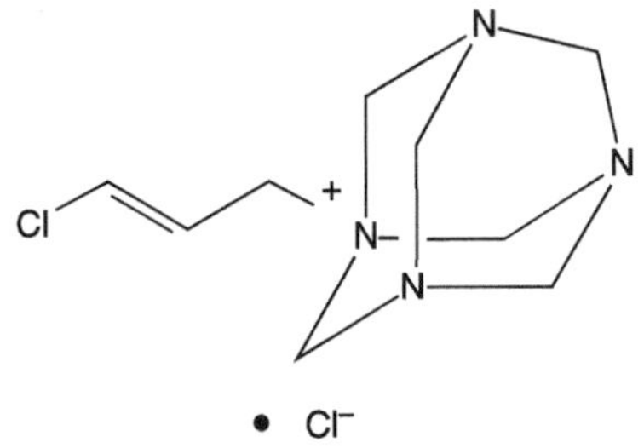

Other names: Methenamine 3-chloroallylochloride
INCI: Quaternium-15
CAS no: 4080-31-3/51229-78-8
Molecular formula: $C_9H_{16}ClN_4.Cl$
Molecular weight: 251.15
Rank of popularity: 224/502
Intended function: Antistatic agent, Preservative
Allergenic potential: Weak sensitizer (max dose = 7.29 μg/cm²/hr)

Resorcinol

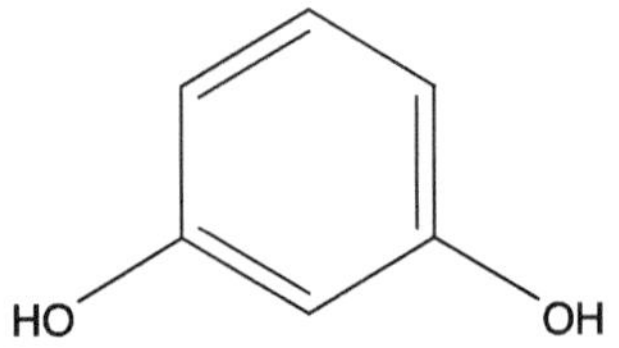

Other names: 1,3-benzenediol, Cl developer 4, m-hydroquinone, Oxidation base 31, Resorcin
INCI: Resorcinol
CAS no: 108-46-3
Molecular formula: $C_6H_6O_2$
Molecular weight: 110.11
Rank of popularity: 312/502
Intended function: Antiacne agent, Antioxidant, Denaturant, External analgesic, Fragrance, Hair colourant
Log P: 0.82
Carcinogenic potential: Category 3 (use with precaution)
Allergenic potential: Weak sensitizer (max dose = 16.7 μg/cm²/hr)

Retinal

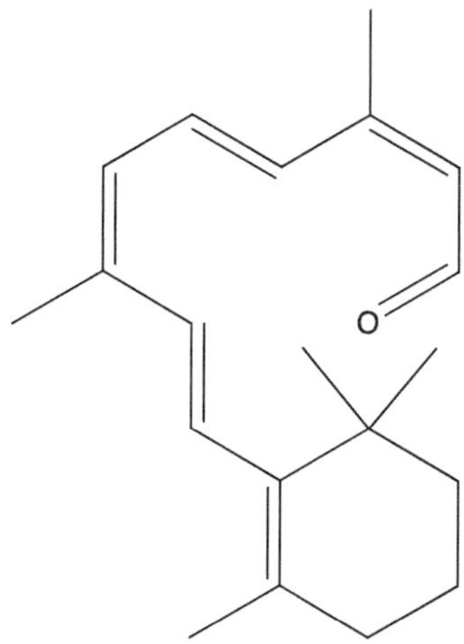

Other names: Retinaldehyde, Trans-retinal, Vitamin A aldehyde
INCI: Retinal
CAS no: 116-31-4
Molecular formula: $C_{20}H_{28}O$
Molecular weight: 284.44
Rank of popularity: 225/502
Intended function: Skin conditioning
Log P: 6.38
Allergenic potential: Moderate sensitizer (max dose = 0.0365 μg/cm²/hr)

Retinol

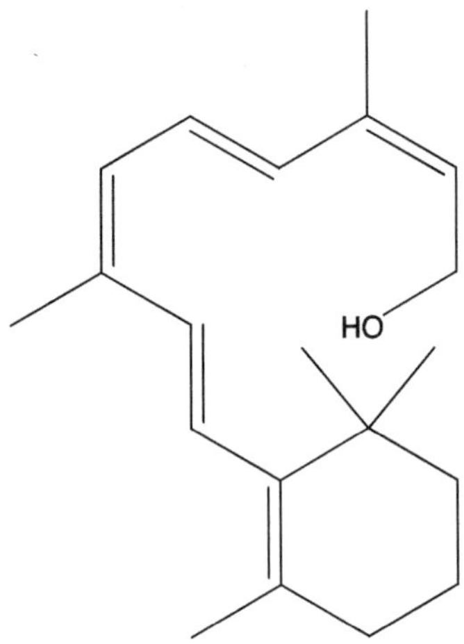

Other names: Dry formed vitamin A, Vitamin A, Vitaminum a
INCI: Retinol
CAS no: 68-26-8/ 11103-57-4
Molecular formula: $C_{20}H_{30}O$
Molecular weight: 286.45
Rank of popularity: 226/502
Intended function: Skin conditioning
Log P: 6.08

Retinyl Palmitate

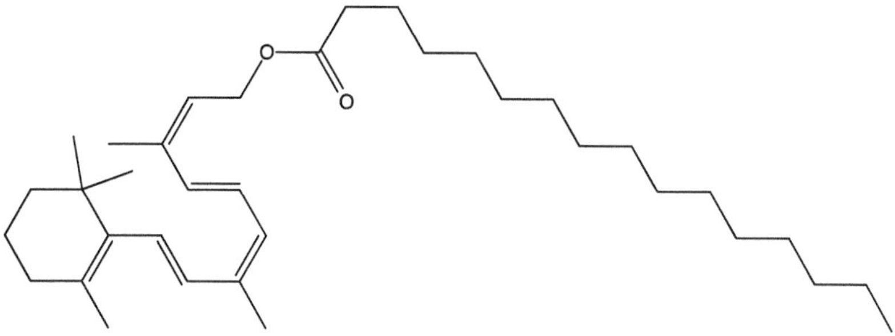

Other names: Axerophthol palmitate, Vitamin A palmitate
INCI: Retinyl Palmitate
CAS no: 79-81-2
Molecular formula: $C_{36}H_{60}O_2$
Molecular weight: 524.86
Rank of popularity: 44/502
Intended function: Skin conditioning
Log P: 14.32
Carcinogenic potential: Category 1 (use within limit on body = 6.2×10^{-4} %w/w; face = 3.8×10^{-2} %w/w; hands = 1.2×10^{-2} %w/w)

Saccharide Isomerate

INCI: Saccharide Isomerate
Rank of popularity: 227/502
Intended function: Humectant
Log P: 6.08

Salicylic Acid

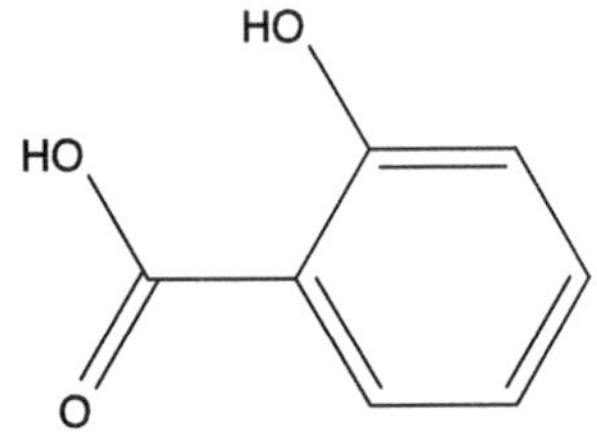

Other names: Acidum salicylicum, Phenol-2-carboxylic acid
INCI: Salicylic Acid
CAS no: 69-72-7
Molecular formula: $C_7H_6O_3$
Molecular weight: 138.12
Rank of popularity: 62/502
Intended function: Antiacne agent, Antidandruff agent, Corn/callus/wart remover, Denaturant, Exfoliant, Hair conditioning, Preservative, Skin conditioning
Log P: 2.01

Sclerotium Gum

Other names: Betasizofiran, Scleroglucan, Sclerogum
INCI: Sclerotium Gum
CAS no: 39464-87-4
Rank of popularity: 313/502
Intended function: Emulsion stabilizer, Skin conditioning, Viscosity increasing agent

Serine

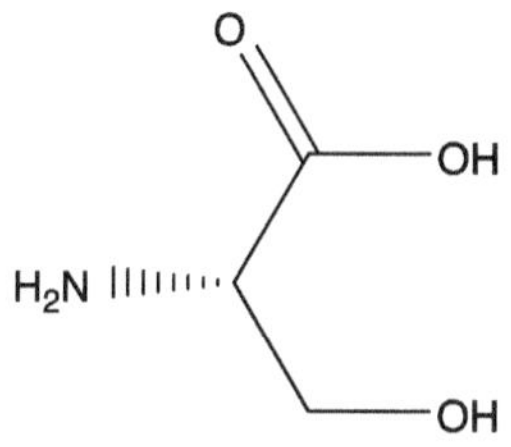

Other names: DL-serine, L-serine, Serinum
INCI: Serine
CAS no: 56-45-1(L-form)
Molecular formula: $C_3H_7NO_3$
Molecular weight: 105.09
Rank of popularity: 228/502
Intended function: Hair conditioning, Skin conditioning
Log P: –1.49
Carcinogenic potential: Category 2 (safe to use)

Silica

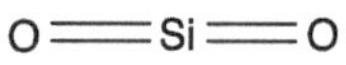

Other names: Amorphous silica, Silicon dioxide, Silicic anhydride
INCI: Silica
CAS no: 7631-86-9/ 60676-86-0/ 112945-52-5
Molecular formula: SiO_2
Molecular weight: 60.08
Rank of popularity: 71/502
Intended function: Abrasive agent, Absorbent, Anticaking agent, Bulking agent, Opacifying agent, Suspending agent
Carcinogenic potential: Category 2 (safe to use)

Silica Dimethyl Silylate

Other names: Dimethylsilyl silicic anhydride
INCI: Silica Dimethyl Silylate
CAS no: 68611-44-9
Rank of popularity: 91/502
Intended function: Anticaking agent, Bulking agent, Slip modifier, Viscosity increasing agent

Silk Protein

Other names: Dimethylsilyl silicic anhydride
INCI: Silk amino acids
CAS no: 65072-01-7
Rank of popularity: 179/502
Intended function: Hair conditioning, Skin conditioning
Allergenic potential: Maximum dose not stated

Simethicone

Other names: Silicone resin
INCI: Simethicone
CAS no: 8050-81-5
Rank of popularity: 229/502
Intended function: Antifoaming agent

Sodium Ascorbate

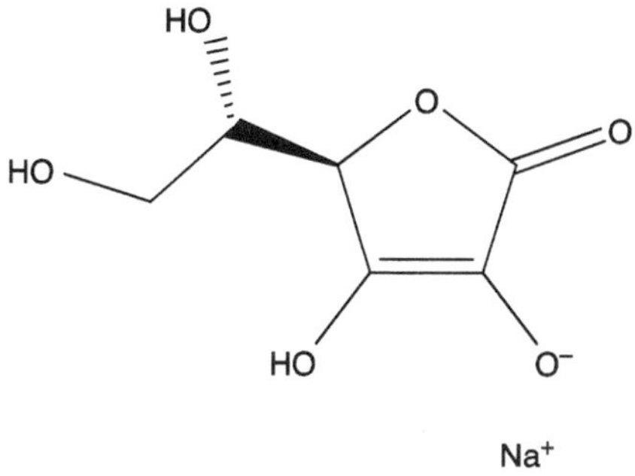

Other names: Vitamin C sodium
INCI: Sodium Ascorbate
CAS no: 134-03-2
Molecular formula: $C_6H_8O_6$. Na
Molecular weight: 199.10
Rank of popularity: 480/502
Intended function: Antioxidant
Carcinogenic potential: Category 3 (use with precaution)

Sodium Ascorbyl Phosphate

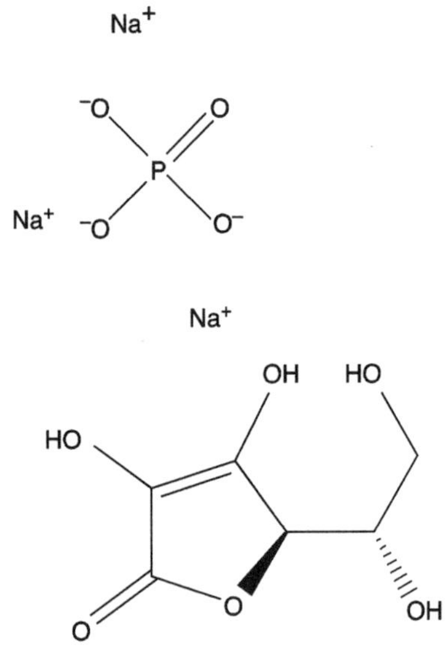

INCI: Sodium Ascorbyl Phosphate
CAS no: 66170-10-3
Molecular formula: $C_6H_6O_9P$. 3Na
Molecular weight: 325.06
Rank of popularity: 230/502
Intended function: Antioxidant

Sodium Benzoate

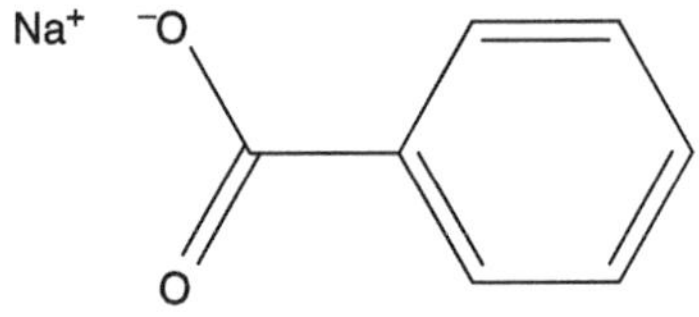

Other names: Natrii benzoas
INCI: Sodium Benzoate
CAS no: 532-32-1
Molecular formula: $C_7H_6O_2$. Na
Molecular weight: 145.10
Rank of popularity: 108/502
Intended function: Corrosion inhibitor, Fragrance, Preservative
Carcinogenic potential: Category 3 (use with precaution)

Sodium Bisulfite

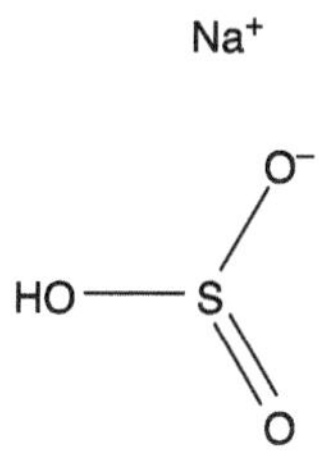

Other names: Sodium acid bisulfite
INCI: Sodium Bisulfite
CAS no: 7631-90-5
Molecular formula: NaH_2SO_3
Molecular weight: 105.06
Rank of popularity: 148/502
Intended function: Antioxidant, Hair curling/straightening agent, Reducing agent
Carcinogenic potential: Category 3 (use with precaution)
Allergenic potential: Weak sensitizer (max dose = 7.29 μg/cm²/hr)

Sodium Carbomer

INCI: Sodium Carbomer
CAS no: 73298-57-4
Rank of popularity: 85/502
Intended function: Emulsion stabilizer, Film former, Viscosity increasing agent

Sodium Cetearyl Sulphate

Other names: Sodium cetostearyl sulfate
INCI: Sodium Cetearyl Sulphate
CAS no: 59186-41-3
Molecular formula: $C_{18} H_{38} O_4 S. C_{16} H_{34} O_4 S. 2 Na$
Molecular weight: 719.04
Rank of popularity: 181/502
Intended function: Cleansing agent

Sodium Cetostearyl Sulphate

Rank of popularity: 314/502

Sodium Chloride

$Na^+ \ Cl^-$

Other names: Halite, Rock salt, Salt
INCI: Sodium Chloride
CAS no: 7647-14-5
Molecular formula: NaCl
Molecular weight: 58.44
Rank of popularity: 86/502
Intended function: Flavouring agent, Oral care agent, Viscosity increasing agent
Carcinogenic potential: Category 2 (safe to use)

Sodium Chondroitin Sulphate

INCI: Sodium Chondroitin Sulphate
CAS no: 9007-28-7/ 9082-07-9
Rank of popularity: 231/502
Intended function: Hair conditioning, Skin conditioning

Sodium Citrate

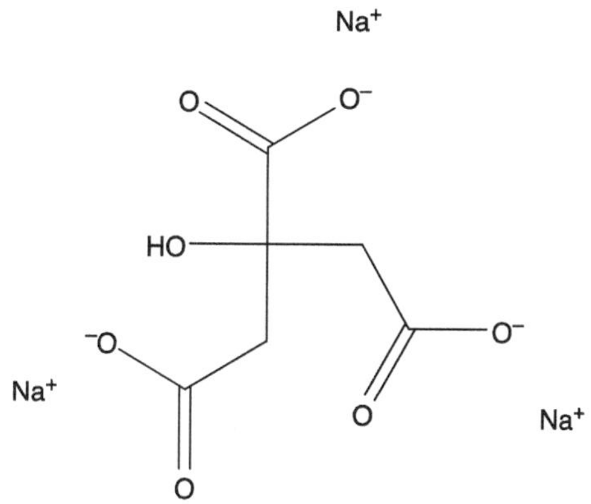

Other names: Trisodium citrate
INCI: Sodium Citrate
CAS no: 68-04-2/ 6132-04-3
Molecular formula: $C_6H_5O_7$. 3Na
Molecular weight: 261.08
Rank of popularity: 43/502
Intended function: Buffering agent, Chelating agent, Fragrance, pH adjuster
Carcinogenic potential: Category 2 (safe to use)

Sodium Cocoyl Isethionate

Other names: Fatty acid coconut oil sulfoethyl esters sodium salt
INCI: Sodium Cocoyl Isethionate
CAS no: 58969-27-0/61789-32-0
Rank of popularity: 315/502
Intended function: Cleansing agent
Allergenic potential: Weak sensitizer (max dose = 0.967 μg/cm^2/hr)

Sodium Cocoyl Sarcosinate

Other names: Amides coconut oil with sarcosine sodium salts
INCI: Sodium Cocoyl Sarcosinate
CAS no: 61791-59-1
Rank of popularity: 180/502
Intended function: Cleansing agent, Hair conditioning

Sodium Dehydroacetate

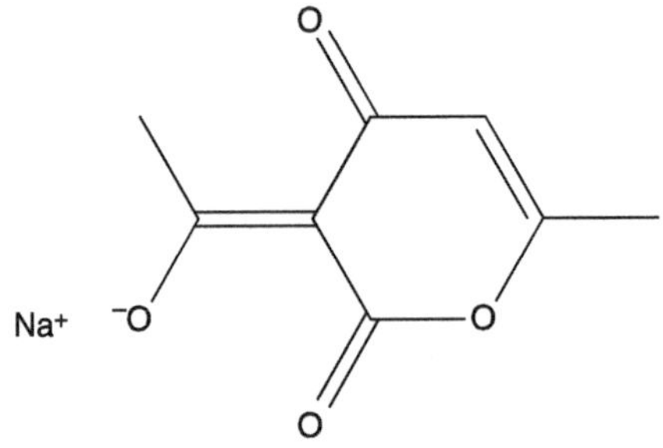

INCI: Sodium Dehydroacetate
CAS no: 4418-26-2
Molecular formula: $C_8H_8O_4$. Na
Molecular weight: 191.13
Rank of popularity: 481/502
Intended function: Preservative
Carcinogenic potential: Category 3 (use with precaution)

Sodium Docusate

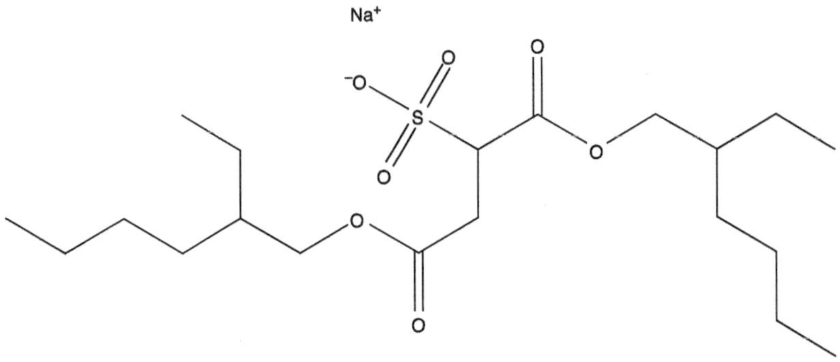

Other names: Diethylhexyl Sodium Sulfosuccinate, Dioctyl Sodium Sulfosuccinate
INCI: Diethylhexyl sodium sulfosuccinate
CAS no: 577-11-7
Molecular formula: $C_{20}H_{38}$O7S. Na
Molecular weight: 445.56
Rank of popularity: 482/502
Intended function: Cleansing agent, Emulsifying agent, Hydrotrope

Sodium Gluconate

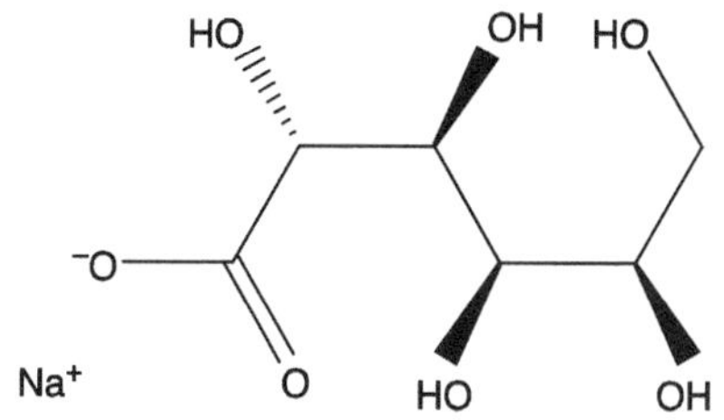

Other names: D-gluconic acid monosodium salt
INCI: Sodium Gluconate
CAS no: 527-07-1/ 14906-97-9
Molecular formula: $C_6H_{12}O_7$. Na
Molecular weight: 219.14
Rank of popularity: 182/502
Intended function: Chelating agent, Skin conditioning

Sodium Hyaluronate

Other names: Hyaluronic acid sodium salt
INCI: Sodium Hyaluronate
CAS no: 9067-32-7
Rank of popularity: 39/502
Intended function: Skin conditioning
Carcinogenic potential: Category 3 (use with precaution)
Allergenic potential: Maximum dose not stated

Sodium Hydroxide

Na^+ OH^-

Other names: Caustic soda, Natrii hydroxidum
INCI: Sodium Hydroxide
CAS no: 1310-73-2
Molecular formula: NaOH
Molecular weight: 39.99
Rank of popularity: 46/502
Intended function: Denaturant, pH adjuster
Carcinogenic potential: Category 3 (use with precaution)

Sodium Hydroxymethylglycinate

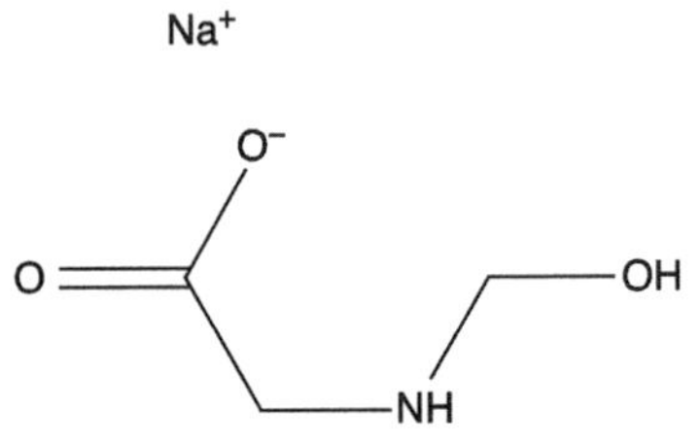

Other names: Glycine, N-(hydroxymethyl)- monosodium salt
INCI: Sodium Hydroxymethylglycinate
CAS no: 70161-44-3
Molecular formula: $C_3H_7NO_3 \cdot$ Na
Molecular weight: 128.07
Rank of popularity: 483/502
Intended function: Hair conditioning, Preservative

Sodium Lactate

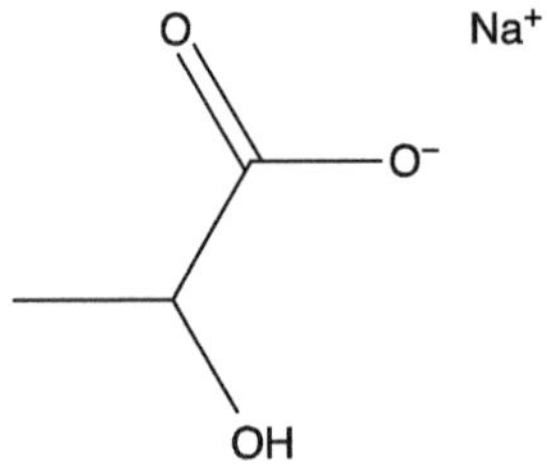

Other names: 2-hydroxypropanoic acid monosodium salt
INCI: Sodium Lactate
CAS no: 72-17-3/ 867-56-1
Molecular formula: $C_3H_6O_3 \cdot$ Na
Molecular weight: 113.06
Rank of popularity: 92/502
Intended function: Buffering agent, Exfoliant, Humectant

Sodium Laureth Sulphate

Other names: Dodecyl sodium sulfate, Sodium PEG lauryl ether sulfate
INCI: Sodium Laureth Sulfate
CAS no: 1335-72-4/ 3088-31-1/ 9004-82-4/ 68585-34-2/ 68891-38-3/ 91648-56-5
Rank of popularity: 484/502
Intended function: Cleansing agent, Emulsifying agent

Sodium Lauroyl Sarcosinate

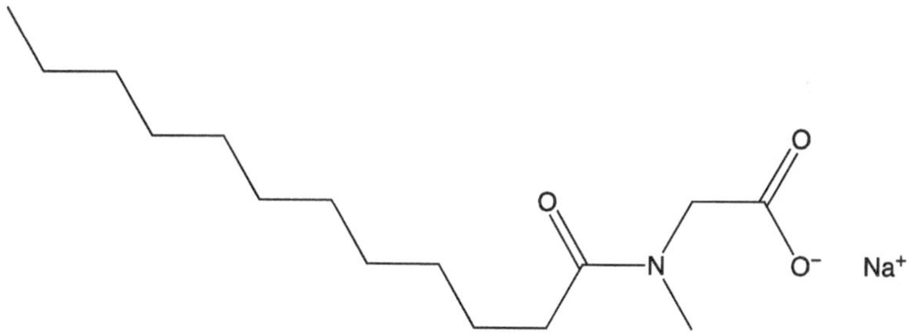

Other names: Sodium N-lauroyl sarcosinate
INCI: Sodium Lauroyl Sarcosinate
CAS no: 137-16-6
Molecular formula: $C_{15}H_{29}NO_3{\cdot}Na$
Molecular weight: 294.38
Rank of popularity: 316/502
Intended function: Cleansing agent, Hair conditioning

Sodium Lauryl Sulphate

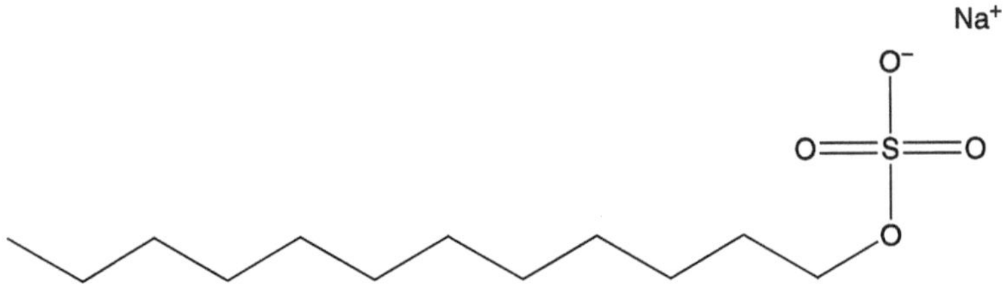

Other names: Natrii laurilsulfas, Sodium dodecyl sulfate
INCI: Sodium Lauryl Sulfate
CAS no: 151-21-3/ 68585-47-7 (generic)/ 68955-19-/ 73296-89-6
Molecular formula: $C_{12}H_{26}O_4S$ .Na
Molecular weight: 289.29
Rank of popularity: 79/502
Intended function: Cleansing agent, Denaturant, Emulsifying agent, Foam booster
Log P: 3.05
Allergenic potential: Moderate sensitizer (max dose = 0.202 μg/cm^2/hr)

Sodium Metabisulfite

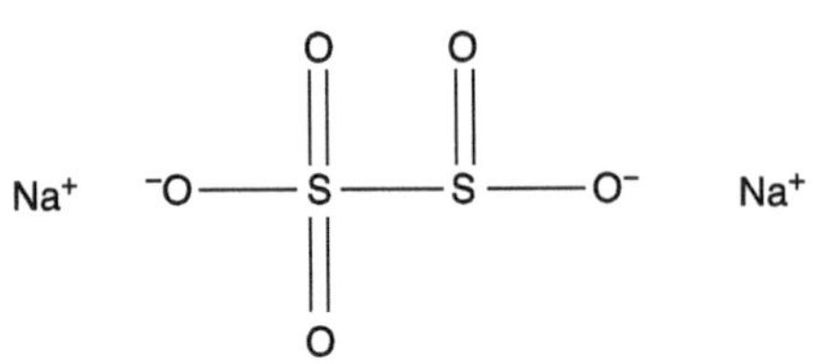

Other names: Disulfurous acid disodium salt, Sodium pyrosulfite
INCI: Sodium Metabisulfite
CAS no: 7681-57-4 / 7757-74-6
Molecular formula: $Na_2S_2O_6$
Molecular weight: 192.33
Rank of popularity: 317/502
Intended function: Antioxidant, Reducing agent
Log P: −3.03
Carcinogenic potential: Category 3 (use with precaution)
Allergenic potential: Weak sensitizer (max dose = 7.29 μg/cm^2/hr)

Sodium Methylparaben

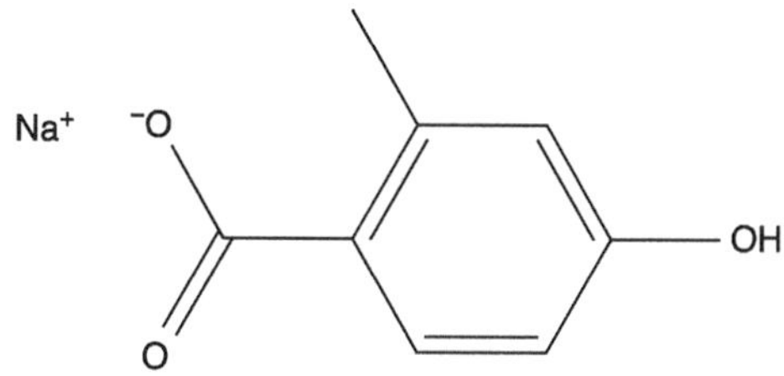

Other names: Sodium 4-carbomethoxyphenolate, Sodium p-methoxycarbonylphenoxide
INCI: Sodium Methylparaben
CAS no: 5026-62-0
Molecular formula: $C_8H_8O_3.Na$
Molecular weight: 175.13
Rank of popularity: 485/502
Intended function: Preservative
Carcinogenic potential: Category 3 (use with precaution)

Sodium Myristoyl Glutamate

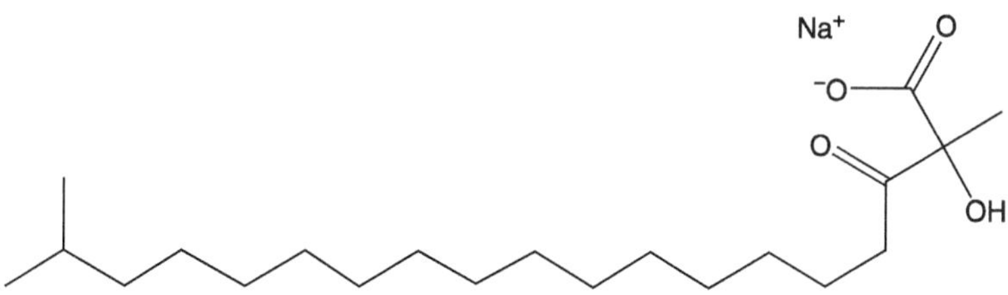

Other names: Sodium N-myristoyl-L-glutamate
INCI: Sodium Myristoyl Glutamate
CAS no: 38517-37-2/ 38754-83-5(dl-alpha)/ 71368-20-2
Molecular formula: $C_{19}H_{35}NO_5$ .Na
Molecular weight: 380.46
Rank of popularity: 486/502
Intended function: Cleansing agent

Sodium PCA

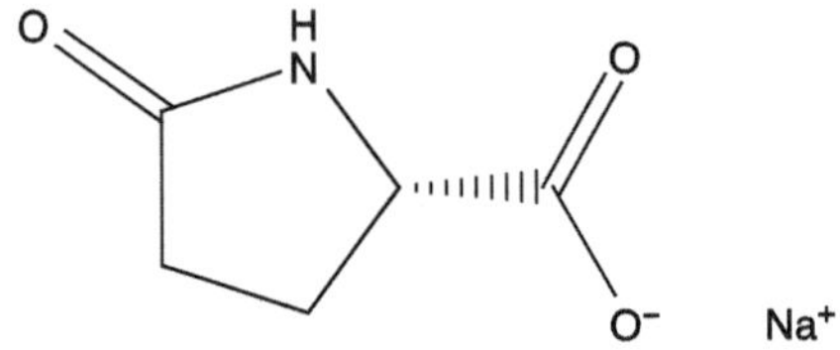

Sodium pyroglutamate

Other names: PCA soda, Sodium pyroglutamate
INCI: Sodium PCA
CAS no: 28874-51-3
Molecular formula: $C_5H_7NO_3 \cdot Na$
Molecular weight: 129.11
Rank of popularity: 72/502
Intended function: Hair conditioning, Humectant

Sodium Polyacrylate Starch

INCI: Sodium Polyacrylate Starch
Rank of popularity: 318/502
Intended function: Absorbent, Binder, Emulsion stabilizer, Film former, Viscosity increasing agent

Sodium Isostearoyl Lactylate

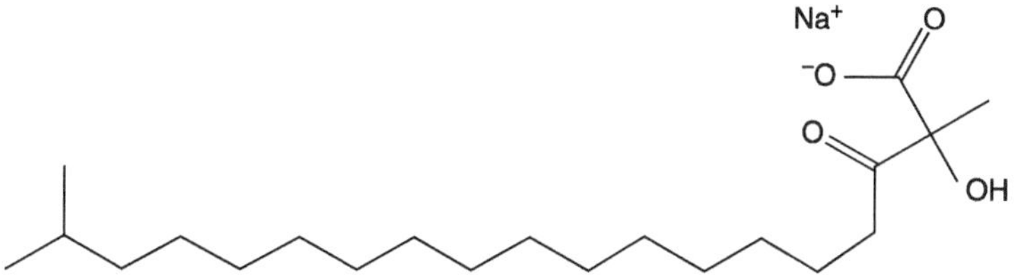

Other names: Sodium 2-(1-carboxylatoethoxy)-1-methyl-2-oxoethyl isooctadecanoate
INCI: Sodium Isostearoyl Lactylate
CAS no: 18200-72-1/25383-99-7
Molecular formula: $C_{24}H_{44}O_6$ .Na
Molecular weight: 379.52
Rank of popularity: 319/502
Intended function: Emulsifying agent
Allergenic potential: Maximum dose not stated

Sodium Sulfite

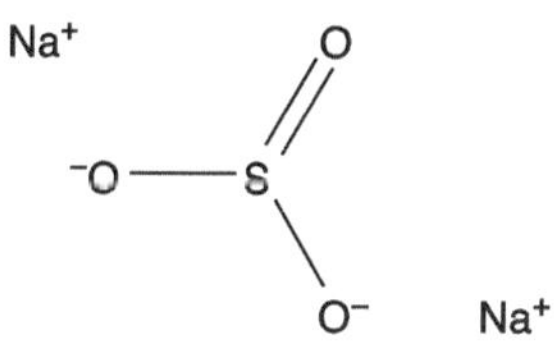

Other names: Anhydrous sodium sulfite, Natrii sulfis (EP), sulforous acid disodium salt
INCI: Sodium Sulfite
CAS no: 7757-83-7
Molecular formula: Na_2SO_3
Molecular weight: 174.27
Rank of popularity: 183/502
Intended function: Antioxidant, Hair curling/straightening agent, Reducing agent
Log P: –3.72
Carcinogenic potential: Category 3 (use with precaution)
Allergenic potential: Weak sensitizer (max dose = 7.29 μg/cm²/hr)

Sodium Sulphate

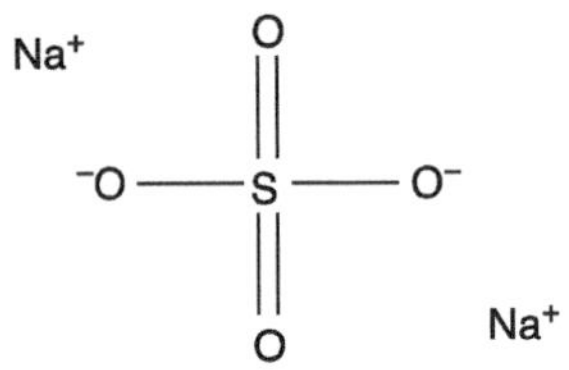

Sodium Sulfate

Other names: Disodium sulfate, Exsiccated sodium sulfate, Natrii sulfas
INCI: Sodium Sulfate
CAS no: 7727-73-3(decahydrate)/ 7757-82-6
Molecular formula: Na_2SO_4
Molecular weight: 144.06
Rank of popularity: 323/502
Intended function: Viscosity increasing agent
Allergenic potential: Maximum dose not stated

Soft White Paraffin

Other names: Mineral jelly, Petrolatum amber, Petrolatum white, Petrolatum jelly, White petrolatum, Yellow petrolatum
INCI: Petrolatum
CAS no: 8009-03-8(NF)
Rank of popularity: 38/502
Intended function: Hair conditioning, Occlusive agent, Skin protectant

Sorbic Acid

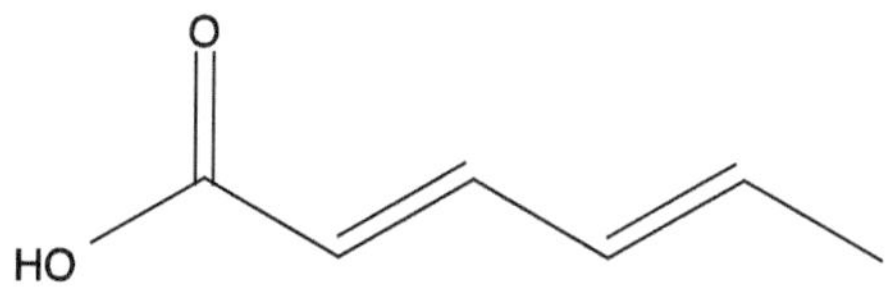

Other names: Acidum sorbicum, 2,4-hexadienoic acid
INCI: Sorbic Acid
CAS no: 110-44-1
Molecular formula: $C_6H_8O_2$
Molecular weight: 112.13
Rank of popularity: 149/502
Intended function: Fragrance, Preservative
Log P: 1.27
Carcinogenic potential: Category 3 (use with precaution)
Allergenic potential: Weak sensitizer (max dose = 8.33 μg/cm^2/hr)

Sorbitan Isostearate

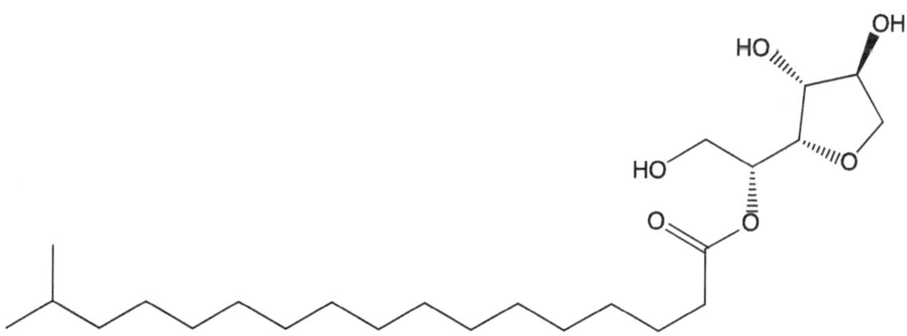

Other names: Sorbitan monoisostearate
INCI: Sorbitan Isostearate
CAS no: 54392-26-6/ 71902-01-7
Molecular formula: $C_{24}H_{46}O_6$
Molecular weight: 430.61
Rank of popularity: 320/502
Intended function: Emulsifying agent

Sorbitan Oleate

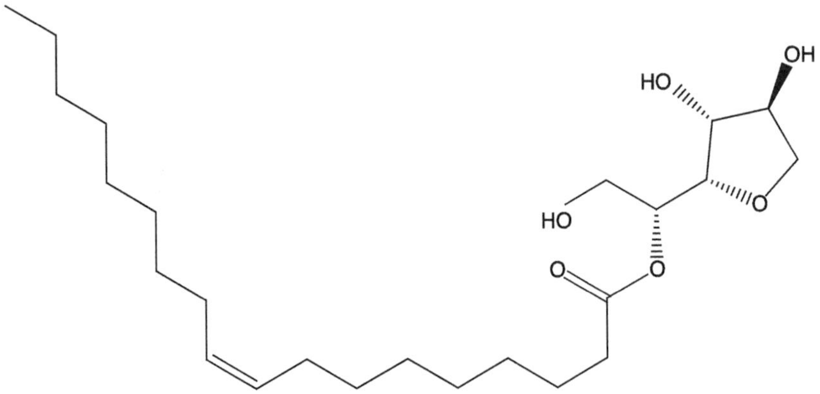

Other names: Alkamuls S80, Sorbitan monooleate
INCI: Sorbitan Oleate
CAS no: 1338-43-8/ 37318-79-9
Molecular formula: $C_{24}H_{44}O_6$
Molecular weight: 428.60
Rank of popularity: 126/502
Intended function: Fragrance, Emulsifying agent
Carcinogenic potential: Category 3 (use with precaution)

Sorbitan Stearate

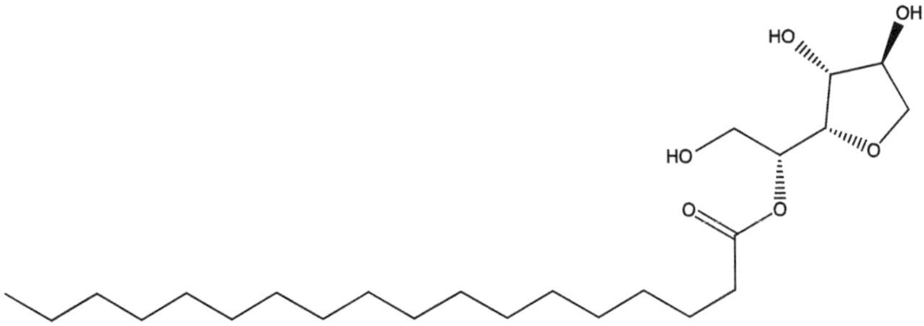

Other names: Sorbitan monostearate
INCI: Sorbitan Stearate
CAS no: 1338-41-6/ 5093-91-4/ 56451-84-4
Molecular formula: $C_{24}H_{46}O_6$
Molecular weight: 430.61
Rank of popularity: 63/502
Intended function: Emulsifying agent, Fragrance

Sorbitan Tristearate

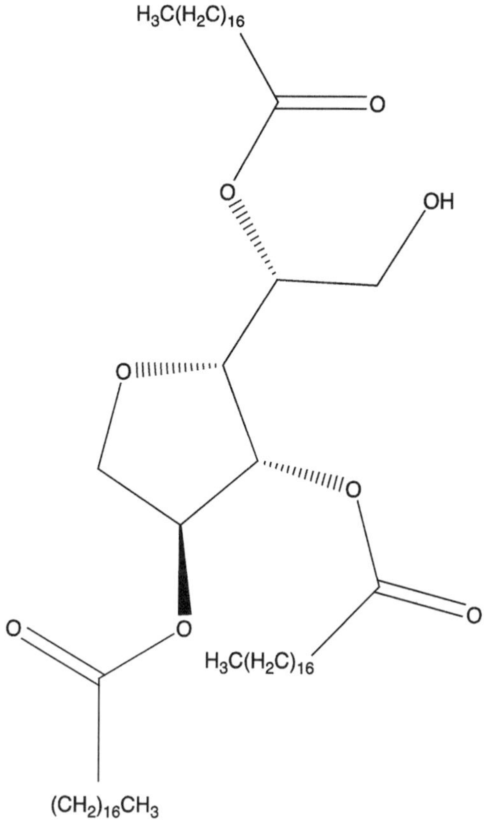

Other names: Anhydrosorbitol tristearate
INCI: Sorbitan Tristearate
CAS no: 26658-19-5
Molecular formula: $C_{60}H_{114}O_8$
Molecular weight: 963.54
Rank of popularity: 321/502
Intended function: Emulsifying agent

Sorbitol

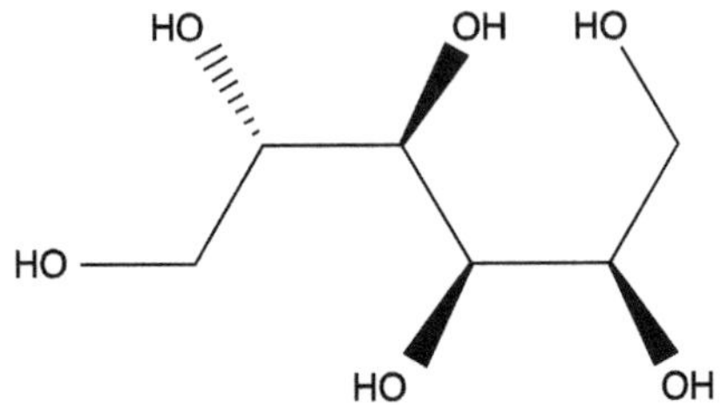

Other names: D-Glucitol, d-sorbitol, Sorbitolum
INCI: Sorbitol
CAS no: 50-70-4
Molecular formula: $C_6H_{14}O_6$
Molecular weight: 182.17
Rank of popularity: 54/502
Intended function: Flavouring agent, Fragrance, Humectant
Log P: −3.26
Allergenic potential: Weak sensitizer (max dose = 72.9 μg/cm²/hr)

Squalane

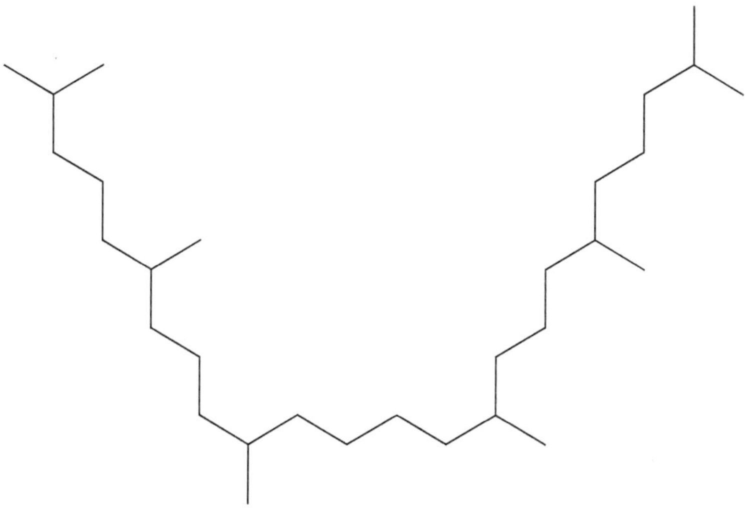

Other names: 2,6,10,15,19,23-Hexamethyltetracosane, Cosbiol, Perhydrosqualene, Robane
INCI: Squalane
CAS no: 111-01-3
Molecular formula: $C_{30}H_{62}$
Molecular weight: 422.81
Rank of popularity: 45/502
Intended function: Hair conditioning, Occlusive agent
Log P: 15.51

Stearalkonium Hectorite

Other names: Benzyldimethylstearylammonium hectorite
INCI: Stearalkonium Hectorite
CAS no: 12691-60-0/ 94891-33-5
Rank of popularity: 232/502
Intended function: Suspending agent
Allergenic potential: Maximum dose not stated

Stearamidopropyl Dimethylamine

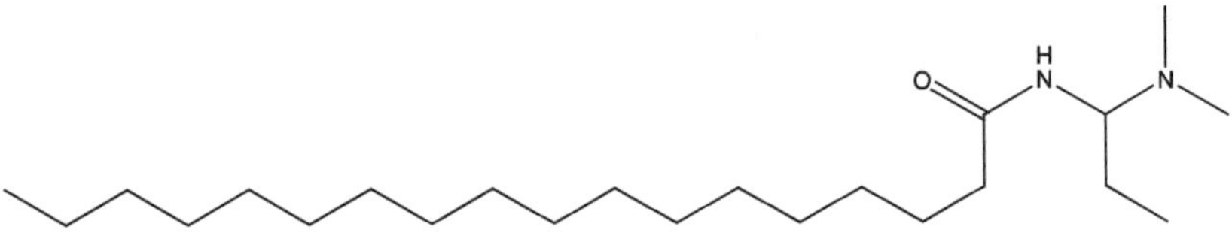

Other names: Dimethylaminopropyl stearamide
INCI: Stearamidopropyl Dimethylamine
CAS no: 7651-02-7/ 20182-63-2
Molecular formula: $C_{23}H_{48}N_2O$
Molecular weight: 368.64
Rank of popularity: 233/502
Intended function: Antistatic agent, Emulsifying agent, Hair conditioning
Log P: 7.62

Steareth-10

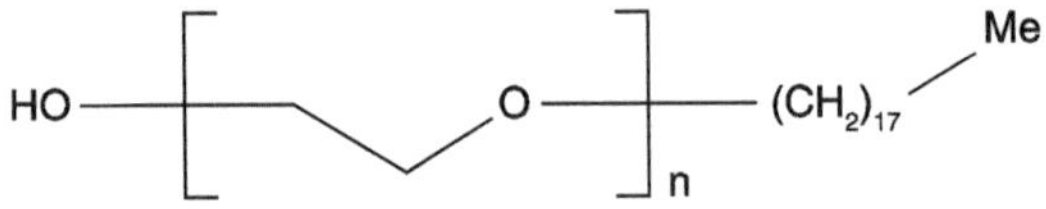

Other names: PEG-10 steryl ether, Polyethylene glycol(500) stearyl ether
INCI: Steareth-10
CAS no: 9005-00-9/ 13149-86-5
Molecular formula: $C_{38}H_{78}O_{11}$
Molecular weight: 711.02
Rank of popularity: 234/502
Intended function: Emulsifying agent
Log P: 5.85

Steareth-100

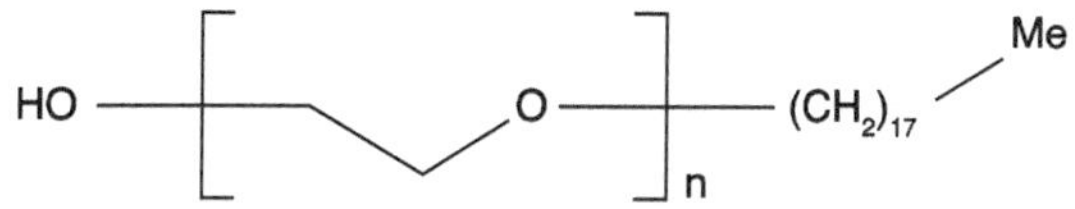

Other names: PEG-100 stearyl ether, Polyethylene glycol (100) stearyl ether
INCI: Steareth-100
CAS no: 9005-00-9
Rank of popularity: 322/502
Intended function: Cleansing agent, Solubilizing agent

Steareth-2

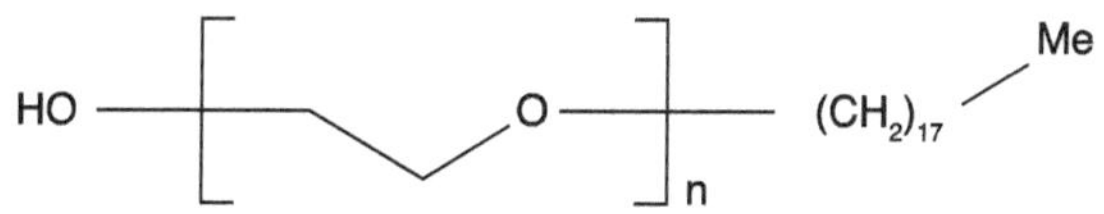

Other names: PEG-2 steryl ether, Polyethylene glycol (2) steryl ether
INCI: Steareth-2
CAS no: 9005-00-9/ 16057-43-5
Molecular formula: $C_{22}H_{46}O_3$
Molecular weight: 358.60
Rank of popularity: 235/502
Intended function: Emulsifying agent
Log P: 7.73

Stereth-21

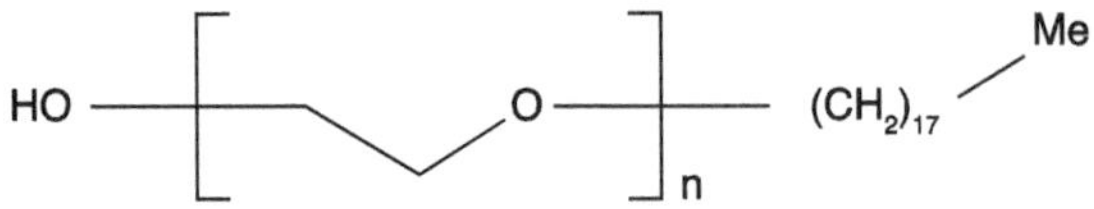

Other names: PEG-21 stearyl ether, Polyethylene glycol (21) stearyl ether
INCI: Steareth-21
CAS no: 9005-00-9
Rank of popularity: 324/502
Intended function: Cleansing agent, Emulsifying agent, Solubilizing agent

Stearic Acid

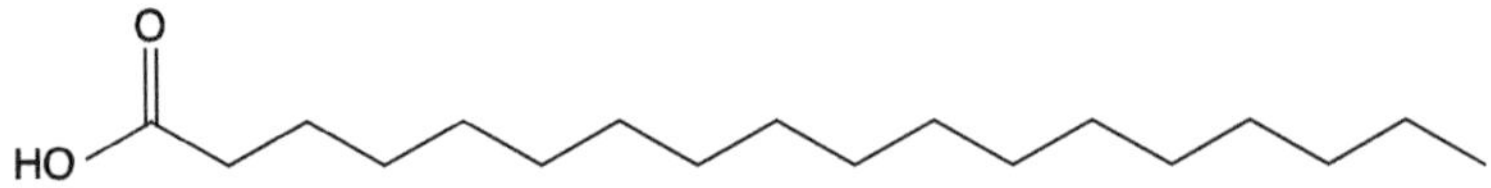

Other names: n-octadecanoic acid
INCI: Stearic Acid
CAS no: 57-11-4
Molecular formula: $C_{18}H_{36}O_2$
Molecular weight: 284.48
Rank of popularity: 12/502
Intended function: Cleansing agent, Emulsifying agent, Fragrance
Log P: 7.83
Allergenic potential: Very weak sensitizer (max dose = 94.8 μg/cm²/hr)

Stearoxytrimethylsilane

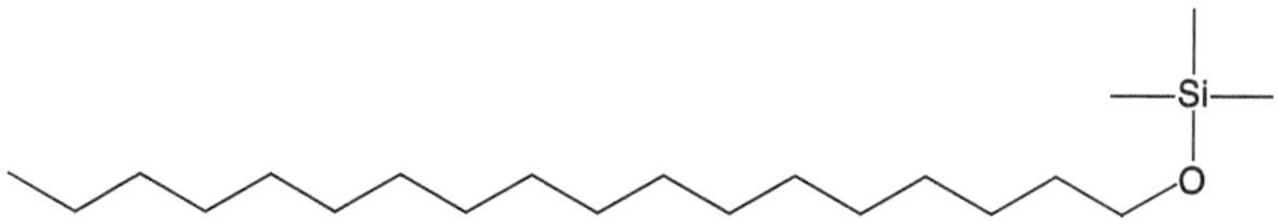

Other names: Trimethyl (octadecyloxy) silane
INCI: Stearoxytrimethylsilane
CAS no: 18748-98-6
Molecular formula: $C_{21}H_{46}OSi$
Molecular weight: 342.67
Rank of popularity: 234/502
Intended function: Emollient
Log P: 10.07

Stearyl Alcohol

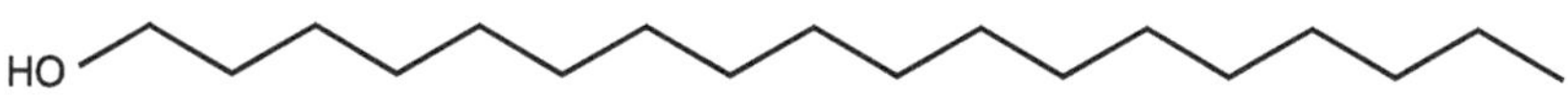

Other names: Alcohol stearylicus, 1 octadecanol
INCI: Stearyl Alcohol
CAS no: 112-92-5
Molecular formula: $C_{18}H_{38}O$
Molecular weight: 270.49
Rank of popularity: 21/502
Intended function: Emulsifying agent, Emulsion stabilizer, Foam booster, Fragrance, Opacifying agent, Viscosity increasing agent
Log P: 7.97
Allergenic potential: Very weak sensitizer (max dose = 218.8 μg/cm^2/hr)

Stearyl Benzoate

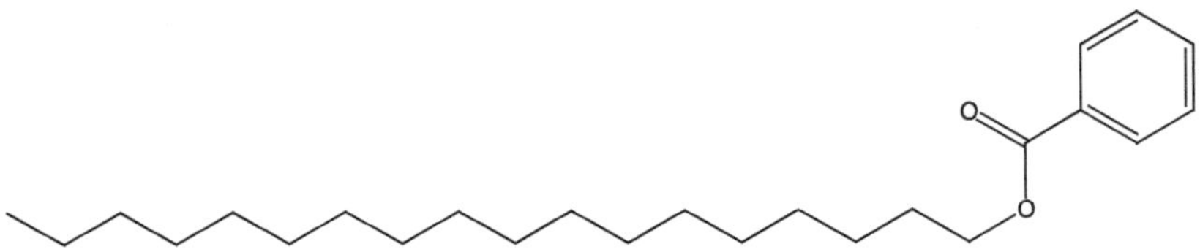

Other names: Octadecyl benzoate
INCI: Stearyl Benzoate
CAS no: 10578-34-4
Molecular formula: $C_{25}H_{42}O_2$
Molecular weight: 374.60
Rank of popularity: 488/502
Intended function: Emollient, Solvent
Log P: 10.79

Stearyl Dimethicone

Other names: Siloxanes and silicones di-Me me stearyl
INCI: Stearyl Dimethicone
CAS no: 67762-83-8
Rank of popularity: 325/502
Intended function: Occlusive agent

Stearyl Stearate

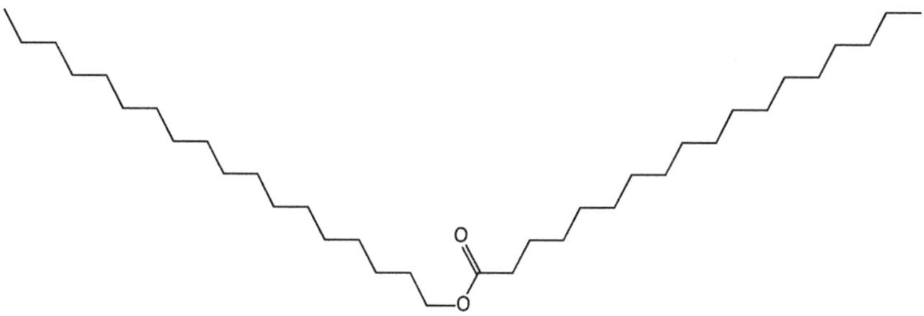

Other names: Octadecanoic acid octadecyl ester
INCI: Stearyl Stearate
CAS no: 2778-96-3
Molecular formula: $C_{36}H_{72}O_2$
Molecular weight: 536.96
Rank of popularity: 326/502
Intended function: Occlusive agent, Viscosity increasing agent
Log P: 17.09

Styrene/Acrylates Copolymer

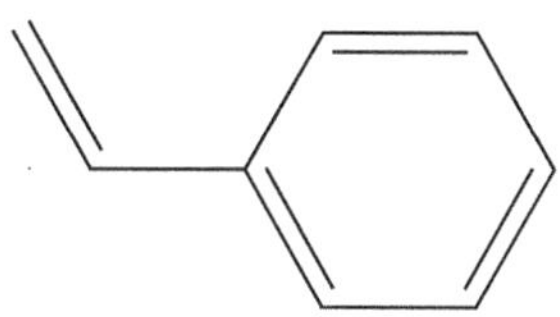

Styrene

INCI: Styrene/Acrylates Copolymer
CAS no: 9010-92-8/25034-86-0
Rank of popularity: 327/502
Intended function: Film former
Allergenic potential: Maximum dose not stated
Note: The structure does not represent the polymer. Only individual components are shown.

Sucrose Distearate

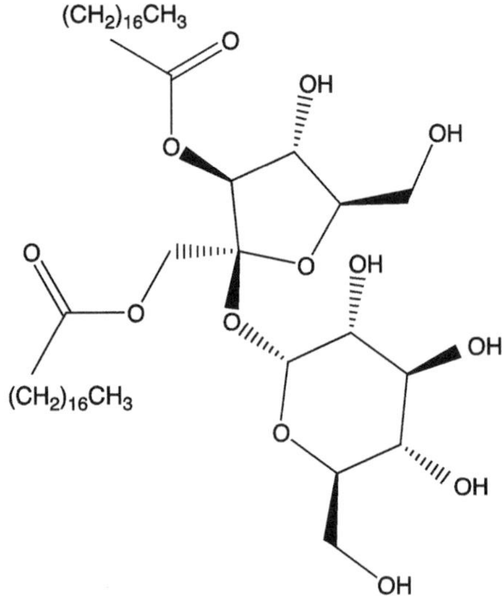

INCI: Sucrose Distearate
CAS no: 27195-16-0
Molecular formula: $C_{48}H_{90}O_{13}$
Molecular weight: 875.22
Rank of popularity: 489/502
Intended function: Emollient, Emulsifying agent

Sucrose Stearate

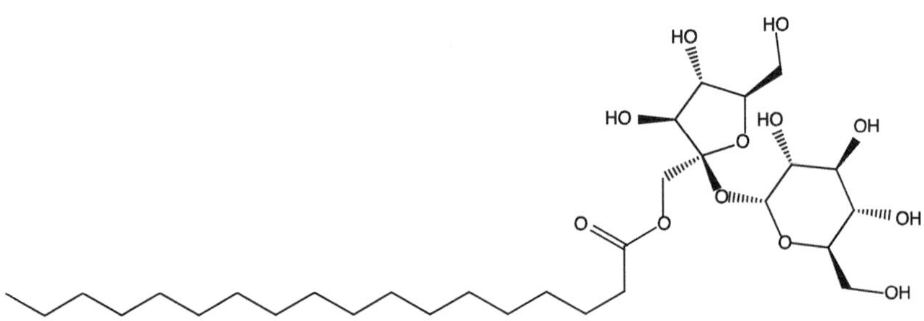

INCI: Sucrose Stearate
CAS no: 25168-73-4/ 37318-31-3
Molecular formula: $C_{30}H_{56}O_{12}$
Molecular weight: 608.75
Rank of popularity: 328/502
Intended function: Emollient, Emulsifying agent

Sulphur

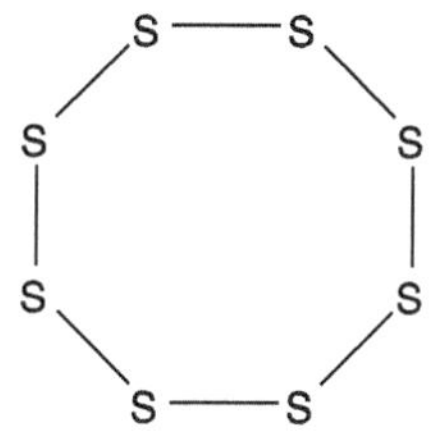

Other names: Flowers of sulfur
INCI: Sulphur
CAS no: 7704-34-9
Molecular formula: S
Molecular weight: 32.07
Rank of popularity: 329/502
Intended function: Antiacne agent, Antidandruff agent, Hair conditioning, Skin conditioning
Allergenic potential: Weak sensitizer (max dose = 72.9 μg/cm^2/hr)

T-butyl Alcohol

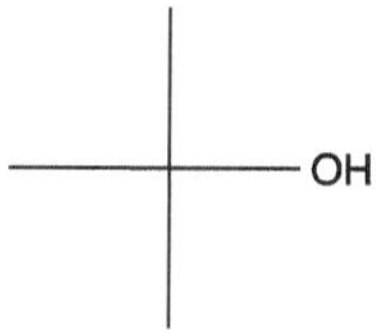

Other names: Tert-butanol, Trimethyl carbinol, Trimethylmenthanol
INCI: T-butyl Alcohol
CAS no: 75-65-0
Molecular formula: $C_4H_{10}O$
Molecular weight: 74.12
Rank of popularity: 490/502
Intended function: Denaturant, Fragrance, Solvent
Log P: 0.58
Carcinogenic potential: Category 1 (use within limit on body = 3.4 %w/w; face >100 % w/w; hands = 72.2 %w/w)
Allergenic potential: Maximum dose not stated

Tetradecanoyl-Octadecanoyl Behenate

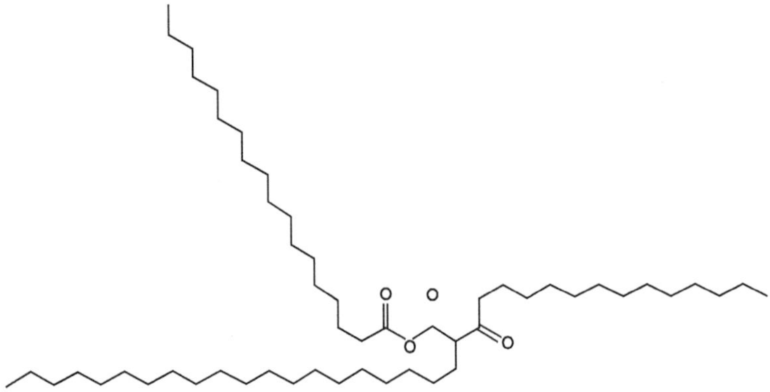

Rank of popularity: 491/502

Tetrahexyldecyl Ascorbate

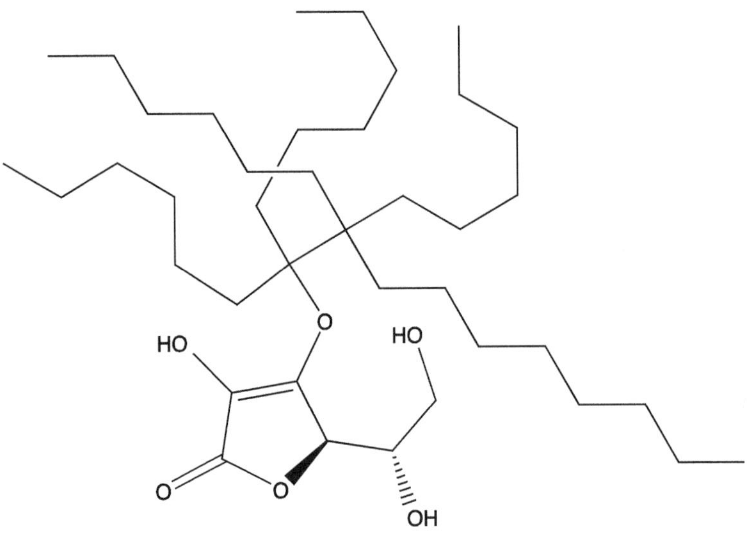

INCI: Tetrahexyldecyl Ascorbate
CAS no: 183476-82-6
Molecular formula: $C_{70}H_{128}O_{10}$
Molecular weight: 1129.76
Rank of popularity: 492/502
Intended function: Antioxidant, Skin conditioning
Log P: 26.15

Tetrasodium EDTA

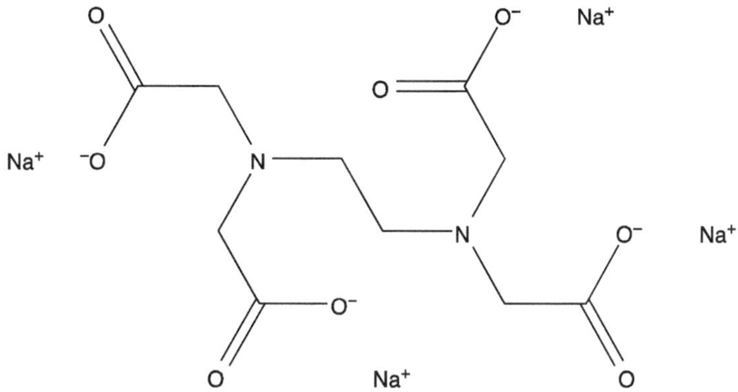

Other names: Edetate sodium, Tetrasodium edetate, Tetrasodium edetate dihydrate, Tetrasodium edetate tetrahydate
INCI: Tetrasodium EDTA
CAS no: 64-02-8
Molecular formula: $C_{10}H_{12}N_2O_8 \cdot 4Na$
Molecular weight: 378.18
Rank of popularity: 36/502
Intended function: Chelating agent

Titanium Dioxide

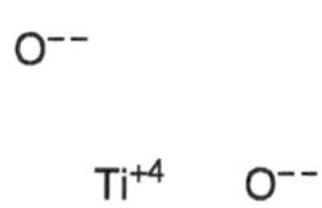

Other names: Amorphous titanium dioxide, Cl77891, Pigment white 6, Titanium oxide
INCI: Titanium Dioxide/ CI77891
CAS no: 13463-67-7
Molecular formula: TiO_2
Molecular weight: 79.86
Rank of popularity: 17/502
Intended function: Colourant, Opacifying agent, UV filter
Carcinogenic potential: Category 2 (safe to use)

Tocopheryl Acetate

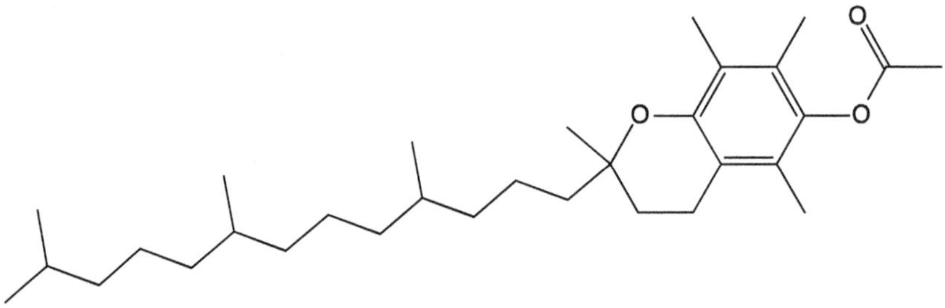

Other names: D-alpha-tocopheryl acetate, Vitamin E acetate
INCI: Tocopheryl Acetate
CAS no: 7695-91-2/ 58-95-7/52225-20-4
Molecular formula: $C_{31}H_{52}O_3$
Molecular weight: 472.74
Rank of popularity: 4/502
Intended function: Antioxidant, Skin conditioning
Log P: 10.69
Allergenic potential: Weak sensitizer (max dose = 29.2 μg/cm²/hr)

Tocopheryl Glucoside

INCI: Tocopheryl Glucoside
Rank of popularity: 184/502
Intended function: Emollient

Tribehenin

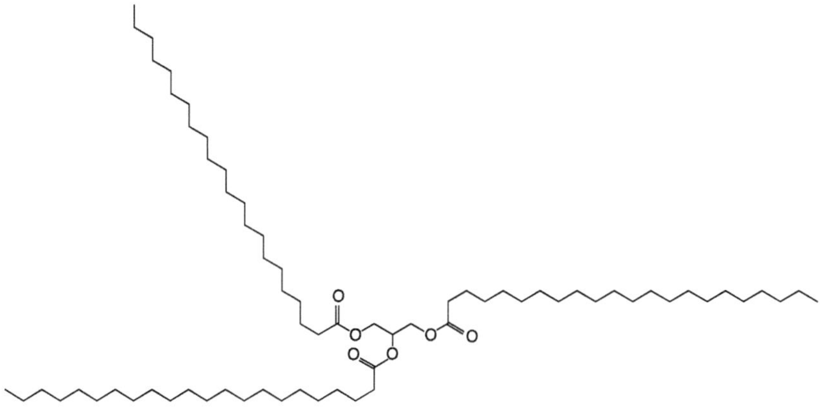

Other names: Glyceryl tribehenate, 1,2,3-propenetriol tridocosanoate
INCI: Tribehenin
CAS no: 18641-57-1
Molecular formula: $C_{69}H_{134}O_6$
Molecular weight: 1059.80
Rank of popularity: 150/502
Intended function: Occlusive agent
Log P: 30.79

Triclosan

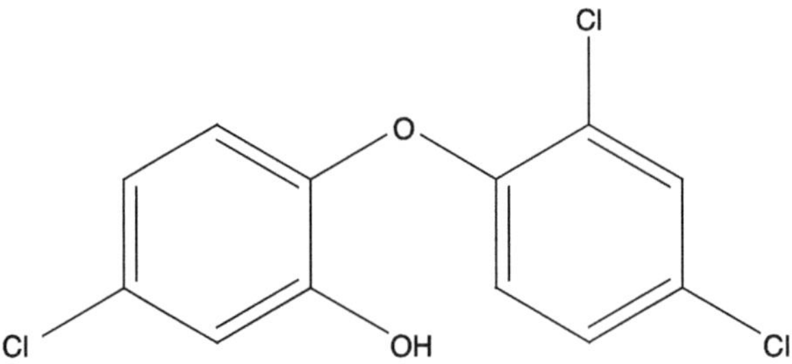

INCI: Triclosan
CAS no: 3380-34-5
Molecular formula: $C_{12}H_7Cl_3O_2$
Molecular weight: 289.54
Rank of popularity: 493/502
Intended function: Cosmetic biocide, Deodorant, Preservative
Log P: 5.34
Carcinogenic potential: Category 3 (use with precaution)
Allergenic potential: Weak sensitizer (max dose = 14.6 μg/cm^2/hr)

Triacontanyl PVP

INCI: Triacontanyl PVP
CAS no: 136445-69-7
Rank of popularity: 339/502
Intended function: Film foamer, Humectant, Viscosity increasing agent
Allergenic potential: Maximum dose not stated

Tridecanoin

Other names: Glceryl tridecanoate, Glyeryl tricaprate
INCI: Tricaprin
CAS no: 621-71-6
Molecular formula: $C_{33}H_{62}O_6$
Molecular weight: 554.84
Rank of popularity: 494/502
Intended function: Fragrance, Occlusive agent
Log P: 12.44

Trideceth-8

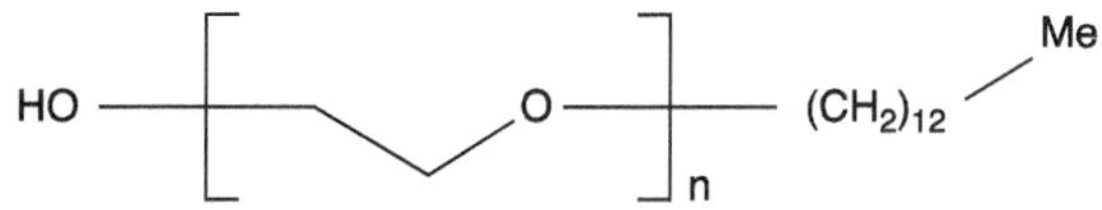

Other names: PEG-8 tridecyl ether, Polyethylene glycol 400 tridecyl ether
INCI: Trideceth-8
CAS no: 24938-91-8
Molecular formula: $C_{29}H_{60}O_9$
Molecular weight: 552.78
Rank of popularity: 495/502
Intended function: Emulsifying agent

Trideceth-9

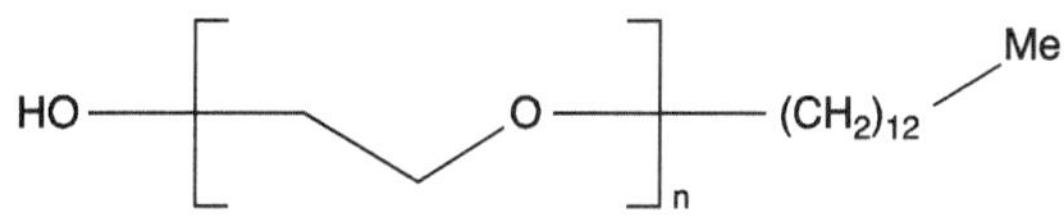

Other names: PEG-9 tridecyl ether, Polyethylene glycol 450 tridecyl ether
INCI: Trideceth-9
CAS no: 24938-91-8
Molecular formula: $C_{31}H_{64}O_{10}$
Molecular weight: 596.83
Rank of popularity: 496/502
Intended function: Emulsifying agent

Tridecyl Neopentanoate

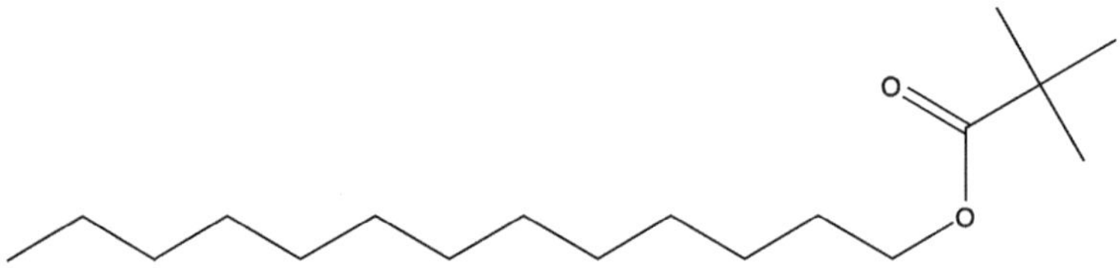

Other names: Neopentanoic acid tridecyl ester
INCI: Tridecyl Neopentanoate
CAS no: 106436-39-9
Molecular formula: $C_{18}H_{36}O_2$
Molecular weight: 284.47
Rank of popularity: 185/502
Intended function: Binder, Emollient

Triethanolamine

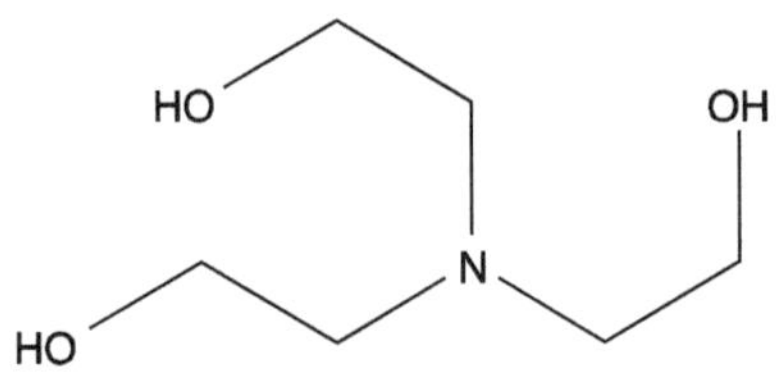

Other names: TEA, Trolamine
INCI: Triethanolamine
CAS no: 102-71-6
Molecular formula: $C_6H_{15}O_3N$
Molecular weight: 149.19
Rank of popularity: 10/502
Intended function: Emulsifying agent, Fragrance, ph adjuster
Log P: −0.99
Carcinogenic potential: Category 1 (use within limit on body = 1.0 %w/w; face = 64.2 %w/w; hands = 21.6 %w/w)
Allergenic potential: Weak sensitizer (max dose = 14.6 μg/cm^2/hr)

Triethoxycaprylylsilane

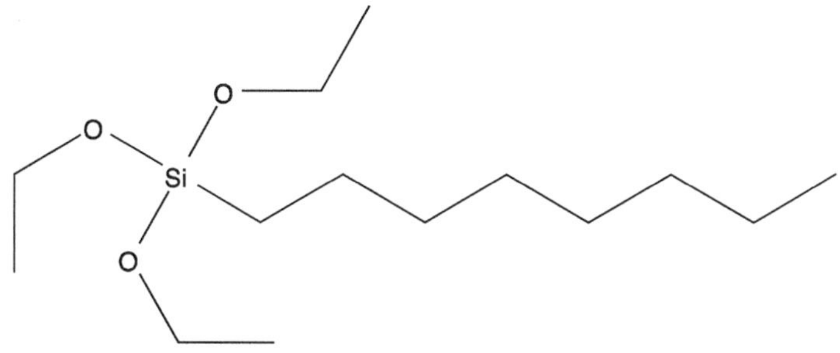

INCI: Triethoxycaprylylsilane
CAS no: 2943-75-1
Molecular formula: $C_{14}H_{32}O_3Si$
Molecular weight: 276.49
Rank of popularity: 151/502
Intended function: Binder
Log P: 6.75

Triethylhexanoin

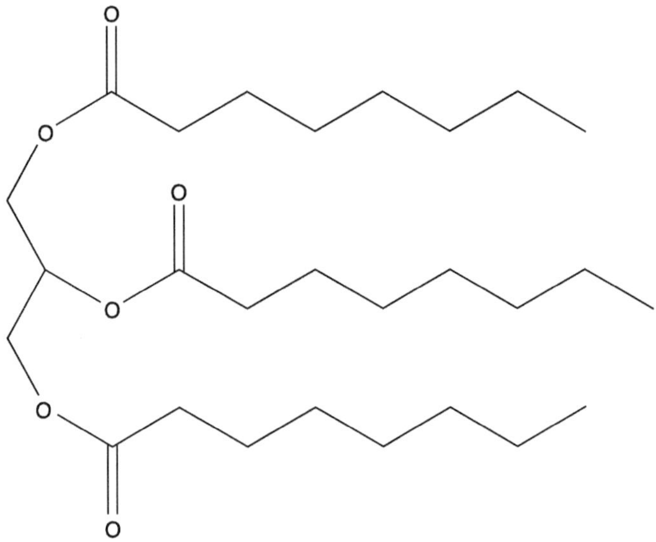

Other names: Trioctanoin
INCI: Triethylhexanoin
CAS no: 7360-38-5
Molecular formula: $C_{27}H_{50}O_6$
Molecular weight: 470.68
Rank of popularity: 497/502
Intended function: Fragrance, Hair conditioning, Occlusive agent
Log P: 8.92

Triglycerides

Rank of popularity: 502/502
Carcinogenic potential: Category 3 (use with precaution)

Triiron Tetraoxide (CI77499)

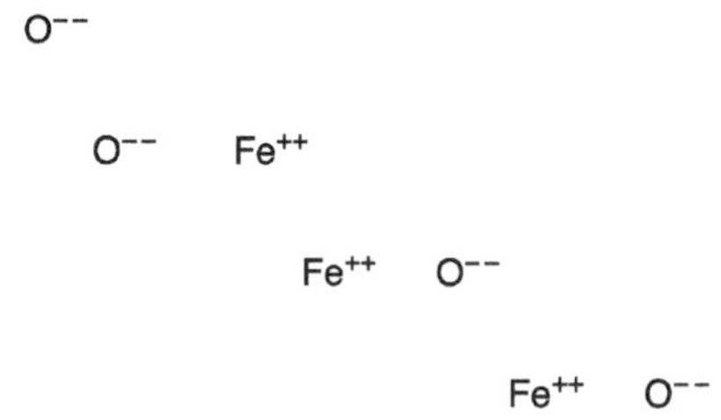

Other names: Iron oxides, Pigment brown 6 and 7, Black iron oxide, Ferrosoferric oxide, Megnetite, Pigment black 11
INCI: Cl77499
CAS no: 1317-61-9/ 1309-37-1/ 1345-25-1/ 1345-27-3/ 52357-70-7/ 12227-89-3
Rank of popularity: 237/502
Intended function: Colourant

Trimethoxycaprylylsilane

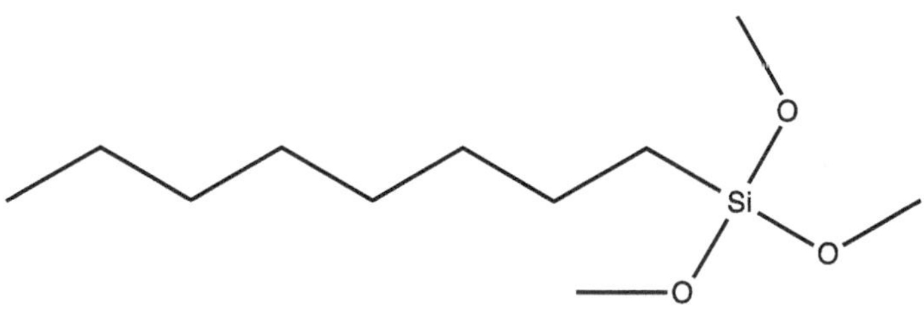

Other names: Trimethoxyoctylsilane
INCI: Trimethoxycaprylylsilane
CAS no: 3069-40-7
Molecular formula: $C_{11}H_{26}O_3Si$
Molecular weight: 234.41
Rank of popularity: 238/502
Intended function: Binder, Surface modifier
Log P: 5.22

Trimethylolpropane Triethylhexanoate

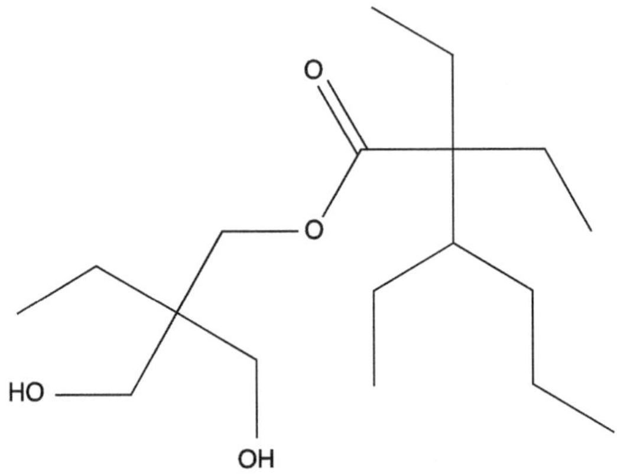

Other names: Trimethylolpropane trioctanoate
INCI: Trimethylolpropane Triethylhexanoate
CAS no: 26086-33-9
Molecular formula: $C_{30}H_{56}O_6$
Molecular weight: 512.76
Rank of popularity: 330/502
Intended function: Occlusive agent
Log P: 10.01

Trisodium EDTA

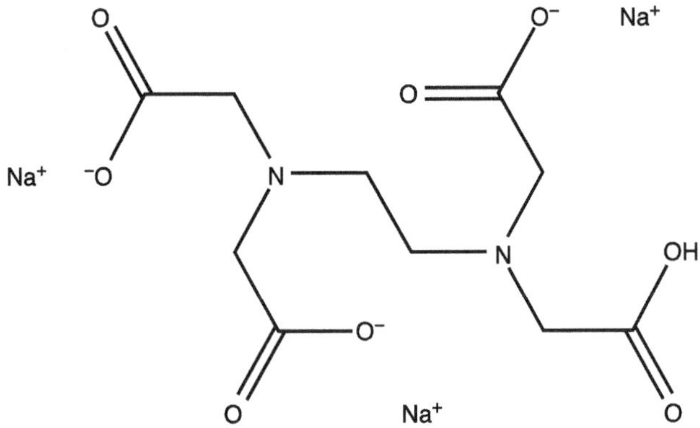

Other names: Edetate trisodium, Trisodium ethylenediamine tetraacetate
INCI: Trisodium EDTA
CAS no: 150-38-9
Molecular formula: $C_{10}H_{16}N_2O_8 \cdot 3Na$
Molecular weight: 355.19
Rank of popularity: 64/502
Intended function: Chelating agent

Tromethamine

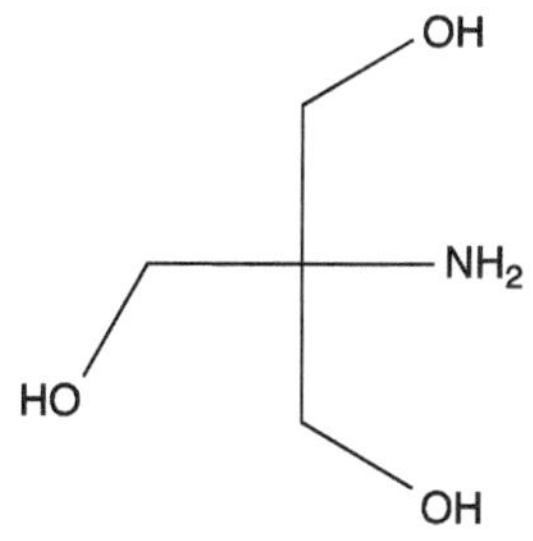

Other names: Tham, Tris (hydroxymethyl) amino methane, Trometamol
INCI: Tromethamine
CAS no: 77-86-1
Molecular formula: $C_4H_{11}NO_3$
Molecular weight: 121.14
Rank of popularity: 186/502
Intended function: Fragrance, pH adjuster
Log P: –2.52

Urea

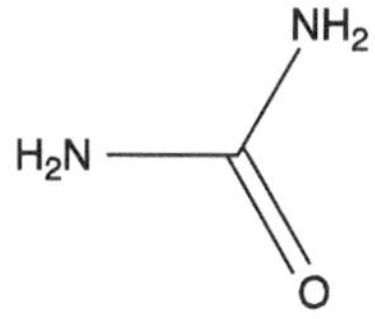

Other names: Carbamide, Urea perhydrate, Ureum
INCI: Urea
CAS no: 57-13-6
Molecular formula: CH_4N_2O
Molecular weight: 60.06
Rank of popularity: 152/502
Intended function: Buffering agent, Humectant
Log P: –1.66
Carcinogenic potential: Category 3 (use with precaution)

Vitamin B6 (Pyridoxine)

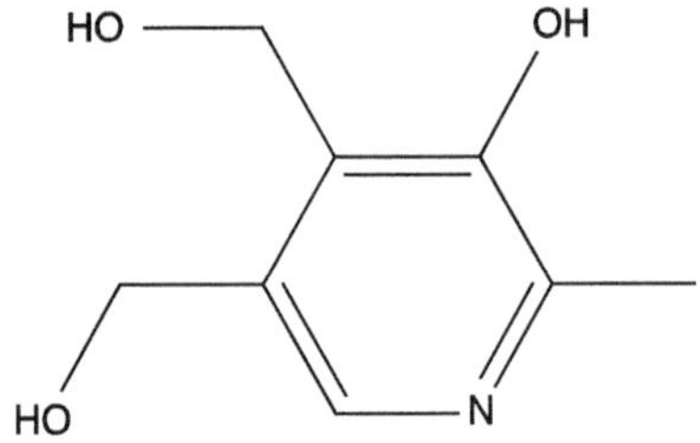

Other names: Pyridoxol, Vitamin B6
INCI: Pyridoxine
CAS no: 8059-24-3/65-23-6
Molecular formula: $C_8H_{11}NO_3$
Molecular weight: 262.12
Rank of popularity: 236/502
Intended function: Hair conditioning, Skin conditioning
Log P: –2.62
Allergenic potential: Weak sensitizer (max dose = 7.29 μg/cm²/hr)

Vitamin C (Ascorbic Acid)

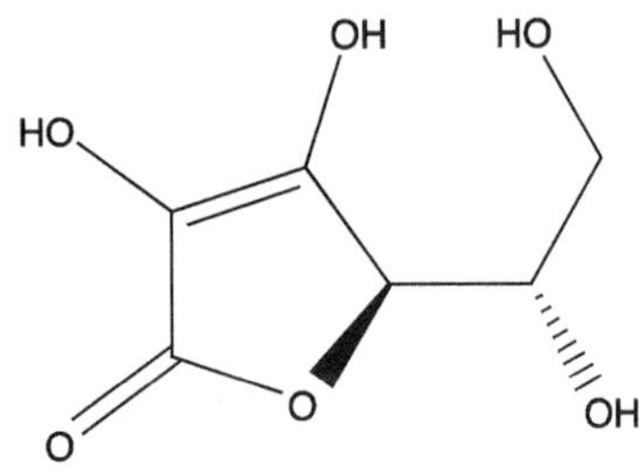

Other names: Vitamin C
INCI: Ascorbic acid
CAS no: 50-81-7 (Lform)/62624-30-0
Molecular formula: $C_6H_8O_6$
Molecular weight: 176.12
Rank of popularity: 128/502
Intended function: Antioxidant, Fragrance, pH adjuster, Skin conditioning
Log P: –2.78
Carcinogenic potential: Category 3 (use with precaution)

Vinyl pyrrolidone/Eicosene Copolymer

Other names: PVP/eicosene copolymer
INCI: VP/Eicosene Copolymer
CAS no: 28211-18-9/77035-98-4
Molecular formula: $(C_6H_9NO \cdot C_{20}H_{40})$
Rank of popularity: 187/502
Intended function: Binder, Film former, Suspending agent, Viscosity increasing agent
Allergenic potential: Maximum dose not stated

Water

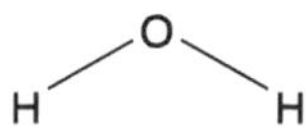

Other names: Aqua, Deionized water, Distilled water, Purified water
INCI: Water
CAS no: 7732-18-5
Molecular formula: H_2O
Molecular weight: 18.01
Rank of popularity: 1/502
Intended function: Skin conditioning, Solvent

Xanthan Gum

Other names: Corn sugar gum, Gummi xanthanum, Xanthan
INCI: Xanthan Gum
CAS no: 11138-66-2
Rank of popularity: 22/502
Intended function: Binder, Emulsifying agent, Emulsion stabilizer, Skin conditioning, Viscosity increasing agent

Xanthophyll

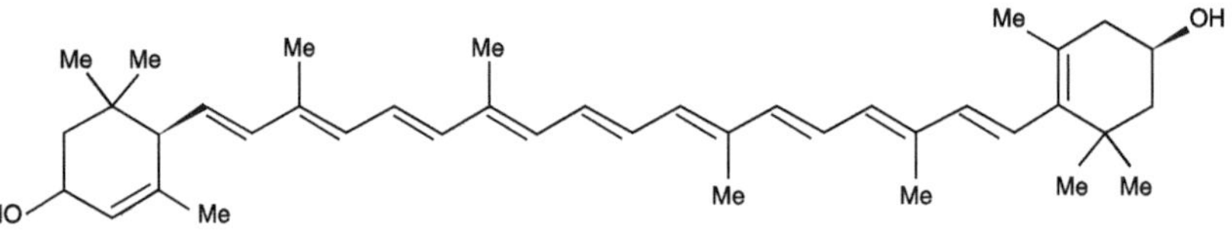

INCI: Xanthophyll
CAS no: 127-40-2
Molecular Formula: $C_{40}H_{56}O_2$
Molecular weight: 568.87
Rank of popularity: 499/502
Intended function: Occlusive agent

Yellow Petroleum Jelly

Other names: Petrolatum
INCI: Petrolatum
CAS no: 8009-03-8(NF)
Rank of popularity: 500/502
Intended function: Hair conditioning, Occlusive agent, Skin protectant

Zinc Gluconate

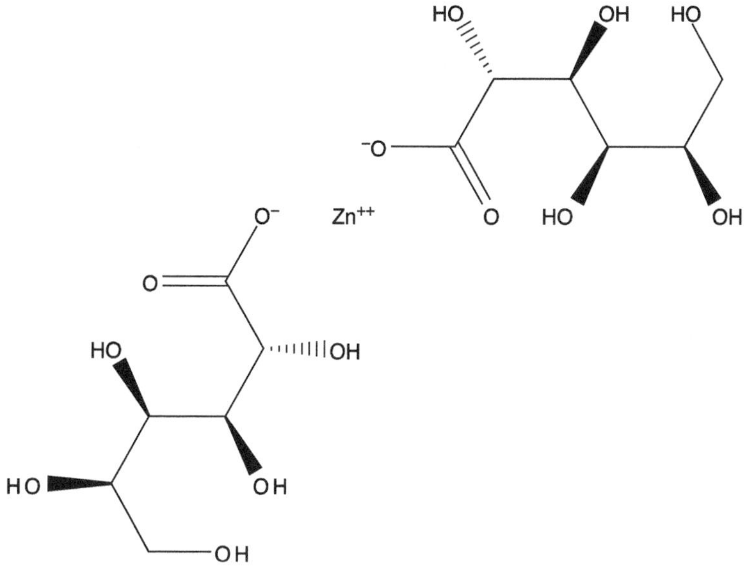

INCI: Zinc Gluconate
CAS no: 4468-02-4
Molecular formula: $C_{12}H_{22}O_{14} \cdot Zn$
Molecular weight: 455.67
Rank of popularity: 109/502
Intended function: Cosmetic biocide, Skin conditioning

Zinc Oxide

$Zn^{++} O^{-}$

INCI: Zinc Oxide
CAS no: 1314-13-2
Molecular formula: ZnO
Molecular weight: 81.37
Rank of popularity: 51/502
Intended function: Bulking agent, Colourant, Skin protectant, UV filter
Carcinogenic potential: Category 2 (safe to use)

Zinc PCA

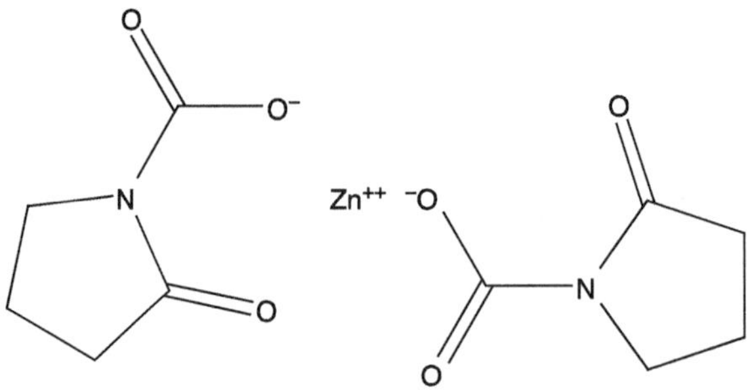

Other names: PCA zinc salt, L-pyrrolidone carboxylic acid zinc
INCI: Zinc PCA
CAS no: 68107-75-5 / 15454-75-8
Molecular formula: $C_5H_7NO_3 \cdot 1/2Zn$
Molecular weight: 161.83
Rank of popularity: 501/502
Intended function: Skin conditioning

Zinc Sulphate

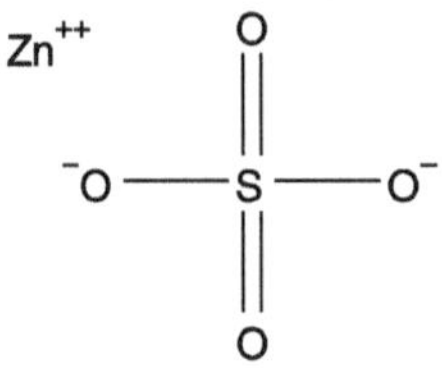

Zinc Sulfate

Other names: Sulfuric acid zinc salt, Zinci sulfas
INCI: Zinc Sulfate
CAS no: 7446-19-7(monohydrate)/ 7446-20-0(heptahydrate)/ 7733-02-0 (anhydrous)
Molecular formula: $ZnSO_4$
Molecular weight: 161.44
Rank of popularity: 502/502
Intended function: Astringent, Cosmetic biocide, Oral care agent
Carcinogenic potential: Category 3 (use with precaution)

Bibliography

Abe, M., Usuda, K., Hayashi, S., Ogawa, I., Furukawa, S., et al. (2008). Carcinogenic risk of copper gluconate evaluated by a rat medium-term liver carcinogenicity bioassay protocol. *Arch Toxicol*, 82, 563–571.

Abraham, M. H., Chadha, H. S. and Mitchell, R. C. (1995). The factors that influence skin penetration of solutes. *J Pharm Pharmacol*, 47, 8–16.

Abraham, M. H., Martins, F. and Mitchell, R. C. (1997). Algorithms for skin permeability using hydrogen bond descriptors: the problem of steroids. *J Pharm Pharmacol*, 49, 858–865.

ACS (1974). Natural Products. *Nomenclature of Organic Compounds*. American Chemical Society. doi:10.1021/ba-1974–0126.ch030.

Adams, R. M., Maibach, H. I., Clendenning, W. E., Fisher, A. A., Jordan, W. J., et al. (1985). A five-year study of cosmetic reactions. *J Am Acad Dermatol*, 13, 1062–1069.

Addo, H. A., Ferguson, J., Johnson, B. E. and Frain-Bell, W. (1982). The relationship between exposure to fragrance materials and persistent light reaction in the photosensitivity dermatitis with actinic reticuloid syndrome. *Br J Dermatol*, 107, 261–274.

Ahn, J. H., Eum, K. H. and Lee, M. (2010). Assessment of the dermal and ocular irritation potential of lomefloxacin by using *in vitro* methods. *Toxicol Res*, 26, 9–14.

Ali, M. A. and Konishi, T. (1998). Enhancement of hydroxyl radical generation in the fenton reaction by alpha-hydroxy acid. *Biochem Mol Biol Int*, 46, 137–145.

And, B. B. and Ros, A.-M. (1998). 7 years experience of photopatch testing with sunscreen allergens in Sweden. *Contact Dermatitis*, 38, 61–64.

Andersen, F. A. (1998). Final Report On the Safety Assessment of Glycolic Acid, Ammonium, Calcium, Potassium, and Sodium Glycolates, Methyl, Ethyl, Propyl, and Butyl Glycolates, and Lactic Acid, Ammonium, Calcium, Potassium, Sodium, and Tea-Lactates, Methyl, Ethyl, Isopropyl, and Butyl Lactates, and Lauryl, Myristyl, and Cetyl Lactates. *Int J Toxicol*, 17, 1–241.

Andersen, F. A. (1999a). Final Report on the Safety Assessment of Bisabolol. *Int J Toxicol*, 18, 33–40.

Andersen, F. A. (1999b). Final Report on the Safety Assessment of Ceteareth-2, -3, -4, -5, -6, -7, -8, -9, -10, -11, -12, -13, -14, -15, -16, -17, -18, -20, -22,

-23, -24, -25, -27, -28, -29, -30, -33, -34, -40, -50, -55, -60, -80, and -100. *Int J Toxicol*, 18, 41–49.

Andersen, K. E. and Goossens, A. (2006). Decyl glucoside contact allergy from a sunscreen product. *Contact Dermatitis*, 54, 349–350.

Andersen, K. E. and Hamann, K. (1984). How sensitizing is chlorocresol? *Contact Dermatitis*, 11, 11–20.

Andersen, K. E., Johansen, J. D., Bruze, M., Frosch, P. J., Goossens, A., et al. (2001). The time–dose–response relationship for elicitation of contact dermatitis in isoeugenol allergic individuals. *Toxicol Appl Pharmacol*, 170, 166–171.

Andrews, C. W., Bennett, L. and Yu, L. X. (2000). Predicting human oral bioavailability of a compound: development of a novel quantitative structure–bioavailability relationship. *Pharm Res*, 17, 639–644.

Anonymous (2005). British Contact Dermatitis Society: summaries of papers. *Br J Dermatol*, 153, 56–63.

Anonymous (2009). British Contact Dermatitis Society. *Br J Dermatol*, 161, 77–87.

Anonymous (2012). Oral Presentations. *Dermatitis*, 23, 134–145. doi:10.1097/DER.0b013e3182592e66.

Aptula, A. O., Roberts, D. W. and Pease, C. K. (2007). Haptens, prohaptens and prehaptens, or electrophiles and proelectrophiles. *Contact Dermatitis*, 56, 54–56.

ASEAN CD (2007a). *Appendix II – ASEAN Cosmetic Labeling Requirements* [Online]. Available: *http://www.hsa.gov.sg/publish/etc/medialib/hsa_library/health_products_regulation/cosmetic_products/files_1.Par.92896.File.dat/Appendix%20II%2004%20September%202007A.pdf* [Accessed 16 July 2013].

ASEAN CD (2007b). *Appendix III – ASEAN Cosmetic Claims Guidelines* [Online]. Available: *http://www.hsa.gov.sg/publish/etc/medialib/hsa_library/health_products_regulation/cosmetic_products/files_1.Par.79982.File.dat/Appendix%20III%2010%20September%202007A.pdf* [Accessed 16 July 2013].

ASEAN CD *Annexes of the ASEAN Cosmetic Directive* [Online]. Available: *http://www.fda.gov.ph/attachments/article/38607/Annex%20II%20revised%20as%20per%2017th%20ACSB.pdf* [Accessed 16 July 2013].

ASEAN CD *Appendix VI – ASEAN Guidelines for Cosmetic Good Manufacturing Practice* [Online]. Available: *http://www.hsa.gov.sg/publish/etc/medialib/hsa_library/health_products_regulation/cosmetic_products/files_1.Par.5910.File.dat/Appendix%20VIA.pdf* [Accessed 16 July 2013].

ASEAN CD *ASEAN Guidelines for safety evaluation of cosmetic products* [Online]. Available: *http://www.hsa.gov.sg/publish/etc/medialib/hsa_library/health_products_regulation/cosmetic_products/files_1.Par.99988.File.dat/* [Accessed 16 July 2013].

Avenel-Audran, M. (2010). Sunscreen products: finding the allergen. *Eur J Dermatol*, 20, 6.

Baan, R. A. (2007). Carcinogenic hazards from inhaled Carbon Black, Titanium Dioxide, and talc not containing asbestos or asbestiform fibers: recent evaluations by an IARC Monographs Working Group. *Inhal Toxicol*, 19, 213–228.

Bárány, E., Lindberg, M. and Lodén, M. (1999). Biophysical characterization of skin damage and recovery after exposure to different surfactants. *Contact Dermatitis*, 40, 98–103.

Barratt, M. D. (1995). Quantitative structure–activity relationships for skin permeability. *Toxicol In Vitro*, 9, 27–37.

Basketter, D. A., Roberts, D. W. and Crown, M. (1992). The value of the local lymph node assay in quantitative structure–activity investigations. *Contact Dermatitis*, 27, 137–142.

Basketter, D. A., Blaikie, L., Dearman, R. J., Kimber, I., Ryan, C. A., et al. (2000). Use of the local lymph node assay for the estimation of relative contact allergenic potency. *Contact Dermatitis*, 42, 344–348.

Basketter, D. A., Clapp, C., Jefferies, D., Safford, B., Ryan, C. A., et al. (2005). Predictive identification of human skin sensitization thresholds. *Contact Dermatitis*, 53, 260–267.

Beck, M. H. and Wilkinson, S. M. (2008). Contact dermatitis: allergic. *Rook's Textbook of Dermatology*. Blackwell Publishing, Inc., Massachusetts, USA. 10.1002/9780470750520.ch20.

Beeby, A. and Jones, A. E. (2000). The photophysical properties of menthyl anthranilate: a UV-A sunscreen. *Photochem Photobiol*, 72, 10–15.

Bindu Nair (1998). Final Report On the Safety Assessment of Polyvinyl Alcohol. *Int J Toxicol*, 17, 67–92.

Blank, I. H. (1964). Penetration of low-molecular-weight alcohols into skin. I. Effect of concentration of alcohol and type of vehicle. *J Invest Dermatol*, 43, 415–420.

Blaut, M., Braune, A., Wunderlich, S., Sauer, P., Schneider, H. and Glatt, H. (2006). Mutagenicity of arbutin in mammalian cells after activation by human intestinal bacteria. *Food Chem Toxicol*, 44, 1940–1947.

Bohle, A., Ruschgerdes, S., Ulmer, A. J., Braasch, H. and Jocham, D. (1996). The effect of lubricants on viability of bacillus Calmette-Guerin for intravesical immunotherapy against bladder carcinoma. *J Urol*, 155, 1892–1896.

Bolognia, J. L., Jorizzo, J. L. and Rapini, R. P. (2003). *Dermatology*, Mosby. Missouri, USA.

Bos, J. D. and Meinardi, M. M. (2000). The 500 Dalton rule for the skin penetration of chemical compounds and drugs. *Exp Dermatol*, 9, 165–169.

Bouwstra, J. A. and Honeywell-Nguyen, P. L. (2002). Skin structure and mode of action of vesicles. *Adv Drug Deliv Rev*, 54, S41–S55.

Brain, K. R., Walters, K. A., and Watkinson, A. C. (1998). Investigation of skin permeation *in vitro*. *Drugs Pharm Sci*, 91, 161–187.

Brisson, P. (1974). Percutaneous absorption. *Can Med Assoc J*, 110, 1182–1185.

Broeckx, W., Blondeel, A., Dooms-Goossens, A. and Achten, G. (1987). Cosmetic intolerance. *Contact Dermatitis*, 16, 189–194.

Bronaugh, R. L. and Stewart, R. F. (1985). Methods for *in vitro* percutaneous absorption studies IV: The flow-through diffusion cell. *J Pharm Sci*, 74, 64–67.

Brown, M. B. (2003). Transdermal drug delivery. In: Jain, K. K. (ed.) *Drug Delivery Systems, Second Edition*. Basel: CRC Press.doi:10.1201/9781420040142.ch6.

Buhrv, J. N. 1980. Photo allergies from benzophenones and beta carotene in sunscreens. *Contact Dermatitis*, 6, 211–239.

Bunge, A. L. and Cleek, R. L. (1995). A new method for estimating dermal absorption from chemical exposure: 2. Effect of molecular weight and octanol–water partitioning. *Pharm Res*, 12, 88–95.

Bunge, A. L., Cleek, R. L. and Vecchia, B. E. (1995). A new method for estimating dermal absorption from chemical exposure. 3. Compared with steady-state methods for prediction and data analysis. *Pharm Res*, 12, 972–982.

Byford, J. R., Shaw, L. E., Drew, M. G. B., Pope, G. S., Sauer, M. J. and Darbre, P. D. (2002). Oestrogenic activity of parabens in MCF7 human breast cancer cells. *J Steroid Biochem Mol Biol*, 80, 49–60.

Cevc, G. (1997). Drug delivery across the skin. *Exp Opin Invest Drugs*, 6, 1887–1937.

CFR (Code of Federal Regulation) 21 C.F.R. Sect. 73(C), 1974. Colourants.

CFR (Code of Federal Regulation) 21 C.F.R. Sect. 700.25, 1983. Tamper-resistant packaging requirements for cosmetic products.

CFR (Code of Federal Regulation) 21 C.F.R. Sect. 740.11, 1996. Cosmetics in self-pressurized containers.

CFR (Code of Federal Regulation) 21 C.F.R. Sect. 701.3, 2004. Designation of ingredients.

CFR (Code of Federal Regulation) 21 C.F.R. Sect. 250.250, 2004. Hexachlorophene, as a component of drug and cosmetic products.

CFR (Code of Federal Regulation) 21 C.F.R. Sect. 700(B), 2008. Requirements for specific cosmetic products.

Chapman, W. H., Kirchhei, D and McRobert, J. (1973). Effect of urine and calculus formation on incidence of bladder tumors in rats implanted with paraffin wax pellets. *Cancer Res*, 33, 1225–1229.

Charles, A. K. and Darbre, P. D. (2009). Oestrogenic activity of benzyl salicylate, benzyl benzoate and butylphenylmethylpropional (Lilial) in MCF7 human breast cancer cells *in vitro*. *J Appl Toxicol*, 29, 422–434.

Chen, W., Weisburger, J. H., Fiala, E. S., Spratt, T. E., Carmella, S. G., et al. (1996). Gastric carcinogenesis: 2-chloro-4-methylthiobutanoic acid, a novel mutagen in salted, pickled Sanma hiraki fish, or similarly treated methionine. *Chem Res Toxicol*, 9, 58–66.

Cheng, S. L., Liu, R. H., Sheu, J. N., Chen, S. T., Sinchaikul, S. and Tsay, G. J. (2006). Toxicogenomics of kojic acid on gene expression profiling of A375 human malignant melanoma cells. *Biol Pharm Bull*, 29, 655–669.

Christfnsen, O. B. and Wall, L. M. (1987). Open, closed and intradermal testing in nickel allergy. *Contact Dermatitis*, 16, 21–26.

Cilurzo, F., Minghetti, P. and Sinico, C. (2007). Newborn pig skin as model membrane in *in vitro* drug permeation studies: a technical note. *AAPS PharmSciTech*, 8.

CIR (2007). Amended final report on the safety assessment of glyceryl dilaurate, glyceryl diarachidate, glyceryl dibehenate, glyceryl dierucate, glyceryl dihydroxystearate, glyceryl diisopalmitate, glyceryl diisostearate, glyceryl dilinoleate, glyceryl dimyristate, glyceryl dioleate, glyceryl diricinoleate, glyceryl dipalmitate, glyceryl dipalmitoleate, glyceryl distearate, glyceryl palmitate lactate, glyceryl stearate citrate, glyceryl stearate lactate, and glyceryl stearate succinate. *Int J Toxicol*, 26 Suppl 3, 1–30.

Clarkeburn, H. (2002). A test for ethical sensitivity in science. *J Moral Educ*, 31, 439–453.

Cleek, R. L. and Bunge, A. L. (1993). A new method for estimating dermal absorption from chemical exposure. 1. General approach. *Pharm Res*, 10, 497–506.

Coronado, M., De Haro, H., Deng, X., Rempel, M. A., Lavado, R. and Schlenk, D. (2008). Estrogenic activity and reproductive effects of the UV-filter oxybenzone (2-hydroxy-4-methoxyphenyl-methanone) in fish. *Aquat Toxicol*, 90, 182–187.

Cronin, M. T. D. and Dearden, J. C. (1997). Correspondence analysis of the skin sensitization potential of organic chemicals. *QSAR Comb Sci*, 16, 33–37.

Culp, S. J., Warbritton, A. R., Smith, B. A., Li, E. E. and Beland, F. A. (2000). DNA adduct measurements, cell proliferation and tumor mutation induction in relation to tumor formation in B6C3F1 mice fed coal tar or benzo[a]pyrene. *Carcinogenesis*, 21, 1433–1440.

De Groot, A. C., Berretty, P. J. M., Van Ginkel, C. J. W., Den Hengst, C. W., Van Ulsen, J. and Weyland, J. W. (1991). Allergic contact dermatitis from tocopheryl acetate in cosmetic creams. *Contact Dermatitis*, 25, 302–304.

De Waard-van der Spek, F. B. and Oranje, A. P. (2009). Patch tests in children with suspected allergic contact dermatitis: a prospective study and review of the literature. *Dermatology*, 218(2), 119–125.

Demir, E., Kocaoglu, S. and Kaya, B. (2008). Genotoxicity testing of four benzyl derivatives in the Drosophila wing spot test. *Food Chem Toxicol*, 46, 1034–1041.

Dick, I. P. and Scott, R. C. (1992). Pig ear skin as an *in vitro* model for human skin permeability. *J Pharm Pharmacol*, 44, 640–645.

Dizon, M., Galzote, C., Estanislao, R., Mathew, N. and Sarkar, R. (2010). Tolerance of baby cleansers in infants: a randomized controlled trial. *Indian Pediatr*, 47, 959–963.

Dromgoole, S. H. and Maibach, H. I. (1990). Sunscreening agent intolerance: contact and photocontact sensitization and contact urticaria. *J Am Acad Dermatol*, 22, 1068–1078.

Dubey, S. and Kalia, Y. N. (2011). Electrically-assisted delivery of an anionic protein across intact skin: cathodal iontophoresis of biologically active ribonuclease T1. *J Control Release*, 152, 356–362.

EC (European Commission) (2009). Regulation No 1223/2009 of the European Parliament and of the Council of 30 November 2009 on Cosmetic Products.

EC (European Commission) (2013). *Regulatory framework* [Online]. Available: *http://ec.europa.eu/consumers/sectors/cosmetics/regulatory-framework/index_en.htm* [Accessed 16 July 2013].

Egles, C., Garlick, J. A. and Shamis, Y. (2010). Three-dimensional human tissue models of wounded skin. *Meth Mol Biol*, 585, 345–359.

El-Kattan, A., Asbill, C. S. and Haidar, S. (2000). Transdermal testing: practical aspects and methods. *Pharm Sci Technol Today*, 3, 426–430.

Esteve, J. (1996). Changes in incidence and mortality from breast cancer in England and Wales since introduction of screening. *Revue D Epidemiologie et de Sante Publique*, 44, 189–191.

European Multicentre Photopatch Test Study, (2012). A European multicentre photopatch test study. *Br J Dermatol*, 166, 1002–1009.

FD and C Act 1993. Listing and certification of colour additives for foods, drugs, devices, and cosmetics.

Fisher, A. A. (1978). Immediate and delayed allergic contact reactions to polyethylene glycol. *Contact Dermatitis*, 4, 135–138.

Flynn, G. L. (1990). Physicochemical determinants of skin absorption. In: *Principles of Route-to-route Extrapolation for Risk Assessment*. T. R. Gerrity and C. J. Henry (eds), Elsevier, New York, 93–127.

Forsbeck, M. and Skog, E. (1977). Immediate reactions to patch tests with balsam of Peru. *Contact Dermatitis*, 3, 201–205.

Fotiades, J., Soter, N. A. and Lim, H. W. (1995). Results of evaluation of 203 patients for photosensitivity in a 7.3-year period. *J Am Acad Dermatol*, 33, 597–602.

Frasch, H. F. (2010). *Skin Permeation Calculator*. US National Institute for Occupational Safety and Health, Education and Information Division. Atlanta, USA.

Friend, D. R. (1992). *In vitro* skin permeation techniques. *J Control Release*, 18, 235–248.

Frum, Y., Eccleston, G. M. and Meidan, V. M. (2007). Evidence that drug flux across synthetic membranes is described by normally distributed permeability coefficients. *Eur J Pharm Biopharm*, 67, 434–439.

Fukushima, S., Thamavit, W., Kurata, Y. and Ito, N. (1986). Sodium citrate: a promoter of bladder carcinogenesis. *Jpn J Cancer Res*, 77, 1–4.

Gallo, R., Sacco, D. D. and Ghigliotti, G. (2004). Allergic contact dermatitis from VP/eicosene copolymer (Ganex® V-220) in an emollient cream. *Contact Dermatitis*, 50, 261.

Gao, A., Song, S. S., Wang, D. L., Peng, W. and Tian, L. (2009). Effect of silicon dioxide on expression of poly (ADP-Ribose) polymerase mRNA and protein. *Cell Biol Int*, 33, 749–754.

Gao, X.-H., Zhang, L., Wei, H. and Chen, H.-D. (2008). Efficacy and safety of innovative cosmeceuticals. *Clin Dermatol*, 26, 367–374.

GCi (2013). *New Research Says Cosmeceuticals Rank as the Fastest Growing Beauty Category* [Online]. Available: *http://www.gcimagazine.com/marketstrends/segments/antiaging/189246721.html?utm_source—ost+Read&utm_medium=website&utm_campaign—ost+Read* [Accessed 17 June 2013].

Gee, R. H., Charles, A., Taylor, N. and Darbre, P. D. (2008). Oestrogenic and androgenic activity of triclosan in breast cancer cells. *J Appl Toxicol*, 28, 78–91.

Gerberick, F. G., Ryan, C. A., Dearman, R. J. and Kimber, I. (2007). Local lymph node assay (LLNA) for detection of sensitization capacity of chemicals. *Methods*, 41, 54–60.

Gerberick, F. G., Ryan, C. A., Kern, P. S., Dearman, R. J., Kimber, I., et al. (2004). A chemical dataset for evaluation of alternative approaches to skin-sensitization testing. *Contact Dermatitis*, 50, 274–288.

Gerberick, F. G., Ryan, C. A., Kern, P. S., Schlatter, H., Dearman, R. J., et al. (2005). Compilation of historical local lymph node data for evaluation of skin sensitization alternative methods. *Dermatitis*, 16, 157–202.

Gilpin, S., Hui, X. and Maibach, H. (2010). *In vitro* human skin penetration of geraniol and citronellol. *Dermatitis*, 21, 41–48.

Giovinazzo, V. J., Harber, L. C., Armstrong, R. B. and Kochevar, I. E. (1980). Photoallergic contact dermatitis to musk ambrette: clinical report of two patients with persistent light reactor patterns. *J Am Acad Dermatol*, 3, 384–393.

Giri, A. K. and Mukherjee, A. (1990). Sister chromatid exchange induced by secondary and tertiary amine containing dyes and in combination with nitrite *in vivo* in mice. *Cancer Letters*, 52, 33–37.

Godin, B. and Touitou, E. (2007). Transdermal skin delivery: predictions for humans from *in vivo*, *ex vivo* and animal models. *Adv Drug Deliv Rev*, 59, 1152–1161.

Gokdemir, G., Ari, S. and Koslu, A. (2008). Assessment of knowledge about skin care among Turkish people. *Turkderm-Archives of the Turkish Dermatology and Venerology*, 42, 60–63.

Goldberg, M. S., Parent, M. E., Siemiatycki, J., Desy, M., Nadon, L., et al. (2001). A case-control study of the relationship between the risk of colon cancer in men and exposures to occupational agents. *Am J Ind Med*, 39, 531–546.

Goossens, A. (2009). Recognizing and testing allergens. *Dermatol Clin*, 27, 219–226.

Goossens, A. (2011). Contact-allergic reactions to cosmetics. *J Allergy*, 2011, 467071.

Goossens, A., Armingaud, P., Avenel-Audran, M., Begon-Bagdassarian, I., Constandt, L., et al. (2002). An epidemic of allergic contact dermatitis due to epilating products. *Contact Dermatitis*, 47, 67–70.

Gore, A. V., Liang, A. C. and Chien, Y. W. (1998). Comparative biomembrane permeation of tacrine using Yucatan minipigs and domestic pigs as the animal model. *J Pharm Sci*, 87, 441–447.

Griem, P., Goebel, C. and Scheffler, H. (2003). Proposal for a risk assessment methodology for skin sensitization based on sensitization potency data. *Regul Toxicol Pharmacol*, 38, 269–290.

Groeber, F., Holeiter, M., Hampel, M., Hinderer, S. and Schenke-Layland, K. (2011). Skin tissue engineering – *in vivo* and *in vitro* applications. *Adv Drug Deliv Rev*, 63, 352–366.

Groot, A. and Frosch, P. (2011). Patch test concentrations and vehicles for testing contact allergens. In: Johansen, J. D., Frosch, P. J. and Lepoittevin, J.-P. (eds.) *Contact Dermatitis*. Springer, Berlin Heidelberg. doi:10.1007/978-3-642-03827-3_56.

Group, E. W. (2013). *EWG Skin Deep® Cosmetics Database* [Online]. Washington, DC. Available: *http://www.ewg.org/skindeep/* [Accessed 5 June 2013].

Gu, X. and Chen, T. (2009). *In vitro* permeation characterization of repellent picaridin and sunscreen oxybenzone. *Pharm Dev Technol*, 14, 332–340.

Gu, X., Kasichayanula, S., Fediuk, D. J. and Burczynski, F. J. (2004). *In vitro* permeation of the insect repellent N,N-diethyl-m-toluamide (DEET) and the sunscreen oxybenzone. *J Pharm Pharmacol*, 56, 621–628.

Guillot, J. P., Giauffret, J. Y., Martini, M. C., Gonnet, J. F. and Soulé, G. (1982). Safety evaluation of gums and thickeners used in cosmetic formulations. *Int J Cosmet Sci*, 4, 53–66.

Gulkac, M. D., Akpinar, G., Ustun, H. and Ozon Kanli, A. (2004). Effects of vitamin A on doxorubicin-induced chromosomal aberrations in bone marrow cells of rats. *Mutagenesis*, 19, 231–236.

Gulston, M. and Knowland, J. (1999). Illumination of human keratinocytes in the presence of the sunscreen ingredient Padimate-O and through an SPF-15 sunscreen reduces direct photodamage to DNA but increases strand breaks. *Mutat Res*, 444, 49–60.

Hadgraft, J. and Lane, M. E. (2005). Skin permeation: the years of enlightenment. *Int J Pharm*, 305, 2–12.

Hannuksela, M. and Salo, H. (1986). The repeated open application test (ROAT). *Contact Dermatitis*, 14, 221–227.

Hansen, K. S. (1983). Occupational dermatoses in hospital cleaning women. *Contact Dermatitis*, 9, 343–351.

Harder, A., Escher, B. I. and Schwarzenbach, R. P. (2003). Applicability and limitation of QSARs for the toxicity of electrophilic chemicals. *Environ Sci Technol*, 37, 4955–4961.

Harris, P. J. and Ferguson, L. R. (1999). Dietary fibres may protect or enhance carcinogenesis. *Mutat Res*, 443, 95–110.

Harvey, P. W. and Darbre, P. (2004). Endocrine disrupters and human health: could oestrogenic chemicals in body care cosmetics adversely affect breast cancer incidence in women? A review of evidence and call for further research. *J Appl Toxicol*, 24, 167–176.

Hatch, K. L. and Maibach, H. I. (1985). Textile fiber dermatitis. *Contact Dermatitis*, 12, 1–11.

Hausen, B. M. (1993). *Centella asiatica* (Indian pennywort), an effective therapeutic but a weak sensitizer. *Contact Dermatitis*, 29, 175–179.

Hausten, U.-F., Tegetmeyer, L. and Ziegler, V. (1985). Allergic and irritant potential of benzoyl peroxide. *Contact Dermatitis*, 13, 252–257.

Hayakawa, R., Matsunaga, K., Suzuki, M., Arima, Y. and Ohkido, Y. (1987). Lipstick dermatitis due to C18 aliphatic compounds. *Contact Dermatitis*, 16, 215–219.

Hayden, C. G. J., Roberts, M. S. and Benson, H. A. E. (1997). Systemic absorption of sunscreen after topical application. *Lancet*, 350, 863–864.

Health Product Act 2008. (Chapter 122D.) Singapore.

Herbst, R. A., Lauerma, A. I. and Maibach, H. I. (1993). Intradermal testing in the diagnosis of allergic contact dermatitis. *Contact Dermatitis*, 29, 1–5.

Herbst, R. A., Uter, W., Pirker, C., Geier, J. and Frosch, P. J. (2004). Allergic and non-allergic periorbital dermatitis: patch test results of the Information Network of the Departments of Dermatology during a 5-year period. *Contact Dermatitis*, 51, 13–19.

Hiasa, Y., Enoki, N., Kitahori, Y., Konishi, N. and Shimoyama, T. (1984). DL-serine – promoting activity on renal tumorigenesis by N-ethyl-N-hydroxyethylnitrosamine in rats. *J Natl Cancer Inst*, 73, 297–299.

Hölzle, E., Lehmann, P. and Neumann, N. (2009). Phototoxic and photoallergic reactions. *JDDG: Journal der Deutschen Dermatologischen Gesellschaft*, 7, 643–648.

HSA (Health Science Authority) (2011). *Regulatory Guidance: Guidelines on the control of cosmetic products* [Online]. Available: *http://www.hsa.gov.sg/*

publish/etc/medialib/hsa_library/health_products_regulation/cosmetic_products/files_1.Par.53868.File.dat/CCU%20GUIDELINES%20Jan%20 2011_Kok%20Ee%20-%2017Jan%2011_Final.pdf [Accessed 16 July 2013].

Huang, S., Zhang, Y., Tang, L., Deng, Z., Lu, W., et al. (2009). Functional bilayered skin substitute constructed by tissue-engineered extracellular matrix and microsphere-incorporated gelatin hydrogel for wound repair. *Tissue Eng A*, 15, 2617–2624.

Hughes, T. M. and Stone, N. M. (2007). Benzophenone 4: an emerging allergen in cosmetics and toiletries? *Contact Dermatitis*, 56, 153–156.

Hui, X., Elkeeb, R., Chan, H. and Maibach, H. I. (2012). Ability to estimate relative percutaneous penetration via a surrogate maker – trans epidermal water loss? *Skin Res Technol*, 18, 108–113.

Illel, B. (1997). Formulation for transfollicular drug administration: some recent advances. *Crit Rev Ther Drug Carr Sys*, 14, 207–219.

Inbaraj, J. J., Bilski, P. and Chignell, C. F. (2002). Photophysical and photochemical studies of 2-phenylbenzimidazole and UVB sunscreen 2-phenylbenzimidazole-5-sulfonic acid. *Photochem Photobiol*, 75, 107–116.

Ishidate Jr, M., Sofuni, T., Yoshikawa, K., Hayashi, M., Nohmi, T., et al. (1984). Primary mutagenicity screening of food additives currently used in Japan. *Food Chem Toxicol*, 22, 623–636.

Jacobi, U., Kaiser, M., Toll, R., Mangelsdorf, S., Audring, H., et al. (2007). Porcine ear skin: an *in vitro* model for human skin. *Skin Res Technol*, 13, 19–24.

Jagiello, G. M., Lin, J. S. and Ducayen, M. B. (1975). SO2 and its metabolite – effects on mammalian eggs chromosomes. *Environ Res*, 9, 84–93.

Jelski, W. and Szmitkowski, M. (2008). Alcohol dehydrogenase (ADH) and aldehyde dehydrogenase (ALDH) in the cancer diseases. *Clinica Chimica Acta*, 395, 1–5.

Jensen, C. D. and Andersen, K. E. (2005). Allergic contact dermatitis from sodium stearoyl lactylate, an emulsifier commonly used in food products. *Contact Dermatitis*, 53, 116.

Jírová, D., Basketter, D., Liebsch, M., Bendová, H., Kejlová, K., et al. (2010). Comparison of human skin irritation patch test data with *in vitro* skin irritation assays and animal data. *Contact Dermatitis*, 62, 109–116.

Johnson, W. (1999). Final Report on the Safety Assessment of Propylene Glycol (PG) Dicaprylate, PG Dicaprylate/Dicaprate, PG Dicocoate, PG Dipelargonate, PG Isostearate, PG Laurate, PG Myristate, PG Oleate, PG Oleate SE, PG Dioleate, PG Dicaprate, PG Diisostearate, and PG Dilaurate. *Int J Toxicol*, 18, 35–52.

Kai, A. C., White, J. M. L., White, I. R., Johnston, G. and Mcfadden, J. P. (2011). Contact dermatitis caused by C30–38 olefin/isopropyl maleate/MA copolymer in a sunscreen. *Contact Dermatitis*, 64, 353–354.

Kang, L., Yap, C. W., Lim, P. F., Chen, Y. Z., Ho, P. C., et al. (2007). Formulation development of transdermal dosage forms: quantitative structure–activity relationship model for predicting activities of terpenes that enhance drug penetration through human skin. *J Control Release*, 120, 211–219.

Karadzovska, D., Brooks, J. D. and Riviere, J. E. (2013b). Modeling the effect of experimental variables on the *in vitro* permeation of six model compounds across porcine skin. *Int J Pharm*, 443, 58–67.

Karadzovska, D., Brooks, J. D., Monteiro-Riviere, N. A. and Riviere, J. E. (2013a). Predicting skin permeability from complex vehicles. *Adv Drug Deliv Rev*, 65, 265–277.

Karlsson, I., Vanden Broecke, K., Mårtensson, J., Goossens, A. and Börje, A. (2011). Clinical and experimental studies of octocrylene's allergenic potency. *Contact Dermatitis*, 64, 343–352.

Karstadt, M. L. (2010). Regulation of cosmetic safety in the United States. *Eur J Oncol*, 15, 111–117.

Kaushik, D., Dureja, H., Gupta, M., Kumar, V. and Lather, V. (2005). Cosmeceuticals: An emerging concept. *Indian J Pharm*, 37, 155–159.

Kawai, K., Nakagawa, M., Kawai, J. and Kawai, K. (1992). Evaluation of skin irritancy of sodium lauryl sulphate: a comparative study between the replica method and visual evaluation. *Contact Dermatitis*, 27, 174–181.

Kimber, I., Basketter, D. A., Berthold, K., Butler, M., Garrigue, J.-L., et al. (2001). Skin sensitization testing in potency and risk assessment. *Toxicol Sci*, 59, 198–208.

Kimber, I., Basketter, D. A., Butler, M., Gamer, A., Garrigue, J. L., et al. (2003). Classification of contact allergens according to potency: proposals. *Food Chem Toxicol*, 41, 1799–1809.

Kimber, I., Dearman, R. J., Basketter, D. A., Ryan, C. A. and Gerberick, G. F. (2002). The local lymph node assay: past, present and future. *Contact Dermatitis*, 47, 315–328.

Kligman, A. M. (1993). Why cosmeceuticals? *Cosmetics and Toiletries*, 108, 37–38.

Kochhar, J. S., Zou, S., Chan, S. Y. and Kang, L. (2012). Protein encapsulation in polymeric microneedles by photolithography. *Int J Nanomedicine*, 7, 3143–3154.

Kochhar, J. S., Goh, W. J., Chan, S. Y. and Kang, L. (2013). A simple method of microneedle array fabrication for transdermal drug delivery. *Drug Dev Ind Pharm*, 39, 299–309.

Kohl, L., Blondeel, A. and Song, M. (2002). Allergic contact dermatitis from cosmetics. *Dermatology*, 204, 334–337.

Korinth, G., Schaller, K. H. and Drexler, H. (2005). Is the permeability coefficient K pa reliable tool in percutaneous absorption studies? *Arch Toxicol*, 79, 155–159.

Kornhauser, A., Wei, R. R., Yamaguchi, Y., Coelho, S. G., Kaidbey, K., et al. (2009). The effects of topically applied glycolic acid and salicylic acid on ultraviolet radiation-induced erythema, DNA damage and sunburn cell formation in human skin. *J Dermatolo Sci*, 55, 10–17.

Kostoryz, E. L., Zhu, Q., Zhao, H., Miller, M. and Eick, J. D. (2006). Assessment of the relative skin sensitization potency of siloranes and bis-GMA using the local lymph node assay and QSAR predicted potency. *J Biomed Mat Res A*, 79A, 684–688.

Kowalzick, L. and Ziegler, H. (2006). Photoallergic contact dermatitis from topical diclofenac in Solaraze® gel. *Contact Dermatitis*, 54, 348–349.

Kreilgaard, M. (2001). Dermal pharmacokinetics of microemulsion formulations determined by *in vivo* microdialysis. *Pharm Res*, 18, 367–373.

Kumar, S. (2005). Exploratory analysis of global cosmetic industry: major players, technology and market trends. *Technovation*, 25, 1263–1272.

Kupczewska-Dobecka, M., Jakubowski, M. and Czerczak, S. (2010). Calculating the dermal flux of chemicals with OELs based on their molecular structure: An attempt to assign the skin notation. *Environ Toxicol Pharmacol*, 30, 95–102.

Kurien, B. T. and Scofield, R. H. (2007). Curcumin/turmeric solubilized in sodium hydroxide inhibits HNE protein modification – an *in vitro* study. *J Ethnopharmacol*, 110, 368–373.

Lammintausta, K., Zimerson, E., Winhoven, S., Susitaival, P., Hasan, T., et al. (2010). Sensitization to dimethyl fumarate with multiple concurrent patch test reactions. *Contact Dermatitis*, 62, 88–96.

Lapczynski, A., Bhatia, S. P., Foxenberg, R. J., Letizia, C. S. and Api, A. M. (2008). Fragrance material review on geraniol. *Food Chem Toxicol*, 46, S160–S170.

Larking, P. W. (1999). Cancer and low levels of plasma cholesterol: the relevance of cholesterol precursors and products to incidence of cancer. *Prev Med*, 29, 383–390.

Lauer, A. C., Elder, J. T. and Weiner, N. D. (1997). Evaluation of the hairless rat as a model for *in vivo* percutaneous absorption. *J Pharm Sci*, 86, 13–18.

Le Coz, C.-J. and Bressieux, A. (2003). Allergic contact dermatitis from cetearyl isononanoate. *Contact Dermatitis*, 48, 343.

Lee, Y. and Hwang, K. (2002). Skin thickness of Korean adults. *Surg Radiol Anat*, 24, 183–189.

Lin, T. J. (2010). Evolution of cosmetics: increased need for experimental clinical medicine. *J Exp Clin Med*, 2, 49–52.

Livingston, E. H. and Lee, S. (2000). Percentage of burned body surface area determination in obese and nonobese patients. *J Surg Res*, 91, 106–110.

Loftsson, T., Konradsdottir, F. and Masson, M. (2006). Development and evaluation of an artificial membrane for determination of drug availability. *Int J Pharm*, 326, 60–68.

Lopez, S., Peláez, A., Navarro, L. A., Montesinos, E., Morales, C. and Carda, C. (1994). Aluminium allergy in patients hyposensitized with aluminium-precipitated antigen extracts. *Contact Dermatitis*, 31, 37–40.

Mah, C. S., Kochhar, J. S., Ong, P. S. and Kang, L. (2013). A miniaturized flow-through cell to evaluate skin permeation of endoxifen. *Int J Pharm*, 441, 433–440.

Mak, V. H. W., Cumpstone, M. B., Kennedy, A. H., Harmon, C. S., Guy, R. H. and Potts, R. O. (1991). Barrier function of human keratinocyte cultures grown at the air–liquid interface. *J Invest Dermatol*, 96, 323–327.

Malaveille, C., Brun, G. and Bartsch, H. (1994). Structure–activity studies in *E. coli* strains on ochratoxin A (OTA) and its analogues implicate a genotoxic free radical and a cytotoxic thiol derivative as reactive metabolites. *Mutat Res*, 307, 141–147.

Mamur, S., Yuzbasioglu, D., Unal, F. and Yilmaz, S. (2010). Does potassium sorbate induce genotoxic or mutagenic effects in lymphocytes? *Toxicol In Vitro*, 24, 790–794.

Mannisto, S., Pietinen, P., Virtanen, M. J., Salminen, I., Albanes, D., et al. (2003). Fatty acids and risk of prostate cancer in a nested case-control study in male smokers. *Cancer Epidemiol Biomarkers Prev*, 12, 1422–1428.

Marieb, E. N. and Hoehn, K. (2007). *Human Anatomy and Physiology*. San Francisco, Pearson Education.

Marks Jr, J. G., Belsito, D. V., Deleo, V. A., Fowler Jr, J. F., Fransway, A. F., et al. (1998). North American Contact Dermatitis Group patch test results for the detection of delayed-type hypersensitivity to topical allergens. *J Am Acad Dermatol*, 38, 911–918.

Marks Jr, J. G., Belsito, D. V., Deleo, V. A., Fowler Jr, J. F., Fransway, A. F., et al. (2000). North American Contact Dermatitis Group patch-test results, 1996–1998. *Arch Dermatol*, 136, 272–274.

Martini, F. H. (2006). *Fundamentals of Anatomy and Physiology*. San Francisco, Pearson Benjamin Cummings.

Marzulli, F. N. and Maibach, H. I. (1975). The rabbit as a model for evaluating skin irritants: a comparison of results obtained on animals and man using repeated skin exposures. *Food Cosmet Toxicol*, 13, 533–540.

Matsumoto, H., Adachi, S. and Suzuki, Y. (2005). Estrogenic activity of ultraviolet absorbers and the related compounds. *Yakugaku Zasshi*, 125, 643–652.

McNamee, P. M., Api, A. M., Basketter, D. A., Frank Gerberick, G., Gilpin, D. A., et al. (2008). A review of critical factors in the conduct and interpretation of the human repeat insult patch test. *Regul Toxicol Pharmacol*, 52, 24–34.

Mehta, S. S. and Reddy, B. S. N. (2003). Cosmetic dermatitis – current perspectives. *Int J Dermatol*, 42, 533–542.

Menné, T. and Hjorth, N. (1988). Routine patch testing with paraben esters. *Contact Dermatitis*, 19, 189–191.

Menon, G. K. (2002). New insights into skin structure: scratching the surface. *Adv Drug Deliv Rev*, 54, S3–S17.

Merch Index (2001). Whitehouse Station, NJ, Merck and Co., Inc.

Merck Millipore. 2012. *Strat-M™* [Online]. Available: *http://www.millipore.com/life_sciences/flx4/stratmandtab1=1#tab1=1* [Accessed 5 March 2013].

Morimoto, Y., Hatanaka, T., Sugibayashi, K. and Omiya, H. (1992). Prediction of skin permeability of drugs: comparison of human and hairless rat skin. *J Pharm Pharmacol*, 44, 634–639.

Morita, T., Takeda, K. and Okumura, K. (1990). Evaluation of clastogenicity of formic acid, acetic acid and lactic acid on cultured mammalian cells. *Mutat Res*, 240, 195–202.

Mortz, C. G., Bindslev-Jensen, C. and Andersen, K. E. (2012). Prevalence, incidence rate and persistence of contact allergy and allergic contact dermatitis in the TOACS cohort: a 15 years follow-up. *Br J Dermatol*, 168, 318–325.

Moser, K., Kriwet, K., Naik, A., Kalia, Y. N. and Guy, R. H. (2001). Passive skin penetration enhancement and its quantification *in vitro*. *Eur J Pharm Biopharm*, 52, 103–112.

Moss, G. P., Wilkinson, S. C. and Sun, Y. (2012). Mathematical modelling of percutaneous absorption. *Curr Opin Colloid Interface Sci*, 17, 166–172.

Moss, G. P., Dearden, J. C., Patel, H. and Cronin, M. T. (2002). Quantitative structure–permeability relationships (QSPRs) for percutaneous absorption. *Toxicol In Vitro*, 16, 299–317.

Msiska, Z., Pacurari, M., Mishra, A., Leonard, S. S., Castranova, V. and Vallyathan, V. (2010). DNA double-strand breaks by asbestos, silica, and titanium dioxide. *Am J Respir Cell Mol Biol*, 43, 210–219.

Mueller, S. O., Kling, M., Arifin Firzani, P., Mecky, A., Duranti, E., et al. (2003). Activation of estrogen receptor [alpha] and ER [beta] by 4-methylbenzylidene-camphor in human and rat cells: comparison with phyto- and xenoestrogens. *Toxicol Lett*, 142, 89–101.

Mura, P., Maestrelli, F., Gonzalez-Rodriguez, M. L., Michelacci, I., Ghelardini, C. and Rabasco, A. M. (2007). Development, characterization and *in vivo* evaluation of benzocaine-loaded liposomes. *Eur J Pharm Biopharm*, 67, 86–95.

Murata, Y., Kumano, K., Ueda, T., Araki, N., Nakamura, T. and Tani, M. (1998). Photosensitive dermatitis caused by pyridoxine hydrochloride. *J Am Acad Dermatol*, 39, 314–317.

Nair, B. (1998). Final Report on the Safety Assessment of Polyvinylpyrrolidone (PVP). *Int J Toxicol*, 17, 95–130.

Nakagawa, M., Kawai, K. and Kawai, K. (1995). Contact allergy to kojic acid in skin care products. *Contact Dermatitis*, 32, 9–13.

Neri, I., Bianchi, F., Giacomini, F. and Patrizi, A. (2006). Acute irritant contact dermatitis due to *Juglans regia*. *Contact Dermatitis*, 55, 62–63.

Nesslany, F., Simar-Meintieres, S., Watzinger, M., Talahari, I. and Marzin, D. (2008). Characterization of the genotoxicity of nitrilotriacetic acid. *Environ Mol Mutagen*, 49, 439–452.

Netzlaff, F., Schaefer, U. F., Lehr, C. M., Meiers, P., Stahl, J., Kietzmann, M. and Niedorf, F. (2006). Comparison of bovine udder skin with human and porcine skin in percutaneous permeation experiments. *Altern Lab Anim*, 34, 499–513.

Nordlind, K. and Liden, S. (1992). Patch test reactions to metal salts in patients with oral mucosal lesions associated with amalgam restorations. *Contact Dermatitis*, 27, 157–160.

Nwaogu, T. A. and Vernon, J. (2004). Comparative Study on Cosmetics Legislation in the EU and Other Principal Markets with Special Attention to so-called Borderline Products. United Kingdom: European Commission.

OECD (2002). Test No. 404: Acute Dermal Irritation/Corrosion. *OECD Guidelines for the Testing of Chemicals*, Section 4. Paris: OECD Publishing.

OECD (2010). *OECD Guidance Notes on Dermal Absorption* [Online]. Available: *http://www.oecd.org/env/ehs/testing/46257610.pdf* [Accessed 5 March 2013].

Ortiz, K. J. and Yiannias, J. A. (2004). Contact dermatitis to cosmetics, fragrances, and botanicals. *Dermatol Ther*, 17, 264–271.

Patel, H. and Cronin, M. T. D. (2001). A novel index for the description of molecular linearity. *J Chem Inf Comput Sci*, 41, 1228–1236.

Patel, H., Schultz, T. W. and Cronin, M. T. D. (2002a). Physico-chemical interpretation and prediction of the dimyristoyl phosphatidyl choline–water partition coefficient. *J Mol Struct*, 593, 9–18.

Patel, H., Ten Berge, W. and Cronin, M. T. (2002b). Quantitative structure–activity relationships (QSARs) for the prediction of skin permeation of exogenous chemicals. *Chemosphere*, 48, 603–613.

Pažoureková, S., Hojerová, J. and Lucová, M. (2011). Evaluation of dermal absorption of coenzyme Q10 and tocopherolacetate by *in vitro* method OECD 428/EU B.45. *Hodnotenie dermálnej absorpcie koenzýmu Q10 a tokoferolacetátu in vitro metódou OECD 428/EU B.45*, 80, 17–22.

Perrenoud, D., Bircher, A., Hunziker, T., Sutter, H., Bruckner-Tuderman, L., et al. (1994). Frequency of sensitization to 13 common preservatives in Switzerland. *Contact Dermatitis*, 30, 276–279.

Pfuhler, S. and Wolf, H. U. (2002). Effects of the formaldehyde releasing preservatives dimethylol urea and diazolidinyl urea in several short-term genotoxicity tests. *Mutat Res*, 502, 133–146.

Philips, N., Keller, T. and Holmes, C. (2007). Reciprocal effects of ascorbate on cancer cell growth and the expression of matrix metalloproteinases and transforming growth factor-beta. *Cancer Lett*, 256, 49–55.

Pifferi, G. and Restani, P. (2003). The safety of pharmaceutical excipients. *Il Farmaco*, 58, 541–550.

Pocza, P., Suli-Vargha, H., Darvas, Z. and Falus, A. (2008). Locally generated VGVAPG and VAPG elastin-derived peptides amplify melanoma invasion via the galectin-3 receptor. *Int J Cancer*, 122, 1972–1980.

Popescu, N. C. and DiPaolo, J. A. (1988). Chromosome alterations in Syrian hamster cells transformed *in vitro* by sodium bisulfite, a nonclastogenic carcinogen. *Cancer Res*, 48, 7246–7251.

Potts, R. O. and Guy, R. H. (1992). Predicting skin permeability. *Pharm Res*, 9, 663–669.

Prausnitz, M. R., Mitragotri, S. and Langer, R. (2004). Current status and future potential of transdermal drug delivery. *Nat Rev Drug Discov*, 3, 115–124.

Preventice (2012). *CARD – A Mobile Health App for Skin Allergy Management Database* [Online]. Available: *www.preventice.com/products/card/* 2012].

Program, N. T. (1992). NTP Toxicology and Carcinogenesis Studies of Polysorbate 80 (CAS No. 9005-65-6) in F344/N Rats and B6C3F1 Mice (Feed Studies). *National Toxicology Program Technical Report Series*, 415, 1–225.

Proksch, E., Brandner, J. M. and Jensen, J. M. (2008). The skin: an indispensable barrier. *Exp Dermatol*, 17, 1063–1072.

Quartier, S., Garmyn, M., Becart, S. and Goossens, A. (2006). Allergic contact dermatitis to copolymers in cosmetics – case report and review of the literature. *Contact Dermatitis*, 55, 257–267.

Rao, H. X. and Zhang, Z. Y. (2012). Preparation, characterization, and permeation property of a liquid crystal/PDMS membrane material. *J Appl Polym Sci*, 123, 191–199.

Reagan-Shaw, S., Nihal, M. and Ahmad, N. (2008). Dose translation from animal to human studies revisited. *Faseb J*, 22, 659–661.

Rein, H. (1924). Experimental electroendosmotic studies on living human skin. *Zeitschrift fur Biologie*, 81, 125–140.

Rencüzogullari, E., Ila, H. B., Kayraldiz, A. and Topaktas, M. (2001). Chromosome aberrations and sister chromatid exchanges in cultured human lymphocytes treated with sodium metabisulfite, a food preservative. *Mutat Res*, 490, 107–112.

Ribeiro, D. A., Bazo, A. P., Franchi, C. A. D., Marques, M. E. A. and Salvadori, D. M. F. (2004). Chlorhexidine induces DNA damage in rat peripheral leukocytes and oral mucosal cells. *J Periodontal Res*, 39, 358–361.

Riva, F., Casasco, A., Nespoli, E., Cornaglia, A. I., Casasco, M., et al. (2007). Generation of human epidermal constructs on a collagen layer alone. *Tissue Eng*, 13, 2769–2779.

Roberts, M. S. and Walters, K. A. (1998). The relationship between structure and barrier function of skin. *Drugs Pharm Sci*, 91, 1–42.

Robinson, M. K., Nusair, T. L., Robert Fletcher, E. and Ritz, H. L. (1990). A review of the Buehler guinea pig skin sensitization test and its use in a risk assessment process for human skin sensitization. *Toxicology*, 61, 91–107.

Ross, G. (2006). A perspective on the safety of cosmetic products: a position paper of the American Council on Science and Health. *Int J Toxicol*, 25, 269–277.

Ross, J. H., Reifenrath, W. G. and Driver, J. H. (2011). Estimation of the percutaneous absorption of permethrin in humans using the parallelogram method. *J Toxicol Environ Health A*, 74, 351–363.

Saghir, S. A., Bartels, M. J. and Snellings, W. M. (2010). Dermal penetration of ethylene glycol through human skin *in vitro*. *Int J Toxicol*, 29, 268–276.

Saint-Leger, D. (2012). 'Cosmeceuticals'. Of men, science and laws. *Int J Cosmet Sci*, 34, 396–401.

Sasaki, Y. F., Kawaguchi, S., Kamaya, A., Ohshita, M., Kabasawa, K., et al. (2002). The comet assay with 8 mouse organs: results with 39 currently used food additives. *Mutat Res*, 519, 103–119.

Sautebin, L. (2008). Understanding the adverse effects of cosmetics – a pilot project in cosmetovigilance. *Drug Safety*, 31, 433–436.

Scheerger, S. B. and Zempleni, J. (2003). Expression of oncogenes depends on biotin in human small cell lung cancer cells NCI-H69. *Internationale Zeitschrift für Vitamin- und Ernährungsforschung. Beiheft.*, 73, 461–467.

Scheuplein, R. J. (1965). Mechanism of percutaneous adsorption. I. Routes of penetration and the influence of solubility. *J Invest Dermatol*, 45, 334–346.

Scheuplein, R. J. and Blank, I. H. (1971). Permeability of the skin. *Physiol Rev*, 51, 702–747.

Schlumpf, M., Cotton, B., Conscience, M., Haller, V., Steinmann, B. and Lichtensteiger, W. (2001). *In vitro* and *in vivo* estrogenicity of UV screens. *Environ Health Perspect*, 109, 239–244.

Schmook, F. P., Meingassner, J. G. and Billich, A. (2001). Comparison of human skin or epidermis models with human and animal skin in *in vitro* percutaneous absorption. *Int J Pharm*, 215, 51–56.

Schwartz, L. (1936). Dermatitis from synthetic resins and waxes. *Am J Public Health Nations Health*, 26, 586–592.

Scibior-Bentkowska, D. and Czeczot, H. (2009). Cancer cells and oxidative stress. *Postępy higieny i medycyny doświadczalnej*, 63, 58–72.

Serpone, N., Dondi, D. and Albini, A. (2007). Inorganic and organic UV filters: their role and efficacy in sunscreens and suncare product. *Inorganica Chimica Acta*, 360, 794–802.

Setala, H. (1956). Tumor promoting and co-carcinogenic effects of some non-ionic and lipophilic-hydrophilic (surface active) agents. An experimental study on skin tumors in mice. *Acta pathologica et microbiologica Scandinavica*, Suppl, 1–93.

Sharma, S. and Sultana, S. (2004). Effect of *Hibiscus rosa sinensis* extract on hyperproliferation and oxidative damage caused by benzoyl peroxide and ultraviolet radiations in mouse skin. *Basic Clin Pharmacol Toxicol*, 95, 220–225.

Shephard, S. E., Hegi, M. E. and Lutz, W. K. (1987). *In vitro* assays to detect alkylating and mutagenic activities of dietary components nitrosated *in situ*. *IARC Sci Publ*, 232–236.

Shibata, M. A., Tamano, S., Shirai, T., Kawabe, M. and Fukushima, S. (1992). Inorganic alkalizers and acidifiers under conditions of high urinary Na+ or K+ on cell-proliferation and 2-stage carcinogenesis in the rat bladder. *Jpn J Cancer Res*, 83, 821–829.

Simon, G. A. and Maibach, H. I. (2000). The pig as an experimental animal model of percutaneous permeation in man: qualitative and quantitative observations – an overview. *Skin Pharmacol Appl Skin Physiol*, 13, 229–234.

Singh, S., Zhao, K. and Singh, J. (2002). *In vitro* permeability and binding of hydrocarbons in pig ear and human abdominal skin. *Drug Chem Toxicol*, 25, 83–92.

Sivak, A. and Tu, A. S. (1980). Cell culture tumor promotion experiments with saccharin, phorbol myristate acetate and several common food materials. *Cancer Lett*, 10, 27–32.

Someya, H., Higo, Y., Ohno, M., Tsutsui, T. W. and Tsutsui, T. (2008). Clastogenic activity of seven endodontic medications used in dental practice in human dental pulp cells. *Mutat Res*, 650, 39–47.

Søsted, H., Basketter, D. A., Estrada, E., Johansen, J. D. and Patlewicz, G. Y. (2004). Ranking of hair dye substances according to predicted sensitization potency: quantitative structure–activity relationships. *Contact Dermatitis*, 51, 241–254.

Stich, H. F., Stich, W., Rosin, M. P. and Powrie, W. D. (1981). Clastogenic activity of caramel and caramelized sugars. *Mutat Res*, 91, 129–136.

Storrs, F. J. and Bell, D. E. (1983). Allergic contact dermatitis to 2-bromo-2-nitropropane-1,3-diol in a hydrophilic ointment. *J Am Acad Dermatol*, 8, 157–170.

Stott, W. T., Radtke, B. J., Linscombe, V. A., Mar, M. H. and Zeisel, S. H. (2004). Evaluation of the potential of triethanolamine to alter hepatic choline levels in female B6C3F1 mice. *Toxicol Sci*, 79, 242–247.

Sugai, T. and Higashi, J. (1975). Hypersensitivity to hydrogenated lanolin. *Contact Dermatitis*, 1, 146–157.

Takano, Y., Okudaira, M. and Harmon, B. V. (1993). Apoptosis induced by microtubule disrupting drugs in cultured human lymphoma-cells – inhibitory effects of phorbol ester and zinc-sulphate. *Path Res Prac*, 189, 197–203.

Takeuchi, H., Mano, Y., Terasaka, S., Sakurai, T., Furuya, A., et al. (2011). Usefulness of rat skin as a substitute for human skin in the *in vitro* skin permeation study. *Exp Anim*, 60, 373–384.

Tan, B., Wang, J. H., Wu, Q. D., Kirwan, W. O. and Redmond, H. P. (2001). Sodium hyaluronate enhances colorectal tumour cell metastatic potential *in vitro* and *in vivo*. *Br J Surg*, 88, 246–250.

Tara, E. G. and John, E. B. (2012). The Personal Care Product Council. *International Cosmetic Ingredient Dictionary and Handbook.*

Toxicology, American College of (1982a). Final Report on the Safety Assessment of Decyl and Isodecyl Oleates. *I J Toxicol*, 1, 85–95.

Toxicology, American College of (1982b). Final Report on the Safety Assessment of Myristyl Myristate and Isopropyl Myristate. *Int J Toxicol*, 1, 55–80.

Toxicology, American College of (1982c). Final Report on the Safety Assessment of Octyl Palmitate, Cetyl Palmitate and Isopropyl Palmitate. *Int J Toxicol*, 1, 13–35.

Toxicology, American College of (1983). Final Report on the Safety Assessment of Laureths 4 and 23. *Int J Toxicol*, 2, 1–15.

Toxicology, American College of (1984a). Final Report on the Safety Assessment of Polysorbates 20, 21, 40, 60, 61, 65, 80, 81, and 85. *Int J Toxicol*, 3, 1–82.

Toxicology, American College of (1984b). Final Report on the Safety Assessment of Butylated Hydroxyanisole. *Int J Toxicol*, 3, 83–146.

Toxicology, American College of (1984c). Final Report on the Safety Assessment of Methylparaben, Ethylparaben, Propylparaben, and Butylparaben. *Int J Toxicol*, 3, 147–209.

Toxicology, American College of (1985a). Final Report on the Safety Assessment of Stearyl Alcohol, Oleyl Alcohol, and Octyl Dodecanol. *Int J Toxicol*, 4, 1–29.

Toxicology, American College of (1985b). Final Report on the Safety Assessment of Propyl Gallate. *Int J Toxicol*, 4, 23–64.

Toxicology, American College of (1985c). Final Report on the Safety Assessment of Butyl Stearate, Cetyl Stearate, Isobutyl Stearate, Isocetyl Stearate, Isopropyl Stearate, Myristyl Stearate, and Octyl Stearate. *Int J Toxicol*, 4, 107–146.

Toxicology, American College of (1985d). Final Report on the Safety Assessment of Butylene Glycol, Hexylene Glycol, Ethoxydiglycol, and Dipropylene Glycol. *Int J Toxicol*, 4, 223–248.

Toxicology, American College of (1987a). Final Report on the Safety Assessment of Propylene Carbonate. *Int J Toxicol*, 6, 23–51.

Toxicology, American College of (1987b). Final Report on the Safety Assessment of Panthenol and Pantothenic Acid. *Int J Toxicol*, 6, 139–162.

Toxicology, American College of (1988a). Final Report on the Safety Assessment of DMDM Hydantoin. *Int J Toxicol*, 7, 245–277.

Toxicology, American College of (1988b). Final Report on the Safety Assessment of Polyquaternium-10. *Int J Toxicol*, 7, 335–351.

Toxicology, American College of (1988c). Final Report on the Safety Assessment of Cetearyl Alcohol, Cetyl Alcohol, Isostearyl Alcohol, Myristyl Alcohol, and Behenyl Alcohol. *Int J Toxicol*, 7, 359–413.

Toxicology, American College of (1990). Final Report on the Safety Assessment of Diazolidinyl Urea. *Int J Toxicol*, 9, 229–245.

Toxicology, American College of (1992). Final Report on the Safety Assessment of Methylisothiazolinone and Methylchloroisothiazolinone. *Int J Toxicol*, 11, 75–128.

Toxicology, American College of (1993a). Final Report on the Safety Assessment of Chlorhexidine/Chlorhexidine Diacetate/Chlorhexidine Dihydrochloride/Chlorhexidine Digluconate. *Int J Toxicol*, 12, 201–223.

Toxicology, American College of (1993b). Final Report on the Safety Assessment of Polyethylene Glycols (PEGs)-6, -8, -32, -75, -150, -14M, -20M. *Int J Toxicol*, 12, 429–457.

Toxicology, American College of (1995). Final Report on the Safety Assessment of Isobutylparaben and Isopropylparaben. *Int J Toxicol*, 14, 364–372.

Toxicology, American College of (1996). Final Report on the Safety Assessment of Methyldibromo Glutaronitrile. *Int J Toxicol*, 15, 140–165.

Toxicology, American College of (1997). Final Report on the Safety Assessment of Cetrimonium Chloride, Cetrimonium Bromide, and Steartrimonium Chloride. *Int J Toxicol*, 16, 195–220.

Toxicology, American College of (2001). Final Report on the Safety Assessment of Benzyl Alcohol, Benzoic Acid, and Sodium Benzoate. *Int J Toxicol*, 20, 23–50.

Toxicology, American College of (2002). Final Report on the Safety Assessment of Acrylates Copolymer and 33 Related Cosmetic Ingredients. *Int J Toxicol*, 21, 1–50.

Toxicology, American College of (2007). Final report on the safety assessment of Glycyrrhetinic Acid, Potassium Glycyrrhetinate, Disodium Succinoyl Glycyrrhetinate, Glyceryl Glycyrrhetinate, Glycyrrhetinyl Stearate, Stearyl Glycyrrhetinate, Glycyrrhizic Acid, Ammonium Glycyrrhizate, Dipotassium Glycyrrhizate, Disodium Glycyrrhizate, Trisodium Glycyrrhizate, Methyl Glycyrrhizate, and Potassium Glycyrrhizinate. *Int J Toxicol*, 26 Suppl 2, 79–112.

Toxicology, American College of (2008). Final report of the Cosmetic Ingredient Review Expert Panel on the safety assessment of Polyisobutene and Hydrogenated Polyisobutene as used in cosmetics. *Int J Toxicol*, 27, 24.

Travassos, A. and Goossens, A. (2012). Potential allergens in moisturizing creams. In: Lodén, M. and Maibach, H. I. (eds.) *Treatment of Dry Skin Syndrome*. Springer Berlin, Heidelberg. doi:10.1007/978-3-642-27606-4_24.

Tupker, R. A., Bunte, E. E., Fidler, V., Wlechers, J. W. and Coenraads, P. J. (1999). Irritancy ranking of anionic detergents using one-time occlusive, repeated occlusive and repeated open tests. *Contact Dermatitis*, 40, 316–322.

Ulmer, H., Borena, W., Rapp, K., Klenk, J., Strasak, A., et al. (2009). Serum triglyceride concentrations and cancer risk in a large cohort study in Austria. *Br J Cancer*, 101, 1202–1206.

U.S. Code (1992). 21 U.S.C. Sect. 362. Misbranded cosmetics. 2006 ed.

U.S. Code (1993). 21 U.S.C. Sect. 361. Adulterated cosmetics. 2006 ed.

USFDA (US Food and Drugs Agency) (1991). *Cosmetic Labeling Guide* [Online]. Available: *http://www.fda.gov/Cosmetics/CosmeticLabelingLabelClaims/CosmeticLabelingManual/ucm126444.htm#clga* [Accessed 16 July 2013].

USFDA (US Food and Drugs Agency) (2005). *FDA Authority Over Cosmetics* [Online]. Available: *http://www.fda.gov/Cosmetics/GuidanceComplianceRegulatoryInformation/ucm074162.htm* [Accessed 16 July 2013].

USFDA (US Food and Drugs Agency) (2008). *Good Manufacturing Practice (GMP) Guidelines/Inspection Checklist* [Online]. Available: *http://www.fda.gov/cosmetics/guidancecomplianceregulatoryinformation/*

goodmanufacturingpracticegmpguidelinesinspectionchecklist/default.htm [Accessed 16 July 2013].

USFDA (US Food and Drugs Agency) (2012a). *Cosmetics Manufacturers, Packagers and Distributors* [Online]. Available: *http://www.fda.gov/Cosmetics/ResourcesForYou/CosmeticsManufacturersPackagersDistributors/default.htm* [Accessed 16 July 2013].

USFDA (US Food and Drugs Agency) (2012b). *Significant Dates in U.S. Food and Drug Law History* [Online]. Available: *http://www.fda.gov/AboutFDA/WhatWeDo/History/Milestones/ucm128305.htm* [Accessed 16 July 2013].

Van De Waterbeemd, H., Camenisch, G., Folkers, G. and Raevsky, O. A. (1996). Estimation of Caco-2 cell permeability using calculated molecular descriptors. *QSAR Comb Sci*, 15, 480–490.

Van Der Valk, P. G. M., Vries, M. H. K.-D., Nater, J. P., Bleu-Mink, E. and De Jong, M. C. J. M. (1985). Eczematous (irritant and allergic) reactions of the skin and barrier function as determined by water vapour loss. *Clin Exp Dermatol*, 10, 185–193.

Van Oosten, E. J., Schuttelaar, M.-L. A. and Coenraads, P. J. (2009). Clinical relevance of positive patch test reactions to the 26 EU-labelled fragrances. *Contact Dermatitis*, 61, 217–223.

Van Ravenzwaay, B. and Leibold, E. (2004). A comparison between *in vitro* rat and human and *in vivo* rat skin absorption studies. *Human Exp Toxicol*, 23, 421–430.

Vena, G. A., Foti, C. and Angelini, G. (1994). Sulfite contact allergy. *Contact Dermatitis*, 31, 172–175.

Vermaat, H., Smienk, F., Rustemeyer, T., Bruynzeel, D. P. and Kirtschig, G. (2008). Anogenital allergic contact dermatitis, the role of spices and flavour allergy. *Contact Dermatitis*, 59, 233–237.

Villa, T. G., Notario, V., Benitez, T. and Villanueva, J. R. (1976). Effect of glucono-delta-lactone on yeast pichia-polymorpha. *Arch Microbiol*, 109, 157–161.

Villela, I. V., De Oliveira, I. M., Da Silva, J. and Henriques, J. A. (2006). DNA damage and repair in haemolymph cells of golden mussel (Limnoperna fortunei) exposed to environmental contaminants. *Mutat Res*, 605, 78–86.

Wagner, H., Kostka, K.-H., Lehr, C.-M. and Schaefer, U. (2000). Drug distribution in human skin using two different *in vitro* test systems: comparison with *in vivo* data. *Pharm Res*, 17, 1475–1481.

Wagner, J. C., Berry, G. and Timbrell, V. (1973). Mesotheliomata in rats after inoculation with asbestos and other materials. *Br J Cancer*, 28, 173–185.

Walles, S. A. (1992). Mechanisms of DNA damage induced in rat hepatocytes by quinones. *Cancer Lett*, 63, 47–52.

Wang, T., Kasichayanula, S. and Gu, X. (2006). *In vitro* permeation of repellent DEET and sunscreen oxybenzone across three artificial membranes. *Int J Pharm*, 310, 110–117.

Wangenheim, J. and Bolcsfoldi, G. (1988). Mouse lymphoma L5178Y thymidine kinase locus assay of 50 compounds. *Mutagenesis*, 3, 193–205.

Webb, R. B. and Hass, B. S. (1984). Biological effects of dyes on bacteria. VI. Mutation induction by acridine orange and methylene blue in the dark with special reference to *Escherichia coli* WP6 (polA1). *Mutat Res*, 137, 1–6.

Weber, J. M. and Villebonne, J. C. D. (2002). Differences in purchase behavior between France and the USA: the cosmetic industry. *Journal of Fashion Marketing and Management*, 6, 396–407.

Wetter, D. A., Davis, M. D. P., Yiannias, J. A., Cheng, J. F., Connolly, S. M., et al. (2005). Patch test results from the Mayo Clinic Contact Dermatitis Group, 1998–2000. *J Am Acad Dermatol*, 53, 416–421.

Whitcomb, D. and Greer, J. (2009). Germ-line mutations, pancreatic inflammation, and pancreatic cancer. *Clin Gastroenterol Hepatol*, 7, S29–S34.

WHO (World Health Organization) (2008). *The Top 10 Causes of Death* [Online]. Available: *http://www.who.int/mediacentre/factsheets/fs310/en/index.html* [Accessed 20 February 2011].

Witschi, H., Malkinson, A. M., Peraino, C., Russell, J. J. and Staffeldt, E. F. (1989). Effects of glycerol on lung and liver tumor development. *Fundam Appl Toxicol*, 13, 174–180.

Yazar, K., Johnsson, S., Lind, M.-L., Boman, A. and Lidén, C. (2011). Preservatives and fragrances in selected consumer-available cosmetics and detergents. *Contact Dermatitis*, 64, 265–272.

Zhang, Z. and Michniak-Kohn, B. B. (2012). Tissue engineered human skin equivalents. *Pharmaceutics*, 4, 26–41.

Zhao, Y. L., Murthy, S. N., Manjili, M. H., Guan, L. J., Sen, A. and Hui, S. W. (2006). Induction of cytotoxic T-lymphocytes by electroporation-enhanced needle-free skin immunization. *Vaccine*, 24, 1282–1290.

Zugerman, C. (1985). Contact dermatitis to yellow iron oxide. *Contact Dermatitis*, 13, 107–109.

Index

Monographs

FSC
www.fsc.org
MIX
Papier | Fördert gute Waldnutzung
FSC® C083411

Kolibri 360 GmbH
Ferdinand-Jühlke-Straße 7
99095 Erfurt, Deutschland
produktsicherheit@kolibri360.de